Pearls and Pitfalls in Cosmetic Oculoplastic Surgery

Pearls and Pitfalls in Cosmetic Oculoplastic Surgery

Edited by

Morris E. Hartstein, MD, FACS

Clinical Associate Professor, Saint Louis University, Department of Ophthalmology and Division of Plastic and Reconstructive Surgery, St. Louis, Missouri

John B. Holds, MD, FACS

Clinical Professor, Saint Louis University, Departments of Ophthalmology and Otolaryngology-Head and Neck Surgery, St. Louis, Missouri

Guy G. Massry, MD

Director, Ophthalmic Plastic and Reconstructive Surgery. American Eye Institute, Cedars Sinai Medical Center, Los Angeles, CA, Spalding Dr. Cosmetic Surgery and Dermatology, Beverly Hills, California, Davidorf Eye Group, West Hills, California

Springer

Morris E. Hartstein, MD, FACS
Clinical Associate Professor
Saint Louis University
Department of Ophthalmology
and Division of Plastic
and Reconstructive Surgery
St. Louis, MO
USA

John B. Holds, MD, FACS
Clinical Professor
Saint Louis University
Departments of Ophthalmology
and Otolaryngology-Head and
Neck Surgery
St. Louis, MO
USA

Guy G. Massry, MD
Director, Ophthalmic Pastic and
Reconstructive Surgery
American Eye Institute
Cedars Sinai Medical Center
Los Angeles, CA
Spalding Dr. Cosmetic Surgery
and Dermatology
Beverly Hills, CA
Davidorf Eye Group
WestHills, CA
USA

Library of Congress Control Number: 2007937487

ISBN: 978-0-387-25389-3 e-ISBN: 978-0-387-25389-3

Printed on acid-free paper.

9 8 7 6 5 4 3 2 1

springer.com

Foreword

Learning oculofacial surgery is a lot like learning to dance. In the beginning, the dance student is consumed with where to put his or her feet. For these new students (or for the rhythmically challenged), dancing is characterized by the struggle to step their feet in imaginary numbered shoeprints, 1–2–3–4, and they barely hear the music. In surgery, the beginning surgeon is preoccupied with steps as well. Their focus is on the mechanical process. Proscribed steps create the paradigm for performing the surgery.

With time, the dance student moves on to the next stage. He does not have to think as much about where he is putting his feet, and can start to listen to the music and feel the rhythm. The advanced surgeon begins to internalize the steps of surgery so that instead of a preoccupation with the next maneuver, she can start to individualize the surgery to the patient and employ flexibilty in the face of unique problems.

The master dancer makes no conscious effort to move his feet; his feet move him. He does not concentrate on rhythm; the rhythm of the music becomes part of him. Freed from the intellectual exercise of dancing and from the technical requirements of keeping time, he is free to break from the restraints of the proscribed steps and invent a new dance as he goes along.

The master surgeon enjoys a similar freedom. The focus is not on maneuvers and, in fact, the surgeon might be temporarily taken aback if asked to explain the mechanical details of what he is doing. Instead, the thought process is conceptual. The surgeon is visualizing a result, is sensitive to the nuances of the patient's individual anatomy, and is always making adjustments to address the unique requirements presented by the case at hand. By approaching the operation conceptually, and having effortless command of anatomy and technique, the master surgeon is freed from the constraints of proscribed operations, and is able to invent new surgeries.

In this book, a high octane collection of master surgeons provide a work that reflects the scope of ophthalmic plastic surgery. There is material here for every type of student. The beginner will appreciate step-by-step instructions and clear anatomic diagrams. The advanced surgeon will be drawn to the delightful tricks and peals that are sprinkled liberally throughout the text. The master surgeon (and the aspiring master) will recognize that they are seeking the same thing that the authors are seeking, and they will be stimulated to continue to search for better treatments and surgeries. The obvious hard work that went into the preparation of this book will pay off handsomely when its readers improve their ability to take care of their patients, and particularly when they are inspired to continue their own journey toward mastery of our discipline.

Robert Alan Goldberg, MD
Karen and Frank Daby Professor of Ophthalmology
David Geffen School of Medicine at UCLA
Chief, Orbital and Ophthalmic Plastic Surgery Division
Jules Stein Eye Institute

Preface

The goal of this book is to help surgeons perform more efficient, productive, and successful surgeries. By sharing our varied experiences, acquired through years of practice, we hope this book will provide insights that can enhance surgical outcomes. In compiling this text, we solicited contributions from experts in cosmetic oculoplastic surgery, as well as surgeons from other related fields, such as facial plastic surgery, plastic surgery, and dermatology. The book is divided into 12 parts, which cover the spectrum of oculofacial procedures. Each section is divided into concise chapters focusing on just one aspect of a given procedure. Within these short chapters, each contributor offers tips on how to achieve optimal results. For example, the section on upper lid blepharoplasty is subdivided as follows:

- Preoperative evaluation
- Incision planning
- Procedure pearls
- Adjunctive procedures
- Wound closure and postoperative care

There are also multiple presentations on the same aspect of a procedure to provide different points of view and approaches. We greatly appreciate the various experts, who have shared their experiences.

Acknowledgments

Roberta D. Sengelmann and Brent R. Moody served as section chiefs for Part IX, Skin Rejuvenation.

Tamara R. Fountain served as section chief for Part XII, Functional Lid Malpositions, Sections 1–2, Ptosis.

We would like to thank Jan Heizer and Chris Kleber, Saint Louis University Department of Ophthamology, for their assistance in preparing this book.

Morris E. Hartstein, MD, FACS
John B. Holds, MD, FACS
Guy G. Massry, MD

Contents

Part III Upper Lid Blepharoplasty

Section One Preoperative Evaluation

Section Two Incision Planning

Section Three Upper Blepharoplasty Procedure Pearls

Part IV Lower Lid Blepharoplasty

Section One Preoperative Considerations

Section Two Lower Blepharoplasty Procedure Pearls

Section Three Fat Repositioning in Lower Blepharoplasty

Section Two Endoscopic Forehead Rejuvenation

Contributors

Richard L. Anderson, MD, FACS
Medical Director, Center for Facial Appearances, Salt Lake City, UT, USA

Sterling S. Baker, MD
Assistant Clinical Professor, Department of Ophthalmology, Adjunct Clinical Professor, Department of Dermatology, University of Oklahoma College of Medicine, Oklahoma City, OK, USA

Leslie Baumann, MD
Professor, University of Miami, Miami Heart Institute, Department of Dermatology, Miami Beach, FL, USA

Kenneth R. Beer, MD
Director, The Palm Beach Esthetic Center, Voluntary Assistant Professor, University of Miami, West Palm Beach, FL, USA

Francesco P. Bernardini, MD
Ospedale Evangelico Internazionale, Department of Ophthalmology, Genova, Italy

Diane S. Berson, MD
Assistant Clinical Professor, Weill Medical College of Cornell University, New York Presbyterian Hospital, Department of Ophthalmology, New York, NY, USA

Evan H. Black, MD
Associate Professor, Wayne State University School of Medicine, Kresge Eye Institute, Department of Ophthalmology, Detroit, MI, USA

Sean M. Blaydon, MD
Ophthalmic Plastic and Reconstructive Surgeon, Texas Oculoplastic Consultants, Austin, TX, USA

Cat Nguyen Burkat, MD
Assistant Professor, Ophthalmic Plastic and Reconstructive Surgery, University of Wisconsin, Madison, WI, USA

John R. Burroughs, MD
Medical Director, Eye and Facial Appearances, Colorado Springs, CO, USA

Kimberly J. Butterwick, MD
Scripps Memorial Hospital, La Jolla, CA, USA

William P.D. Chen, MD, FACS
Clinical Professor, UCLA School of Medicine, Harbor-UCLA Medical Center, Department of Ophthalmology, Long Beach, CA, USA

Howard Conn, MD
Private Practice, Irvine, CA, USA

Philip L. Custer, MD
Professor, Washington University School of Medicine, Department of Ophthalmology and Visual Sciences, St. Louis, MO, USA

Roger A. Dailey, MD, FACS
Lester Jones Chair, Oculofacial Plastic Surgery, Oregon Health and Sciences University, Division of Oculofacial Plastic & Reconstructive Surgery, Portland, OR, USA

Sheri L. DeMartelaere, MD, FACS
Assistant Professor, Uniformed Services, University of the Health Sciences, Director, Ocular and Orbital Trauma Service, Brooke Army Medical Center, Department of Surgery, San Antonio, TX, USA

Martin H. Devoto, MD
Director, Consultores Oftalmologicos, Division of Oculoplastic and Orbital Surgery, Buenos Aires, Argentina

Lisa M. Donofrio, MD
Associate Clinical Professor, Yale University School of Medicine, Department of Dermatology, New Haven, CT, USA

Jeffrey S. Dover, MD
SkinCare Physicians, Chestnut Hill, MA, USA

Steven C. Dresner, MD
Associate Clinical Professor, University of Southern California, Department of Ophthalmology, Los Angeles, CA, Eyesthetica Inc., Santa Monica, CA, USA

Kathleen M. Duerksen, MD, FACS
Private Practice, Tuscon, AZ, USA

Jeffrey P. Edelstein, MD
Private Practice, Chandler, AZ, USA

Andrew S. Eiseman, MD
Assistant Professor, Uniformed Services University of the Health Sciences, Chief, Oculoplastics and Orbit Disease Center, Department of Surgery, Walter Reed Army Medical Center, Eye Clinic, Washington D.C., USA

Yoash R. Enzer, MD
Assistant Clinical Professor, Warren Albert School of Medicine of Brown University, Rhode Island Hospital, Department of Surgery, Division of Ophthalmology, Providence, RI, USA

Melanie H. Erb, MD
Assistant Clinical Professor, University of California at Irvine, Department of Ophthalmology, Irvine, CA, University of Southern California, Department of Ophthalmology, Los Angeles, CA, Eyesthetica Inc., Santa Monica, CA, USA

Robert G. Fante, MD
Clinical Associate Professor, University of Colorado, Departments of Ophthalmology and Otolaryngology, Denver, CO, USA

Jill A. Foster, MD
Associate Clinical Professor, The Ohio State University, The Eye Center of Columbus, Department of Ophthalmology, Columbus, OH, USA

Raf Ghabrial, MBBS, FRANZCO
Senior Lecturer, University of Sydney, Sydney Oculoplastic Surgery, Sydney, Australia

Geoffrey J. Gladstone, MD
Co-director of Oculofacial Surgery, William Beaumont Hospital, Department of Ophthalmology, Southfield, MI, USA

Mark J. Glasgold, MD
Clinical Assistant Profesor, Robert Wood Johnson Medical School, Department of Surgery, Highland Park, NJ, USA

Robert A. Glasgold, MD
Clinical Assistant Professor, Robert Wood Johnson Medical School, Department of Surgery, Highland Park, NJ, USA

Herbert J. Glatt, MD
University of Tennessee Medical Center, Department of Surgery, Knoxville, TN, USA

Russell S. Gonnering, MD, FACS
Clinical Professor, The Medical College of Wisconsin, Department of Ophthalmology, Brookfield, WI, USA

Andrea N. Hass, MD
Hass Plastic Surgery and Medispa, Palm Beach Gardens, FL, USA

Morris E. Hartstein, MD, FACS
Clinical Associate Professor, Saint Louis University, Department of Ophthalmology and Division of Plastic and Reconstructive Surgery, St. Louis, MO, USA

R. Jeffrey Hofmann, MD
Assistant Clinical Professor, Brown University, Rhode Island Eye Institute, Department of Ophthalmology, Providence, RI, USA

David E.E. Holck, MD
Chairman, Department of Ophthalmology, The University of Texas at San Antonio, Health Sciences Center, Director, Oculofacial Plastics and Orbital Service, Wilford Hall Medical Center, Department of Ophthalmology, San Antonio, TX, USA

John B. Holds, MD, FACS
Clinical Professor, Saint Louis University, Departments of Ophthalmology and Otolaryngology-Head and Neck Surgery, St. Louis, MO, USA

Erin L. Holloman, MD
Private Practice, Oklahoma City, OK, USA

David F. Horne, MD
Assistant Clinical Professor, Cornell University, New York Presbyterian Hospital, Department of Dermatology, New York, NY, USA

Edsel Ing, MD, FRCSC
Assistant Professor, University of Toronto, Toronto East General Hospital, Toronto, Ontario, Canada

Derek H. Jones, MD
Clinical Assistant Professor, David Geffen School of Medicine at UCLA, Department of Dermatology, Los Angeles, CA, USA

Kevin A. Kalwerisky, MD
Fellow, Oculofacial Plastic Surgery, The University of Texas at San Antonio, Health Sciences Center, Wilford Hall Medical Center, Department of Ophthalmology, San Antonio, TX, USA

Michael S. Kaminer, MD
Assistant Professor, Yale Medical School, New Haven, CT, Dartmouth Medical School, Hanover, NH, Department of Dermatology, SkinCare Physicians of Chestnut Hill, Chestnut Hill, MA, USA

Andrew J. Kaufman, MD, FACP
Assistant Clinical Professor, David Geffen School of Medicine at UCLA, Center for Dermatology Care, Los Angeles, CA, USA

Jemshed A. Khan, MD
Clinical Professor, Kansas University School of Medicine, Kansas University Medical Center, Department of Ophthalmology, Kansas City, MO, USA

Don O. Kikkawa, MD
Clinical Professor, Chief, Division of Oculofacial Plastic and Reconstructive Surgery, University of California, San Diego, Department of Ophthalmology, La Jolla, CA, USA

Bobby S. Korn, MD, PhD
Assistant Professor, University of California, San Diego School of Medicine, Shiley Eye Center, Department of Ophthalmology, Division of Oculofacial Plastic & Reconstructive Surgery, La Jolla, CA, USA

Bradley T. Kovach, MD
Florida Coastal Dermatology Associates, Naples, FL, USA

Samuel M. Lam, MD, FACS
Facial Plastic Surgeon, Lam Facial Plastics, Plano, TX, USA

Gustavo H. Leibaschoff, MD
President, ICAM USA, Inc., Director, International School of Mesotherapy, Dallas, TX, USA

James Leong, MBBS, MMed
Clinical Associate Lecturer, University of Sydney, Sydney Eye Hospital, Sydney, Australia

Peter S. Levin, MD
Clinical Adjuvant Professor, Stanford University School of Medicine, Department of Ophthalmology, Mountain View, CA, USA

Don Liu, MD
Professor, University of Missouri, Department of Ophthalmology, Columbia, MO, USA

Manuel A. Lopez, MD
Director, Facial Plastics Service, The University of Texas at San Antonio, Health Sciences Center, Wilford Hall Medical Center, Department of Otolaryngology, San Antonio, TX, USA

Mark J. Lucarelli, MD
Associate Professor, University of Wisconsin, Director, Oculoplastics Service, Department of Ophthalmology and Visual Sciences, Madison, WI, USA

William P. Mack, MD
Clinical Assistant Professor, University of South Florida, Department of Ophthalmology, Tampa, FL, USA

Geva Mannor, MD, MPH
Head, Oculoplastic Surgery, SCRIPPS Clinic, Department of Ophthalmology, La Jolla, CA, USA

Guy G. Massry, MD
Director, Ophthalmic Plastic and Reconstructive Surgery, American Eye Institute, Cedars Sinai Medical Center, Los Angeles, CA, Spalding Dr. Cosmetic Surgery and Dermatology, Beverly Hills, CA, Davidorf Eye Group, West Hills, CA, USA

Seth L. Matarasso, MD
Clinical Profesor, University of California, San Francisco, Department of Dermatology, San Francisco, CA, USA

Joseph A. Mauriello Jr., MD
Ophthalmic Plastic and Reconstructive Surgeon, University of Medicine and Dentistry of New Jersey, Summit, NJ, USA

Robert A. Mazzoli, MD, FACS
Consultant in Ophthalmology to the Surgeon General, Director, Ophthalmic Plastic, Reconstructive and Orbital Surgery, Associate Professor, Uniformed Services University of the Health Sciences, Bethesda, MD, Madigan Army Medical Center, Tacoma, WA, USA

John D. McCann, MD, PhD
Medical Director, The Center for Facial Appearances, Salt Lake City, UT, USA

Clinton D. McCord, Jr., MD
Associate Clinical Professor, Emory University School of Medicine, Paces Plastic Surgery and Recovery Center, Atlanta, GA, USA

Michael E. Migliori, MD, FACS
Clinical Associate Professor, The Warren Alpert School of Medicine at Brown University, Rhode Island Hospital, Department of Ophthalmology, Providence, RI, USA

Yasaman Mohadjer, MD
Washington University in St. Louis, Department of Ophthalmology and Visual Sciences, St. Louis, MO, USA

Brent R. Moody, MD
Assistant Professor, Vanderbilt University, Department of Dermatology, Nashville, TN, USA

Asa D. Morton, III, MD
Director, Ophthalmic and Facial Plastic Surgery, Eye Care Center of San Diego, San Diego, CA, USA

Shoib Myint, DO, FAACS, FACO
Ophthalmic and Facial Plastic Surgeon, Co-director, Beaumont Eye Institute, William Beaumont Hospital, Department of Ophthalmology, Southfield, MI, USA

Paul S. Nassif, MD, FACS
Spalding Drive Cosmetic Surgery & Dermatology, Beverly Hills, CA, USA

Frank A. Nesi, MD
Associate Clinical Professor, Kresge Eye Institute, Wayne State University School of Medicine, William Beaumont Hospital, Department of Ophthalmology and Otolaryngology, Royal Oak, MI, USA

Russell W. Neuhaus, MD
Ophthalmic Plastic and Reconstructive Surgeon, Texas Oculoplastic Consultants, Austin, TX, USA

Joseph Niamtu, III, DMD
Private Practice, Cosmetic Facial Surgery, Richmond, VA, USA

John Pak, MD, PhD
Oculoplastic Surgeon, Wheaton Eye Clinic, Department of Ophthalmology, Wheaton, IL, USA

Allen M. Putterman, MD
Professor of Ophthalmology, Co-Director, Oculofacial Plastic Surgery, University of Illinois School of Medicine, Michael Reese Hospital and Medical Center, Chicago, IL, USA

Oscar M. Ramirez, MD, FACS
Clinical Assistant Professor, The John's Hopkins University School of Medicine, Baltimore, MD, Esthetique Internationale, Timonium, MD, USA

Camilo O. Reyes, MD
Clinical Fellow, Esthetique Internationale, Timonium, MD, USA

O. Bailey Robertson, DDS
Director, Facial Plastics Services, Wilford Hall Medical Center, Department of Oral and Maxillofacial Surgery, San Antonio, TX, USA

Thomas E. Rohrer, MD
SkinCare Physicians of Chestnut Hill, Chestnut Hill, MA, USA

Elizabeth F. Rostan, MD
Private Practice, Dermatology and Cosmetic Surgery Center of Charlotte, Charlotte, NC, USA

Vivian Schiedler, MD
Oculoplastics and Orbital Consultants, Charlottesville, VA, USA

Stuart R. Seiff, MD
Emeritus Professor, University of California, San Francisco, Chief, San Francisco General Hospital, Department of Ophthalmology, San Francisco, CA, USA

Todd R. Shepler, MD
Ophthalmic Plastic and Reconstructive Surgeon, Texas Oculoplastic Consultants, Austin, TX, USA

John W. Shore, MD
Ophthalmic Plastic and Reconstructive Surgeon, Texas Oculoplastic Consultants, Austin, TX, USA

John D. Siddens, DO
Ophthalmic Plastic Surgery Clinical Instructor, University of South Carolina School of Medicine, Department of Ophthalmology, Columbia, SC, USA

Rona Z. Silkiss, MD
Chief, Division of Ophthalmic Plastic Reconstructive and Orbital Surgery, California Pacific Medical Center, Department of Ophthalmology, San Francisco, CA, USA

Guy Ben Simon, MD
Tel Aviv University, Goldschleger Eye Institute, Department of Ophthalmology, Ramat Gan, Israel

David J. Singer, MD, FACS
Associate Clinical Professor, University of Miami School of Medicine, Anne Bates Leach Eye Hospital of Bascom Palmer Eye Institute, Department of Ophthalmology, Miami, FL, Aspen Valley Hospital, Aspen, CO, USA

Bryan S. Sires, MD, PhD
Allure Laser Center and Medispa, Kirkland, WA, USA

Charles B. Slonim, MD, FACS
Clinical Professor, University of South Florida College of Medicine, Department of Ophthalmology, Tampa, FL, USA

Eric A. Steele, MD
Assistant Professor, Oregon Health & Sciences University, Department of Oculofacial Plastic and Reconstructive Surgery, Portland, OR, USA

William L. Walter, MD
Emeritus Staff, Washington University Medical Department, Barnes Hospital, Private Practice, St. Louis Eye Clinic, St. Louis, MO, USA

John J. Woog, MD
Professor, Mayo Clinic, Department of Ophthalmology, Rochester, MN, USA

Michael T. Yen, MD
Associate Professor, Baylor College of Medicine, Department of Ophthalmology, Houston, TX, USA

Part I

Preoperative Evaluation

1

Preoperative Evaluation of the Cosmetic Patient

Jemshed A. Khan

First and foremost, the surgeon should elicit from the patient those specific topographic facial features that the patient wants to have improved. Patients often express concern that their periocular facial features are communicating unintended signals such as disapproval (glabellar frown lines), tiredness (lower eyelid fat pad herniation or upper eyelid ptosis), worry, or ageing (crow's feet). The face, as an organ of communication, is malfunctioning.[1]

After eliciting and documenting the patient's concerns and taking photographs, the surgeon can evaluate the facial features for the anatomic basis of the patient's concerns. Patient's concerns are often related to familial, gravitational, or age-related facial changes.

Patients who cannot accept a "marked definite and noticeable improvement" as opposed to a "perfect result" may be considered poor candidates for aesthetic surgery. Informed consent includes discussing with the patient the risks, consequences, benefits, and alternatives of surgery as well as a signed document.

Finally, keep in mind that properly informed patients will not and should not always choose the surgical option that most effectively addresses their physical concerns. Other considerations factor in, including cost, invasiveness, surgical risk, location and visibility of surgical incisions, recovery times, postoperative morbidity, and procedure length. The goal is not to invariably create the best aesthetic improvement, but rather to educate the patient to the point where the patient can select the procedures which best meet their aesthetic goals while at the same time considering financial and psychological constraints, tolerance for surgical risk, and desires regarding rapidity of recovery.

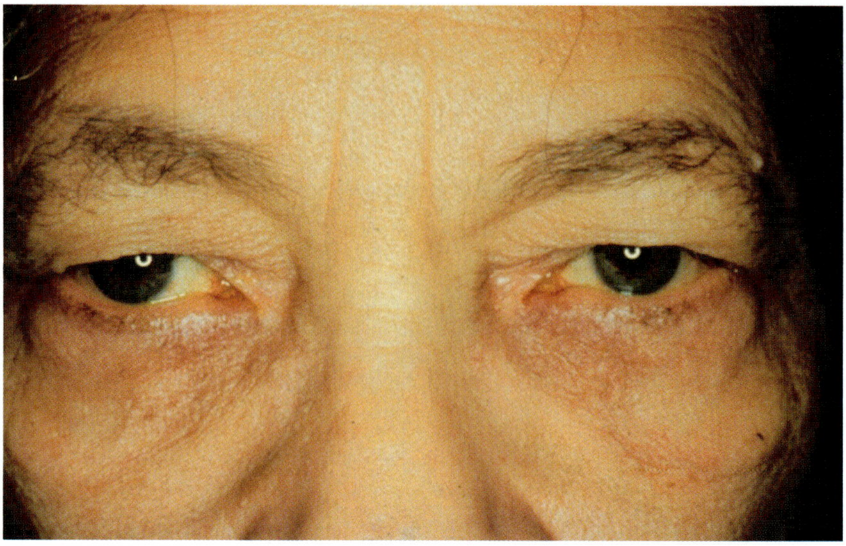

Figure 1.1. Preoperative appearance of upper eyelid dermatochalasis communicates unintended facial signals of anger, skepticism, or disapproval.

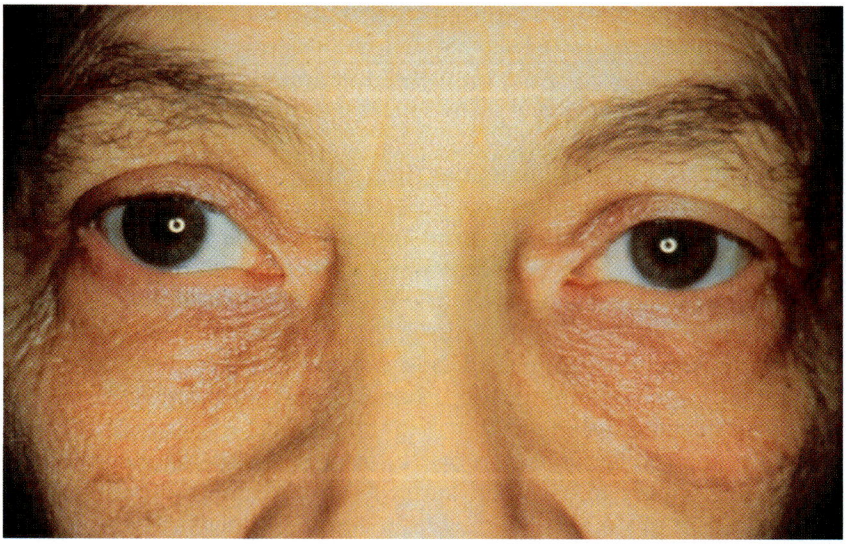

Figure 1.2. Postoperative appearance communicates a more neutral and friendly appearance.

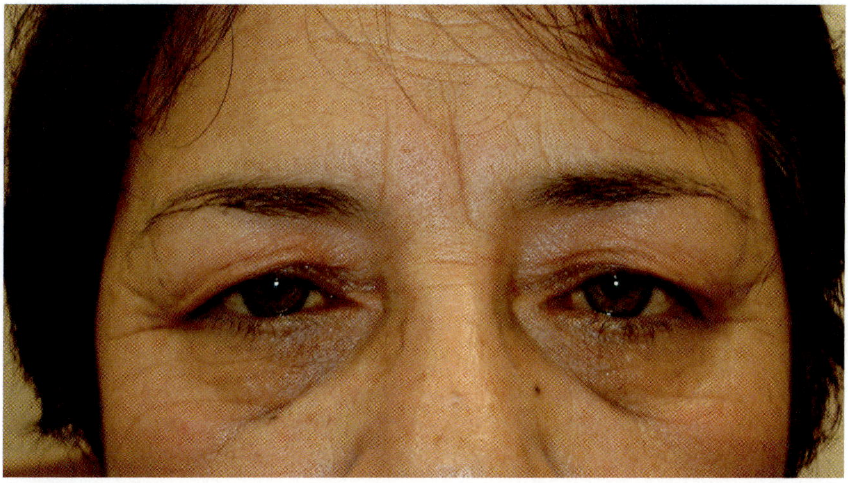

Figure 1.3. Note the tired unfriendly facial expression due to upper eyelid dermatochalasis.

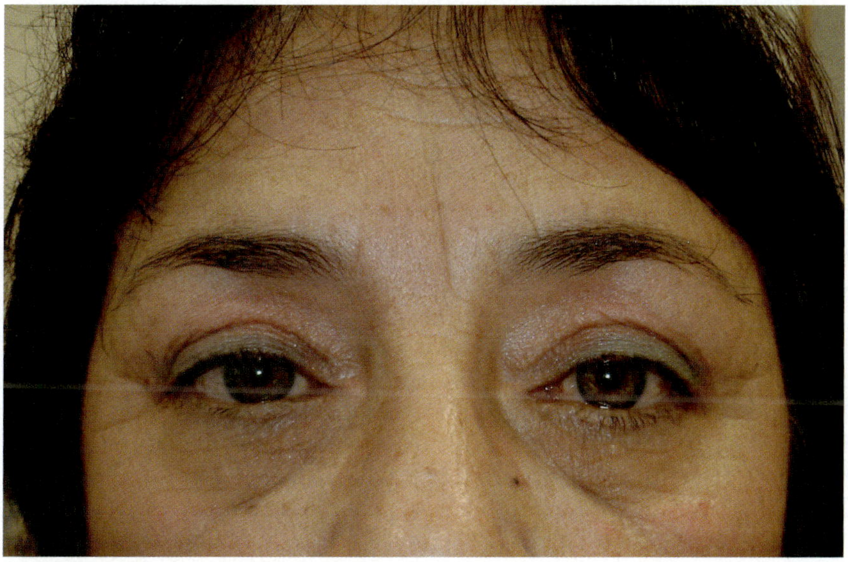

Figure 1.4. Note the improvement of facial appearance and signaling following upper eyelid blepharoplasty.

Reference

1. Khan JA. Aesthetic surgery: diagnosing and healing the miscues of human facial expression. Ophthal Plast Reconstr Surg 2001;17(1):4–6.

Reprinted with permission from: Chen WPD, Khan JA, McCord, Jr, CD. Color Atlas of Cosmetic Oculofacial Sugery. Philadelphia: Butterworth Heinemann/ Elsevier, 2004.

2

Evaluation of the Cosmetic Patient

Rona Z. Silkiss

The Eightfold Path to Patient Happiness

1. Manage the balance of power
2. Listen to the patient
3. Ensure appropriate patient motivation
4. Determine realistic surgical goals
5. Screen out the difficult patient
6. Conduct thorough informed consent
7. Avoid surgical overcorrection
8. Create an aesthetic environment

Manage the Balance of Power Between Doctor and Patient

The relationship between the doctor and patient must be bilateral and balanced. Both the patient and surgeon must be willing to walk away from the "contract" that exists prior to surgery if signs of imbalance exist. If the balance of power lies too heavily with either the patient or the surgeon, the potential for an unhappy patient is high.

The patient must take responsibility for the initial objectives of the cosmetic surgery. In order for the surgeon to meet the patient's expectations, they must be established by the patient to him- or herself preoperatively. There must be an established metric for surgical success. If there is no defined endpoint, vague dissatisfaction or even litigation is a possible outcome.

Additionally, the decision to recommend surgery by the surgeon should not be based on whether you "can" perform surgery, but whether you "should." Patients may be asking for reassurance and may not be ready for surgery either physically or emotionally. A patient may be reacting to the increasing pressure of early surgery perpetuated by the media. Cosmetic surgery procedures may change the patient's perception of self and lead to an unhappy patient. A patient may already be unhappy and be sublimating this into a "surgical fix."

In general, surgeons may advertise but should avoid "selling" their services. A patient will appreciate honesty. Surgical integrity will be rewarded many times over. What is rare and withheld is valued more highly.

Listen to Your Patient Before Surgery (or you will surely have to listen to them after)

In the course of a consultation with a patient, surgeons should specifically ask patients what they wish to achieve. Ask to see old photographs and remind the patient of his or her youthful configuration. Allow the patient to bring in photos of the desired or anticipated outcome.

The contrast between target and actual configuration serves as the basis of a discussion about what surgery can and cannot provide. This defines the "envelope of the possible" for the patient. Remind the patient that "perfection is not part of the equation" for results no matter how perfect the surgery or procedure.

Document and Demonstrate

Photograph the patient during the consultation and demonstrate preoperative asymmetry. Patients may not be aware of their own preoperative asymmetry. In contrast, with certainty, they will be aware of any postoperative asymmetry. Preoperative awareness and documentation may prevent the patient from ascribing their underlying preoperative asymmetry to the surgery or surgeon.

Ensure Appropriate Patient Motivation

Often patients will be motivated to seek cosmetic surgery in the event of a recent job loss, divorce, or life crisis. It is critical that the surgeon assess the patients' motivation for surgery to decide if they are appropriate surgical candidates. Do not give the patient the opportunity to transfer his or her unhappiness to the recent surgery or surgeon. It may be useful to advise the patient to return after an interval of time when life circumstances have become more stable.

A patient's surgical goals should be appropriate and self-generated. The patient must be personally committed to the surgery and accept the risks of surgery and the physical alteration. Patients may be seeking reassurance from a consultant that surgery is optional at a particular point in time. Reassurance alone may be the best medicine. A patient trying to reestablish his or her own self-esteem, advised to postpone surgical intervention, may be your most grateful and happy patient.

Determine Realistic Surgical Goals

Both the surgeon and patient must be realistic. The surgeon needs a clear understanding of what a technique can optimally and usually provides. He or she needs to communicate this knowledge to patients so that their expectations can be adjusted to an informed reality. In advising patients, do not assume that the patient shares your personal aesthetic or style. Be aware of misguided surgical goals such as:

1. An attempt by the patient to match a distant image ideal (celebrity).
2. An attempt by the patient to achieve arbitrary standards of perfection through more surgery.
3. An attempt by the patient to heal psychological pain by body alteration or wounding.

Misguided surgical goals may lead the patient "driving to imperfection." This is a situation where the patient's fervent desire to achieve an impossible ideal may lead to surgical outcomes that are quite the opposite of beauty.

Screen Out the Difficult Patient

Learn to recognize the warning signs of a difficult patient. This is a limited list of signs of the potentially difficult patient:

1. The patient's chief complaint is one concerning prior surgeons.
2. The patient has already received multiple procedures and is still not satisfied.
3. The patient manifests an obsessive/compulsive approach to small or invisible suboptimalities. This may be demonstrated by overt self-intolerance or disdain or overly detailed, lengthy questions or email prior to considering the procedure.
4. The patient complains of pain or an abnormal feeling related to the cosmetic concern.
5. The patient continues to critically self-evaluate and primp in the mirror, despite your initiation of a conversation.
6. The patient appears to have an unrealistic expectation for the surgical outcome.
7. The patient refuses to "hear" the limitations of surgery and reiterates a desired outcome despite your explanation regarding the improbability or impossibility of same.
8. The patient displays an inappropriate level of familiarity or flattery, especially during the initial consultation.
9. The patient is inappropriately aggressive or hostile during the consultation or is inappropriately demanding or demeaning to the office staff.
10. The patient consultation takes an unusually lengthy period of time, making the surgeon uncomfortable with the degree of self-absorption and detail demanded.
11. There is excessive "negotiating" about price, location, or insurance prior to surgery.
12. Repeated cancellation of the surgical date.
13. Insistence by the cosmetic patient that "their friend's surgery was covered by insurance."
14. The patient seeks urgent or emergent cosmetic surgery unrealistically close to an important social event such as a wedding or reunion.

15. Your intuition informs you that this patient is likely to be difficult, yet your ego struggles with your desire to "fix the problem" other surgeons have been unable to correct, leading to your own internal tension and turmoil.

Determine whether a potentially difficult patient is someone for whom you wish to care in the event of a problem. The consultation is the honeymoon phase. The relationship is unlikely to get easier. Ask whether the patient will later insist, should there be a suboptimal outcome in his mind, that he or she was not given alternatives, appropriate time to make an informed decision, or that the surgeon "rushed" to operate?

There are several psychiatric syndromes associated with difficult patients. The two most common are narcissism and body dysmorphic syndrome.

Narcissism is a condition in which the individual expresses an extreme need to be the center of attention. They make an inappropriate attempt to control the social environment. The etiology of narcissism is an underlying deep insecurity.

Body dysmorphic syndrome is manifest by an inaccurate, inappropriate assessment of body appearance. Patients manifest severe distress regarding their physical appearance despite numerous cosmetic procedures, irrespective of their actual appearance.

Surgery does not cure these conditions. The experiment has been done again and again and again. There is no need to repeat the experiment.

As a surgeon, you are not obligated to care for a cosmetic patient whom you view as litigious, threatening, or difficult or for whom you believe the surgery is unlikely to satisfy—independent of result.

Conduct a Thorough Informed Consent

It is critical that the operative surgeon obtain a thorough informed consent prior to surgery. In addition to the specifics of the procedure, the consent discussion must emphasize that "function trumps form" every time. The potential risks and suboptimalities of surgery should be discussed openly. The most common risk is "expectation risk," and this should be discussed explicitly. Patients need to be reminded that that "perfection is not part of the equation" for surgery and if they will be satisfied with improvement they will likely be happy. If they are seeking perfection, they will not be happy.

During the patient consultation and consent, the patient should be educated regarding the aesthetic surgeon's understanding of rejuvenation. In years past, more surgery, more excavation, more hollowness or tautness was considered the standard of care and sometimes even proof of getting "one's money's worth" in surgery. This provided patients with an unnatural, obvious, surgical alteration leading one to look "lost in time." In contrast, the current understanding of rejuvenation emphasizes that fullness is a sign of youth and that youthful individuals are not taut, hollow, or skeletonized. Additionally, youthful individuals are not overly frozen, plump, or exaggerated in configuration.

It is important it remind patients that form follows function, and that a maximally aesthetic result will follow from the appropriate management of the target tissue. These tissues should not be overcorrected. Aesthetic results are always relative to age and native configuration. Patients and surgeons need to keep the correction in context to the patient's age, ethnicity, and natural appearance in youth.

Create an Aesthetic Environment

As an aesthetic surgeon, it is beneficial to create an environment in the office which expresses your ability to understand the nature of aesthetics. One should develop a clean, comfortable space with current décor. There should be health and fashion magazines in the patient lounge. Although the medical profession may receive its cosmetic information from peer-reviewed scientific journals, your patients are receiving their information and misinformation from mass media. The surgeon should be somewhat familiar with the current "lore or buzz" in the media.

The aesthetic environment should extend to the operating room. Here, the surgeon should provide for a calm, controlled, relaxing experience. "Handesthesia" goes a long way to reassuring an anxious patient during a procedure.

Patients always like to receive something more than expected. Send your patients home with sunglasses, gel packs, ointment, etc. Make the postoperative period easy. Send patients home with their postoperative medication or prescriptions, a postoperative appointment, and easy to read, explicit instructions. Ensure comfortable suture removal. In the event of a need for revision, be explicit about your revision policy. Make certain this is well known to the staff in advance to avoid unnecessary confusion or conflict. Finally, and above all, be available, affable, and able to follow through in resolving patient issues before and after a procedure.

The ultimate secret to a happy patient is communication, expectation management, and informed surgical and procedural judgment. Perhaps "The Eightfold Path to Patient Happiness" can help guide your way.

3

Preoperative Patient Counseling for Cosmetic Blepharoplasty

William P.D. Chen

Cosmetic blepharoplasty is one of the most popular forms of aesthetic surgery of the face. The surgical outcome is intimately related to the interaction of the upper eyelids with the forehead and brows, as well as the lower eyelids, lateral canthi, and the mid-face and cheek's topography. Therefore, in any discussion and examination of a patient with regard to this form of surgery, an astute clinician should be attentive to the entire face and not confine his or her attention to the superficial upper and lower eyelid skin layers. This awareness of surrounding as well as deeper structures will ultimately yield much better surgical outcome and a happier patient.

In my first office consultation with new patients, I listen first to their complaints, and mentally classify the complaints into relative orders (or wish list) including those that can be improved upon versus transient improvement or no improvement at all. I then assess from their personality and temperament what degree of enthusiasm or tolerance to surgery they possess. Ultimately, the surgeon and the patient need to mutually agree on what is comfortable, beneficial, and worthwhile for the patient to undertake. This may include financial matters, time commitment as to postoperative healing course, as well as overall general medical conditions that may have a bearing on the type of surgery and anesthesia recommended.

I always try to encourage patients to speak their mind, even if they may be embarrassed, and I try to facilitate this in an environment free of stress. Very often patients may be overly self-conscious about an issue that matters very little to anyone they interact with, or one may need to point out an extreme condition that needs to be corrected before the aesthetic outcome can be achieved, for example, involutional ptosis in conjunction with upper eyelid hooding. It is important to customize individual aspects of your particular technique for that patient. For example, I have not performed two exactly identical procedures among any of my patients who came to me to have Asian blepharoplasty.

After an adequate prioritization of goals with the patient, I then explain what the procedure involves before, during and after the surgery and what is expected of the patient.

In the office chart for the patient, I jot down particular aspects of their facial structure (like ptosis, ectropion, entropion, lateral canthal dehiscence, thinning of levator and aponeurosis, forehead brow overaction, prominent sulcus), what was mentioned to them (for example, one upper lid margin is half a millimeter lower than the other, one eye is more sunken and shows a more prominent sulsus), what were the patient's response and preferences (high crease, low crease, shape of crease line selected as well as skin texture and preexistent thining of lower lid skin and telangiectatic blood vessels observed) as well as whether I told the patient that despite their stated preference, whether it can be achieved. If a patient has thick dry skin, an oily complexion, superficial furuncles, or rosacea—these are all noted onto my plan of management for this patient.

If a patient seems extremely nervous, I usually try to call them the night before the procedure to make sure all is well. On the day of surgery in the preoperative area, I greet the patient again and reiterate the goal(s) of the surgery. If there is any discrepancy between what I told them and what they think and expect of the surgery, I will always defer the surgery until another day, although this is extremely rare.

Reprinted with permission from: Chen WPD, Khan JA, McCord, Jr, CD. Color Atlas of Cosmetic Oculofacial Sugery. Philadelphia: Butterworth Heinemann/ Elsevier, 2004.

Part II

Anesthesia

4

Guide to Local Anesthetic Medications

Vivian Schiedler and Bryan S. Sires

Topical Ocular Anesthetics

Proparacaine or tetracaine drops can be applied to the ocular surface to help minimize the discomfort of subconjunctival injections. Facial prep solutions, bright lights, and repeated opening of eyes intraoperatively to adjust lid height may cause drying and ocular irritation. Treating both eyes helps increase patient comfort and cooperation. Tetracaine is the most potent topical agent[1] and can be used directly on the tarsal plate during procedures such as ptosis repair in which anesthetic use is minimized to avoid levator muscle paralysis. Use of topical anesthetic drops should be limited in all patients to prevent iatrogenic corneal epitheliopathy. The postoperative analgesic regimen should never include topical ocular anesthetic agents.

Lidocaine

Lidocaine is the most commonly used local anesthetic. As an amide, it is hepatically metabolized and has a longer duration of action than ester anesthetics, which are locally metabolized by esterases. Lidocaine is available in 0.5, 1, 2, and 4% concentrations with or without epinephrine. The lowest concentration is preferable in infants and young children secondary to the risk of systemic toxicity. It has a rapid onset of action (30–60 seconds) but a relatively short duration (30–120 minutes).[1] Its duration of action is shortened without epinephrine since it is the most potent vasodilator of all local anesthetics. The maximum recommended dose of lidocaine with epinephrine is 7 mg/kg, which is equivalent to 50 ml of a 1% lidocaine concentration for a 70-kg person.[2] Without epinephrine, the maximum recommended lidocaine dose should be halved.

Bupivacaine

Bupivacaine is also an amide local anesthetic. It is four times as potent as lidocaine and has a longer onset of action (5 minutes) as well as a longer duration of action (120–180 minutes).[1] Therefore, it is commonly mixed with lidocaine in order to provide continuous analgesia during longer procedures as well as some postoperative analgesia. The maximal recommended dose of bupivacaine with epinephrine is 2.5–3 mg/kg.[2] This is equivalent to 35–40 ml of a 0.5% bupivacaine concentration for a 70-kg person.

Epinephrine

Local anesthetics cause vasodilation secondary to paralysis of vascular smooth muscle. This can be counteracted by epinephrine. This limits absorption of the local anesthetic into the bloodstream, thereby preventing systemic side effects. Vasoconstriction also increases the local anesthetic duration of action by slowing its removal. Due to its vasoconstrictive effect, epinephrine should be used cautiously in the penis, digits,[3] and ears to avoid tissue necrosis.

Epinephrine should be used cautiously in young children and patients with cardiac conditions as it raises heart rate and blood pressure and can cause arrhythmias. The maximal recommended dose for cardiac patients is 0.2 mg in 40 ml of a 1:200,000 dilution.[4,5] The optimal concentration to prolong the duration of local anesthesia is 1:200,000. Higher concentrations do not significantly enhance anesthetic duration and can increase the risk of side effects. It can be diluted to 1:400,000 by using a 50:50 mixture of lidocaine with a 1:200,000 concentration of epinephrine and bupivacaine without epinephrine. Of note, the epinephrine concentration can be unpredictable in the premixed form and is usually much lower than labeled. For a more reliable 1:100,000 dilution, one can add 5 ml of 8.4% sodium bicarbonate to a 50-ml bottle of 2% lidocaine and 0.55 ml of epinephrine 1:1000 (John B. Holds, MD, personal communication).

EMLA

Topical anesthetic creams can increase patient tolerance of local anesthetic injections. EMLA cream is a mixture of 2.5% lidocaine and 2.5% proparacaine applied to intact skin with an overlying occlusive dressing to enhance absorption.[6] For minor procedures, including venipuncture or anesthetic injection, EMLA should be applied 1 hour ahead of time. For split thickness skin graft harvesting or laser treatment, it should be applied for 2 hours. Presurgical planning with a prescription and careful instructions on the amount, site, and time of application are necessary for maximal efficacy. The upfront effort involved on behalf of the patient and the staff giving the instructions can outweigh the analgesic benefit of EMLA cream as compared to other quicker analgesic approaches. Although systemic side effects are rare, bloodstream levels are directly related to area and duration of application and body weight. Local but transient side effects include skin blanching, edema, and erythema. Periocular use is contraindicated since contact with the ocular surface causes severe irritation and requires copious irrigation.

Other Topical Anesthetics

A number of other topical skin anesthetics are available, including Ela-Max, Topicaine, and topical tetracaine gel. These topical agents all have limitations, as well as a maximum surface area that can be treated if toxicity is to be avoided.

The editors have had particular success with Betacaine LA ointment, which is compounded from lidocaine, prilocaine, and phenylephrine and is available from Custom Scripts Pharmacy in Tampa, Florida. This compounded ointment has the advantage of being applied without occlusion and providing superior anesthesia in 10 to 20 minutes.

Bicarbonate

To reduce the pain of local anesthetic injection, bicarbonate 8.4% can be added to the mixture in a 1:4 to 1:10 ratio. By buffering the slightly acidic pH of the anesthetic (lidocaine pH is 6.4), pain is significantly reduced without affecting the onset or duration of action of the anesthetic.[7,8]

Benzyl Alcohol

An alternative to bicarbonate for pain reduction of local anesthetic injection is saline with 0.9% benzyl alcohol. It is a bacteriostatic agent with local anesthetic properties.[9] The authors use a 1:1:1 mixture of 2% lidocaine with 1:100,000 epinephrine, 0.75% bupivacaine, and saline with 0.9% benzyl alcohol for direct infiltration of local periocular and facial anesthesia.

References

1. Benz JD. Injectable local anesthetics. AORN J 1992;55:274–284.
2. Tetzlaff JE. The pharmacology of local anesthetics. Anesthesiol Clin North Am 2000;18:217–233.
3. Krunic AL, Wang LC, Soltani K, Weitzul S, Taylor RS. Digital anesthesia with epinephrine: an old myth revisited. J Am Acad Dermatol 2004;51: 755–759.
4. Brown RS, Rhodus NL. Epinephrine and local anesthesia revisited. Oral Surg Oral Med Oral Pathol Oral Radiol Endod 2005;100(4):401–408.
5. New York Heart Association. Use of epinephrine in connection with procaine in dental procedures. J Am Dent Assoc 1955;50:108.
6. Lidocaine and prilocaine. Available at: http://www.rxlist.com/cgi/generic2/emla.htm. Accessed November 19, 2005.
7. Davies RJ. Buffering the pain of local anaesthetics: a systematic review. Emerg Med 2003;15:81–88.
8. Parham SM, Pasieka JL. Effect of pH modification by bicarbonate on pain after subcutaneous lidocaine injection. Can J Surg 1996;39:31–35.
9. Yuen VH, Dolman PJ. Comparison of three modified lidocaine solutions for use in eyelid anesthesia. Ophth Plast Reconstr Surg 1999;15:143–147.

5

Motor Nerve Blocks in Oculofacial Surgery

Vivian Schiedler and Bryan S. Sires

Facial akinesia is most useful for intraocular surgery to prevent forceful eyelid closure. It may also be useful in select patients undergoing cosmetic or functional procedures, such as those with hemifacial spasm or blepharospasm.

Facial Nerve Blocks

The Van Lint block prevents eyelid closure by anesthetizing only the distal branches of the facial nerve. The needle is inserted at the intersection between a line drawn parallel to the lateral orbital rim and a line drawn parallel to the inferior orbital rim. Approximately 2 ml of local anesthetic is injected along the lateral orbital rim to affect the temporal branches innervating the upper lid. Another 2 ml is injected along the inferior orbital rim to affect the zygomatic branches innervating the lower lid (Figures 5.1 and 5.2). Because buccal branches may overlap with zygomatic branches to innervate the medial lower eyelid from below, the van Lint approach may not fully block this area. Several advantages of the van Lint block include ease of application, anatomic selectivity of branches that innervate only the eyelids, and a lower risk of iatrogenic facial nerve injury than the more proximal blocks.[1,2]

The Atkinson block is more proximal than the van Lint. About 5 ml of local anesthetic is administered just inferior to the zygomatic arch and directed over the bone toward the top of the ear as well as in the opposite direction (Figures 5.3 and 5.4). It may not be entirely effective at producing full eyelid akinesia due to the multiple anastomoses between the temporal, zygomatic, and buccal branches of the facial nerve.[2]

The O'Brien block is the most proximal of the aforementioned facial nerve blocks. Approximately 5 ml of local anesthetic is infiltrated just anterior to the tragus of the ear over the condyloid process of the mandible at a depth of 1.0 cm (Figure 5.5). As with the Atkinson block, there is some degree of unpredictability in achieving full facial akinesia due to anatomic variability of the course of the facial nerve and its major branches.[1]

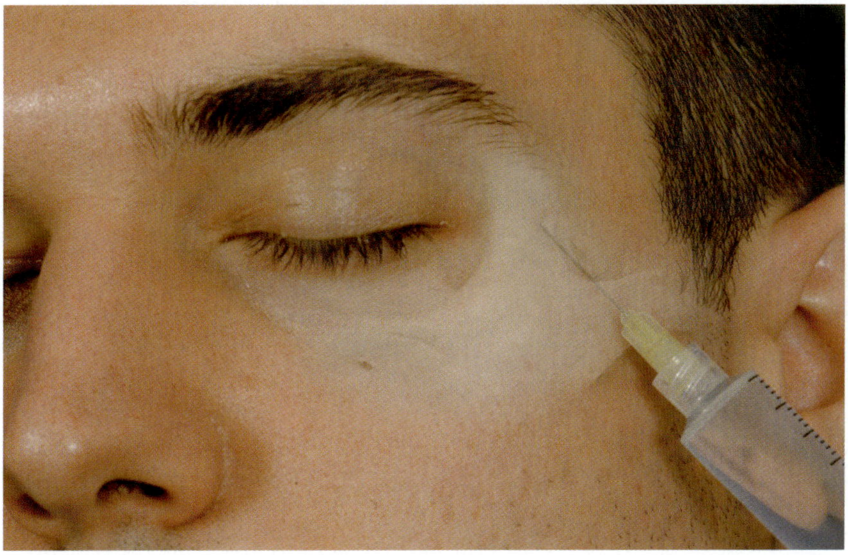

Figure 5.1. A Van Lint block involves two injection tracts. The superior eyelid contributes more to forceful eyelid closure than the inferior lid. Blocking the superior lid is accomplished by injecting local anesthetic along the superotemporal orbital rim to anesthetize the distal branches of the facial nerve that supply the superior eyelid.

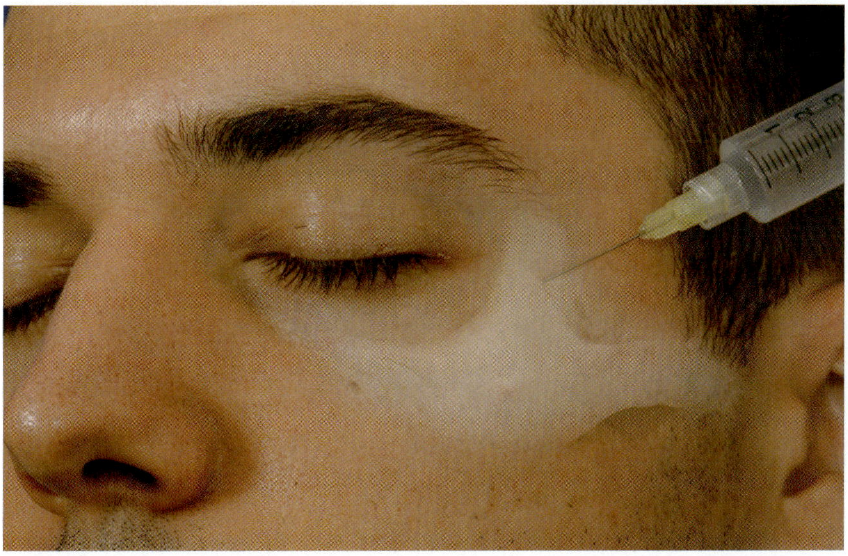

Figure 5.2. The inferior eyelid is blocked in Van Lint fashion by injecting local anesthetic along the inferotemporal orbital rim.

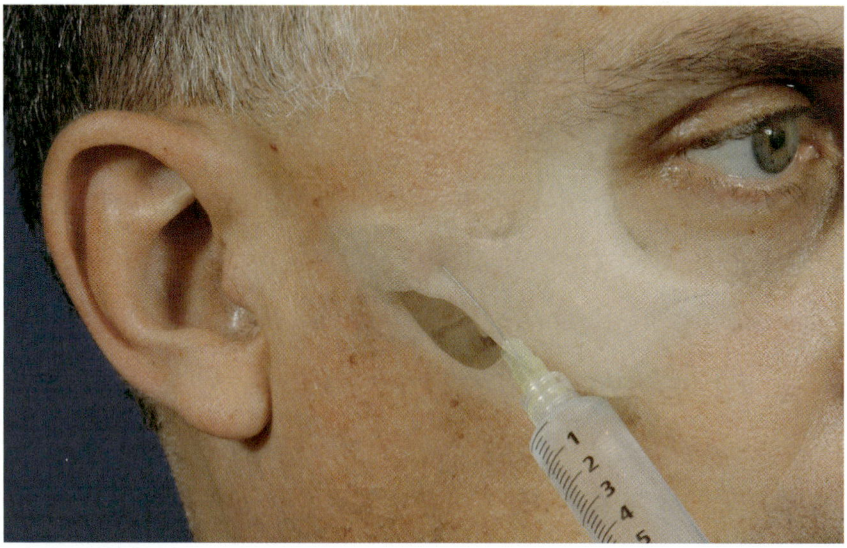

Figure 5.3. The Atkinson block is a two-tract procedure. Approximately 2–3 ml of local anesthetic is injected along a linear tract over the zygomatic arch toward the top of the ear.

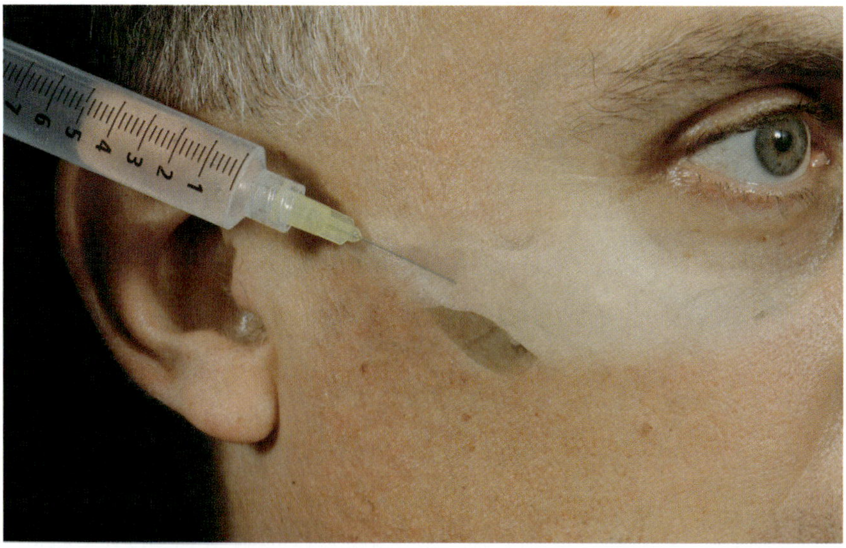

Figure 5.4. Another 2–3 ml of local anesthetic is injected in a linear tract over the zygomatic arch in the opposite direction as the first tract.

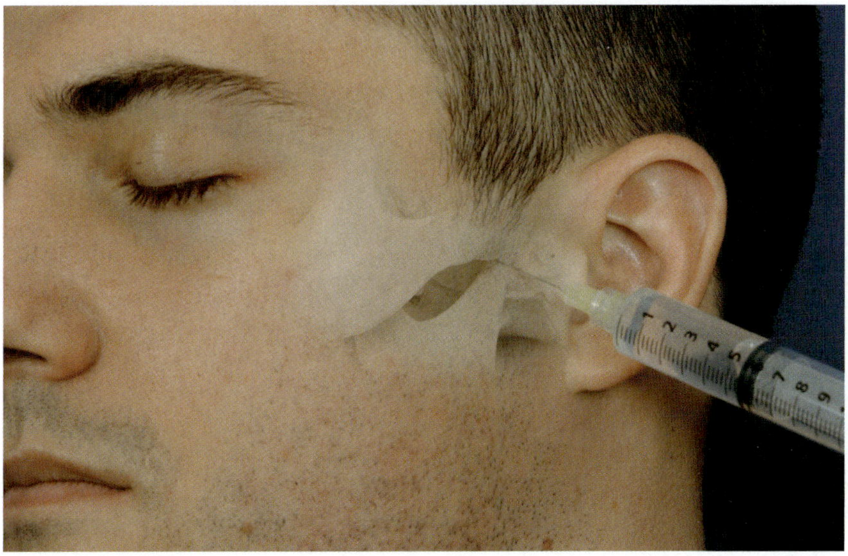

Figure 5.5. The O'Brien block anesthetizes the facial nerve at a proximal location. Approximately 5 ml of local anesthetic is injected over the condyloid process at a depth of 1.0 cm just anterior to the tragus of the ear.

Retrobulbar and Peribulbar Blocks

Socket reconstruction usually has cosmetic as well as reconstructive goals. To provide anesthesia to this area, an injection of local anesthetic is given in either the intraconal or extraconal space. In the enucleated socket, epinephrine can be used for hemostasis without concern for central retinal artery spasm. However, caution must still be used to avoid intravascular or subarachnoid space injection. After extensive orbital tissue manipulation with an ocular implant, postoperative analgesia can be given locally with a longer-acting anesthetic such as bupivacaine. However, the volume injected in the retrobulbar space should be kept under 3.5 ml to avoid seizures if accidentally injected into the cerebrospinal fluid space. In the peribulbar space, the volume injected should be kept under 7 ml to allow retention of a conformer under fully closed eyelids.

References

1. Greenbaum S. Anesthesia for eye surgery. In: Tasman W, Jaegar EA (eds.). Duane's Clinical Ophthalmology on CD-ROM. Philadelphia: Lippincott, Williams, and Wilkins, 2005: Vol 6, Ch 1.
2. Schimek F, Fahle M. Techniques of facial nerve block. Br J Ophthalmol 1995;79:166–173.

6

Regional Nerve Blocks in Oculofacial Surgery

Vivian Schiedler and Bryan S. Sires

Regional nerve blocks are useful when tissue distortion from anesthetic volume is to be avoided. They are also useful for patients undergoing more invasive procedures such as dacryocystorhinostomy who are poor candidates for general anesthesia.

Sensory Nerve Blocks

Sensory innervation to the orbit and periocular tissues is provided by the ophthalmic and maxillary divisions of the trigeminal nerve. The ophthalmic division enters the orbit through the superior orbital fissure and has three branches: the lacrimal, frontal, and nasociliary nerves. The maxillary division enters the orbit through the inferior orbital fissure and has two branches: the infraorbital and zygomatic nerves.

Lacrimal Nerve Block

This nerve supplies the lateral aspect of the superior eyelid and the lacrimal gland. To block the lacrimal nerve, 1–2 ml of anesthetic is injected close to the internal superotemporal orbital wall approximately 2 cm posterior to the orbital rim behind the lacrimal gland (Figure 6.1).

Frontal Nerve Block

This nerve branches into the supraorbital and supratrochlear nerves. The supraorbital nerve supplies the middle aspect of the superior eyelid, brow, and forehead extending to past the mid-coronal plane. The supratrochlear nerve supplies the medial aspect of the superior eyelid and brow. To block the supraorbital nerve, local anesthetic is injected over the supraorbital notch. It is palpable at the junction of the medial one-third with the lateral two thirds of the superior orbital rim (Figure 6.2). To block the supratrochlear nerve, the needle is inserted along the superomedial orbital wall just above the trochlea to a depth of 1.5 cm (Figure 6.3).

Nasociliary Nerve Block

This nerve branches into the posterior and anterior ethmoidal nerves and the infratrochlear nerve. It innervates the lacrimal sac, inner canthus, and lateral aspect of the nose. To block the infratrochlear nerve, the needle is inserted just above the medial canthal ligament along the medial wall of the orbit to a depth of 1.0 cm (Figure 6.4). If performing local anesthesia for dacryocystorhinostomy, the anterior ethmoidal nerve with its distal external nasal branch should be blocked using the same procedure but to a depth of 2.0 cm posterior to the anterior lacrimal crest.

Infraorbital Nerve Block

The maxillary nerve courses through the inferior orbital canal, giving off the anterior superior alveolar nerve branch within the canal, which supplies the superior incisors, canines, first molar, and gingiva. As it exits the inferior orbital canal through the infraorbital foramen, it becomes the infraorbital nerve, which supplies the skin and conjunctiva of the inferior eyelid, the cheek overlying the maxilla, the lateral nasal skin and septum, and the superior lip skin and mucosa. To block the infraorbital nerve, local anesthetic is injected over the foramen, which is palpable approximately 1.0 cm below the inferior orbital rim at the junction of the medial one third with the lateral two thirds of the rim. This can be done either percutaneously (Figure 6.5) or intraorally (Figure 6.6).

Zygomaticofacial Nerve Block

The zygomaticofacial nerve passes along the inferolateral orbit and exits the foramen by the same name to supply the the skin of the malar eminence and lateral cheek. The foramen can be located over the inferolateral rim below the lateral canthus and blocked with direct infiltration (Figure 6.7).

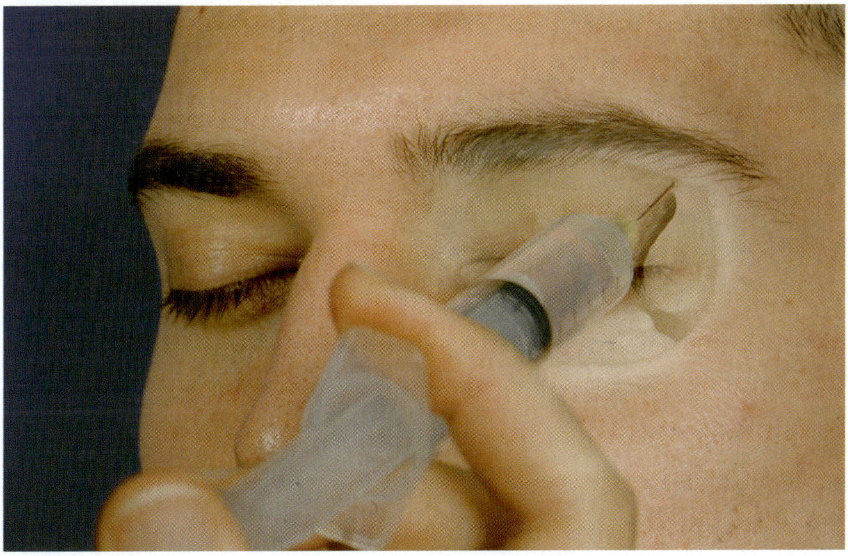

Figure 6.1. The lacrimal nerve is blocked by advancing the needle along the superotemporal orbital wall and injecting 1–2 ml of local anesthetic behind the lacrimal gland at a depth of approximately 2.0 cm.

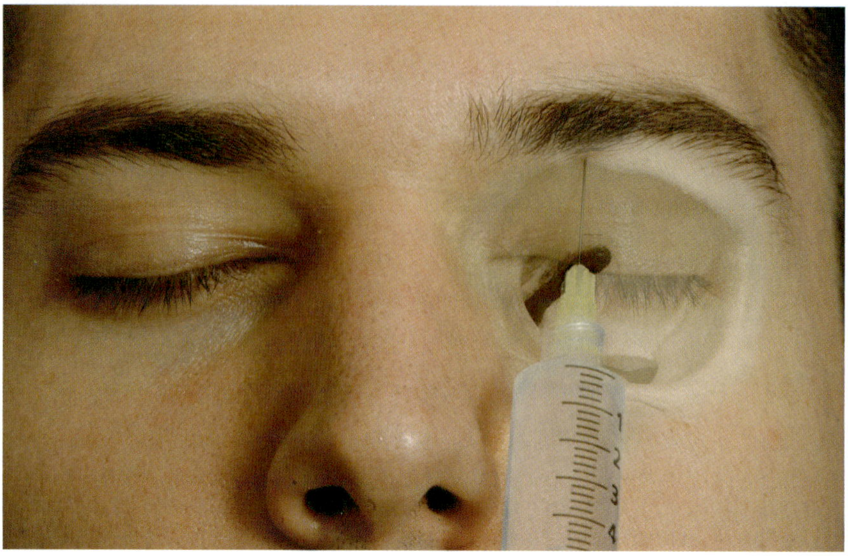

Figure 6.2. Injection of 1–2 ml of local anesthetic over the supraorbital notch will block the supraorbital nerve.

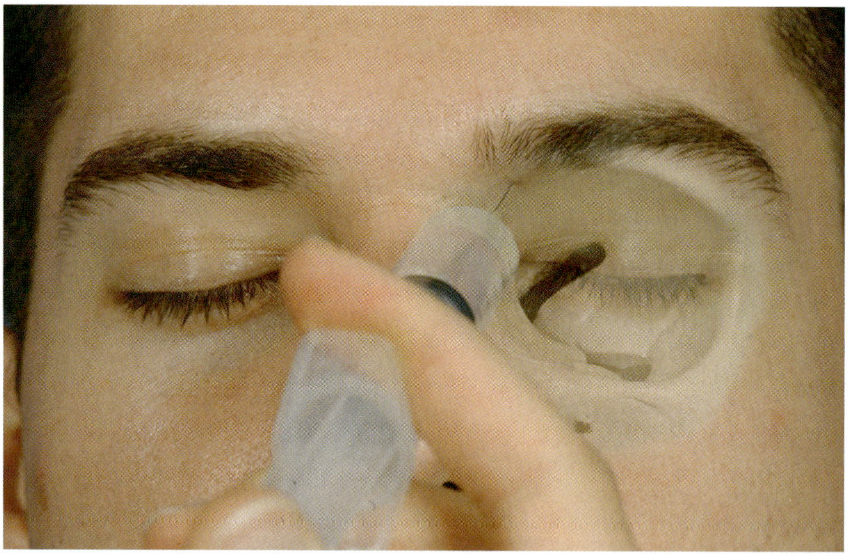

Figure 6.3. The supratrochlear nerve is blocked with local anesthetic by inserting a needle just above the trochlea to a depth of approximately 1.5 cm.

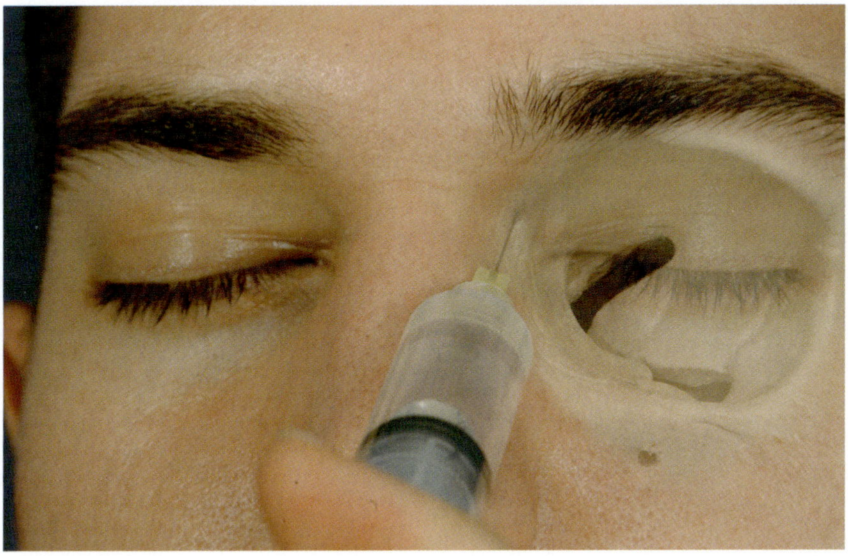

Figure 6.4. Local anesthetic injection just superior to the medial canthal ligament and along the medial orbital wall to a depth of 1.0 cm will block the infratrochlear nerve.

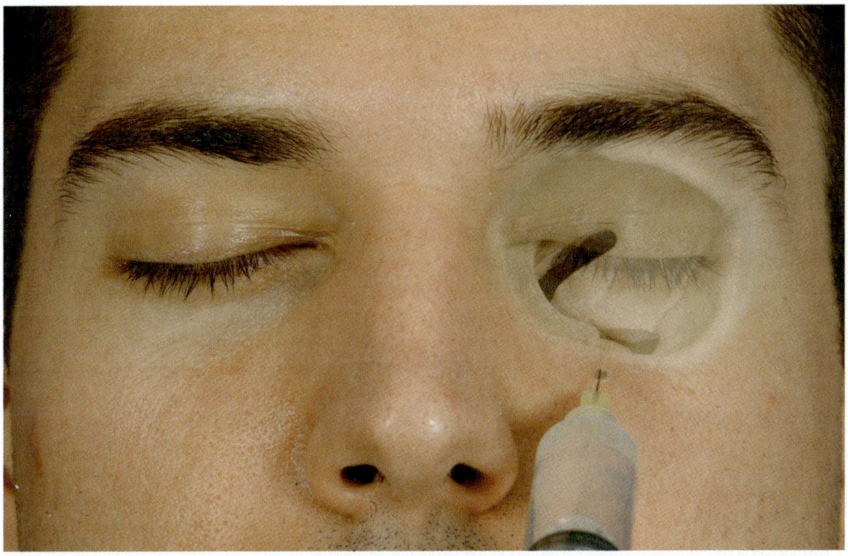

Figure 6.5. The infraorbital nerve can be blocked percutaneously by direct injection over the infraorbital foramen at the junction of the medial one third and lateral two thirds of the lower lid and 1.0 cm below the orbital rim.

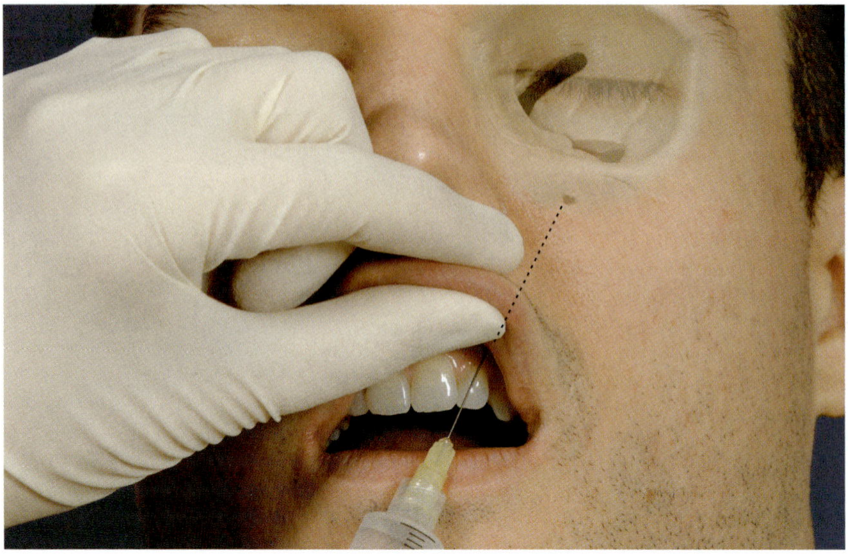

Figure 6.6. Alternatively, the infraorbital nerve can be blocked via an intraoral approach by inserting the needle through the gingiva superior to the canine and aiming toward the infraorbital foramen.

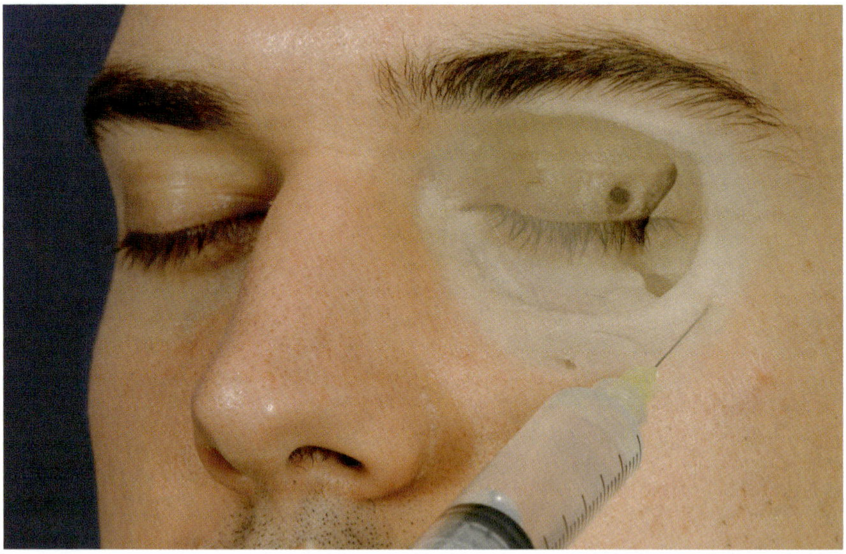

Figure 6.7. The zygomaticofacial nerve can be blocked at the inferotemporal rim inferior to the lateral canthus.

7

Procedural Sedation in Oculofacial Surgery

Vivian Schiedler and Bryan S. Sires

Staff

States, hospitals, and ambulatory surgery centers may have different credentialing and privileging requirements for those who administer sedative agents. The surgeon should be aware of these regulations. In general, only licensed independent practitioners such as medical doctors, dentists, registered nurses, physician assistants, or nurse practitioners who have undergone specific training are qualified to evaluate patients for and administer conscious sedation. They should be certified to give advanced life support and trained to rescue a patient who has lost protective reflexes from a deeper level of sedation. They should also be familiar with the pharmacology of the various sedative agents as well as reversal agents. In order to enhance patient safety, the person administering sedation and monitoring the patient for adverse events should not have any other responsibilities during the procedure. The surgeon should be free to fully concentrate on the technical aspects of the procedure.

Risk factors for complications related to conscious sedation include poor cooperation, extremes of age, severe cardiac, pulmonary, hepatic, renal, or central nervous system disease, morbid obesity, sleep apnea, pregnancy, chemical dependence, history of difficult intubation, and inadequate spontaneous ventilation. Care of such patients should be handled instead by qualified anesthesia personnel.

Monitoring

A patient under sedation should be able to tolerate unpleasant stimuli while maintaining adequate cardiorespiratory function and the ability to respond purposefully to verbal or tactile commands. Monitoring is critical to ensure this goal is met throughout the procedure and recovery period. Baseline vital signs (heart rate, respiratory rate, blood pressure, and oxygen saturation) and level of consciousness should be assessed. They are reevaluated at specific intervals during surgery and should return to baseline prior to discharge. Despite return of baseline vitals and level of consciousness, effects of sedative agents can linger and impair coordination and alertness. Therefore, in no circumstance should a patient who has received sedative agents be sent home alone or allowed to drive for 24 hours.[1]

Minimal Sedation

Oral benzodiazepines can provide good anxiolysis, relaxation, and amnesia. Cognitive function and coordination may be impaired, but cardiopulmonary function remains unaffected. Diazepam (Valium) is administered in 5- to 10-mg doses. It has a long half-life and active metabolites that can accumulate, especially in patients with poor renal function. Lorazepam (Ativan) is given in 1- or 2-mg doses. Its advantage is a somewhat shorter half-life than diazepam, and no active metabolites. Age, medical conditions, and drug clearance factors (renal or hepatic dysfunction) should be considered when dosing benzodiazepines.[1]

Moderate Sedation

Typically intravenous opiates or benzodiazepines are used to achieve a state of depressed consciousness during which the patient can respond purposefully to verbal and tactile commands. Cardiopulmonary function may be slightly affected and require oxygen administration, but should be maintained independently. Pulse oximetry and vital signs should be monitored every 15 minutes until recovery of baseline function. The combination of midazolam (Versed) and fentanyl is most commonly used for conscious sedation. Midazolam provides more profound amnesia and sedation than its oral benzodiazepine counterparts. It is given intravenously in 0.5-mg increments, not exceeding a total dose of 5 mg for young patients and 3 mg for patients older than 60 years.[2] It must be carefully titrated because the response may be unpredictable. This depends on hepatic acetylation and other medication use. Fentanyl crosses the blood–brain barrier more rapidly than any other opiate and therefore has a quick onset of action with excellent analgesia and sedation. It is given intravenously in 25-μg doses incrementally, with a maximal dose of 5 μg/kg (2 μg/kg in patients older than age 60 or debilitated patients).[2] Administration should be slow to avoid skeletal muscle rigidity and impaired ventilation seen with rapid injection. For most conscious sedation procedures, these agents are administered solely for pain reduction during local anesthetic infiltration or nerve block. Once the surgical site is adequately anesthetized, there should be no need for continuous administration of sedative agents.[1]

Antagonists/Reversal Agents

Occasionally patients may need to be rescued pharmacologically from a deeper stage of sedation. Cardiopulmonary function needs to be supported in these stages. Reversal agents return the patient to a greater level of consciousness by directly competing for and displacing the agonist from its receptors. Flumazenil is a benzodiazepine antagonist given in 0.2-mg increments intravenously over 15 seconds. If the desired level of consciousness is not obtained after waiting 45 seconds, the same dose can be repeated once every minute for a total of 1 mg.[3] Naloxone is an opiate antagonist that must be used with extreme caution. Except for cases of life-threatening respiratory depression, naloxone should be given in very small doses (0.04 mg). It can be repeated every 2 minutes to titrate the reversal of opiate side effects.[4] Larger doses can cause severe cardiovascular complications, including pulmonary edema, ventricular fibrillation, and death. Recurrent respiratory depression can occur due to the longer half-life of most agonist sedative agents. Therefore, patients must be monitored carefully for an extended period.

References

1. American Society of Anesthesiologists. Practice guidelines for sedation and analgesia for non-anesthesiologists: a report by the American Society of Anesthesiologists Task Force on Sedation and Analgesia by Non-Anesthesiologists. Anesthesiology 1996;84:459–471.
2. Shields RE. A comprehensive review of sedative and analgesic agents. Crit Care Nurs Clin North Am 1997;9:281–287.
3. O'Donnell J, Bragg K, Sell S. Procedural sedation: safely navigating the twilight zone. Nursing 2003;33:36–44.
4. Burke DF, Dunwoody CJ. Naloxone: a word of caution. Orthopaedic Nurs 1990;9:44–46.

8

Preoperative Preparation and Anesthesia

William P.D. Chen

Preoperative Regimen

For cosmetic blepharoplasty I rountinely prescribe Diazepam 10 mg 1 tab at 60–90 minutes prior to the procedure. This allows a good period of time for the sedation as well as analgesic effect to take place. Patients may often have been nervous and sleepless the night prior to coming in, or they may have traveled a bit before getting there and most can use the premedication.

About 10 minutes before the scheduled time, I greet my patient and go through the following checklist:

1. Reaffirm the physical findings previously observed and discussed with the patient.
2. Reaffirm the goals of the patient for the surgery that day.
3. Ask if there are any unanswered questions.
4. Take photos.

Intraoperative Regimen

I use 1 ml of 2% xylocaine (1:100,000 concentration epinephrine), which is first mixed with 9 ml of sterile saline injection as a diluted preparation. 0.25 ml of this diluted injection is then given subcutaneously over each eyelid. Clinical blanching of the skin is noted after a couple of minutes. Further infiltration of 0.5–1 ml of regular 2% xylocaine (with 1:100,000 epinephrine) per eyelid is then given submuscularly.

I apply 0.5 ml subcutaneously per eyelid; I then wait 2 minutes. Clinical blanching of the skin is observed. Futher infiltration of about 0.5–1.5 ml per eyelid is then given submuscularly.

A drop of Proparacaine is applied per eye for topical anesthesia of the cornea, conjunctiva, and inner surface of the eyelids.

Intravenous aliquots of Midazolam 0.5 mg are given as needed should futher sedation be necessary. Room air may be supplied via nasal cannula.

Surgical drapes are applied. I use paper drapes as well as an operculated 3M #1020 adhesive drape to minimize any potential communication between the operative field and the rest of the face under the paper drape. A drop of tetracaine is appled per eye.

A black corneo-scleral shell that conforms to the curvatures of the cornea and sclera is lubricated with sterile Lacrilube ophthalmic ointment and then applied over the eye to be operated on. The procedure commences.

Ice-cold saline solution is used on the operative field.

In select patients or those who prefer a deeper level of conscious sedation or general anesthesia, the use of an anesthesiologist may be preplanned.

Reprinted with permission from: Chen WPD, Khan JA, McCord, Jr, CD. Color Atlas of Cosmetic Oculofacial Sugery. PhiladelphiaL Butterworth Heinemann/ Elsevier, 2004.

9

"Digital Diffusion" Technique for the Administration of Local Anesthetic in Eyelid Surgery

Rona Z. Silkiss

My preferred technique for the administration of local anesthetic has been dubbed "digital diffusion." This technique involves the administration of a 50/50 mixture of 2% xylocaine with 1:100,000 epinephrine, 0.5% marcaine with 1:200,000 epinephrine combined with $NaHCO_3$ and hyaluronidase. We add 0.5 ml of $NaHCO_3$ to 9 ml of the local mixture and 0.5 ml or less of the hyaluronidase to a total of 10 ml.

The local is injected in a single point in the lateral aspect of the eyelid, just below the skin. The needle is directed away from the globe in the event the patient moves his or her head or sneezes unexpectedly. One to 2 ml of local is placed into the eyelid at the single injection site. Using a gauze pad around a digit, the local is slowly wiped across the eyelid. This local then diffuses into the eyelid in a uniform distribution, without residual tissue distortion. Additionally, because the lid has only been injected in a single point, the risk of ecchymosis formation drops significantly. This is known as the "digital diffusion" of the local anesthetic.

10

Anesthesia for In-Office Oculoplastic Surgery: How We Do It

Brent R. Moody and John B. Holds

The effective use of local anesthesia combined with minimal oral sedation can obviate the need for intravenous sedation or general anesthesia in many common oculoplastic procedures. We routinely perform upper and lower blepharoplasty, fat pad repositioning, ptosis correction, tumor removal and reconstruction, and entropion and ectropion repair without the use of intravenous or general anesthesia.

We have implemented a system of local anesthesia administration that is nearly painless for the patient. We add oral sedation only for prolonged procedures to enhance patient comfort or to alleviate significant anxiety. When oral sedation is employed, we strive for minimal sedation. Our goal is an awake but relaxed patient.

Selection of Local Anesthesia

Local anesthesia involves topical agents for superficial conjunctival anesthesia combined with injectable agents for skin and soft tissue use. Occasionally, a topical skin anesthetic such as Betacaine (Medical Center Pharmacy, Tampa, FL) or lidocaine will be used as an adjuvant to injectable local anesthesia. The instillation of proparacaine 0.5% causes less discomfort than tetracaine 0.5%; therefore, it is the preferred agent for conjunctival anesthesia.[1,2] The duration of action of proparacaine is limited to approximately 15 minutes; therefore, the surgeon must instill the agent as needed during the procedure.[2]

Lidocaine and bupivacaine serve all injectable anesthesia requirements. A low pH and rapid injection of the solution are associated with increased discomfort. Controlled slow infiltration and a neutral or nearly neutral solution is a simple technique that the surgeon can employ.[3] Our preferred local anesthetic consists of a fresh mixture of the following: 50 mL lidocaine 2%, 5 mL sodium bicarbonate 8.4%, and 0.5 mL epinephrine 1:1000. The use of commercially available lidocaine 2% with epinephrine 1:100,000 is acceptable as long as the solution is neutralized. The addition of 8.4% sodium bicarbonate in a nine-part lidocaine and one-part sodium bicarbonate mixture will effectively raise the pH of the solution into the neutral range. For prolonged local anesthetic effect, we favor bupivicaine 0.75% with epinephrine added at 1:100,000.

Selection of Oral Sedative Agent

The selection of an oral sedative agent is based primarily on surgeon familiarity with a given agent. We typically employ diazepam or occasionally lorazepam. The benzodiazepine sedative agent zolpidem is an acceptable alternative. Diazepam dosage ranges from 5 to 20 mg and lorazepam from 0.5 to 2 mg depending on age, weight, expressed anxiety, and previous experience with benzodiazepine medications. With zolpidem, we typically administer a 10-mg dose, although a 5-mg dose can be administered in selected patients.[4] Flumazenil, a benzodiazepine reversal agent, is available. We rarely find it necessary to use narcotics for oculoplastic surgery. Apprehension and pain contribute to one another, so adequate preoperative counseling to decrease anxiety will make patients tolerate the procedure much better. A calm and reassuring manner from the surgeon and staff, as well as a sense of orderliness to the process, will help alleviate patient stress.

Procedure

1. Final preoperative counseling occurs, and questions are answered. The patient undergoes informed consent, and appropriate permission forms are signed before any oral agent is given. The patient is then administered a sedative agent, if one is to be employed. The recommended application time for the topical skin anesthetics ranges from 30 to 60 minutes so they should be applied promptly.[5] Topical skin anesthetic can be applied by the nursing staff as soon as the patient arrives at the office.
2. Conjunctival anesthesia—one to two drops of proparacaine are instilled in the eye. For cutaneous topical anesthesia, Betacaine ointment may be applied to the sites of needle entry. Next, we perform preoperative surgical marking; once complete, the proparacaine will have achieved its effect. Next, a pledget is created by saturating a cotton-tipped swab with proparacaine. The pledget is placed in the inferior fornix for approximately 5 minutes. Before local anesthesia injection, the pledgets are removed. Using a dilute form of the fresh local anesthetic mixture and a 1.25-inch 27-gauge needle, the lower eyelid is anesthetized through a conjunctival approach. The dilute form of the anesthetic is prepared by combining 0.5 mL of the fresh anesthetic mix and 2.5 mL of sterile saline. We find that this very dilute form of local anesthetic is well tolerated and nearly painless. By injecting slowly through the area of pledget contact, most patients are completely unaware of this injection. If an upper eyelid procedure is also planned, the upper eyelids are anesthetized. The use of the 1.25-inch 27-gauge needle allows the entire upper eyelid to be anesthetized with two needle insertions. Approximately

1.5 cc of the initial anesthetic is instilled in each eyelid. The patient is then prepared, and this sequence allows time for the maximal vasoconstrictive effects of epinephrine to occur.

3. A second injection of local anesthesia is performed with a higher concentration agent to ensure effective anesthesia in the operative site. We use the fresh mix lidocaine 2% with epinephrine and/or bupivacaine 0.75% for the second local anesthetic injection. The patient will not feel this additional injection.

4. Local anesthetic is kept on the surgical field should the patient require any additional anesthesia.

We have found that this systematic approach to local anesthesia consistently provides effective anesthesia, minimal patient discomfort, and a high level of patient acceptance.[6,7] The major advantages of this approach are decreased cost of surgery, decreased need for postoperative observation, and decreased risk of an untoward event from intravenous agents. Patients who receive oral sedation are generally alert immediately postoperatively and can be safely released from the office or surgical suite without any prolonged observation period. Many patients appreciate having their procedure in the familiar office environment as opposed to an unfamiliar location, if the surgery occurred outside the office setting. Advantages to the surgeon are greater use of office-based surgery, minimizing the amount of nonproductive time spent traveling to an operating room or surgical center, and better control of costs. It is easy to see other patients while office staff are preparing the next surgical patient. Potential disadvantages include the need to train office staff to perform many functions that traditionally were performed in the hospital or surgery center, the staff must be familiar with the handling of surgical instruments and biohazardous waste and be prepared to handle the rare allergic reaction. Of course, appropriate resuscitation equipment should be on hand and operational. Finally, surgery on an awake patient forces the surgeon to be highly attentive to patient needs during the procedure. The surgeon may need to pay extra attention to the operative environment because the patient will be aware of all activity and conversation.

References

1. Bartfield JM, Holmes TJ, Raccio-Robak N. A comparison of proparacaine and tetracaine eye anesthetics. Acad Emerg Med 1994;1:364–367.
2. Havener WH. Anesthesia. In: Ocular Pharmacology. St. Louis: CV Mosby; 1983:72–119.
3. Scarfone RJ, Jasani M, Gracely EJ. Pain of local anesthetics: rate of administration and buffering. Ann Emerg Med 1998;31:36–40.
4. Terzano MG, Rossi M, Palomba V, et al. New drugs for insomnia: comparative tolerability of zopiclone, zolpidem and zalepon. Drug Saf 2003;26:261–282.
5. Friedman PM, MaFong EA, Friedman ES, Geronemus RG. Topical anesthetics update: EMLA and beyond. Dermatol Surg 2001;27:1019–1026.

6. Matarasso SL, Glogau RG. Local anesthesia. In: Lask GP, Moy RL, (eds.). Principles and Techniques of Cutaneous Surgery. New York: McGraw-Hill, 1996:63–76.
7. Moody BR, Holds JB. Anesthesia for office-based ocuplastic surgery. Dermatol Surg 2005;31:766–769.

Part III

Upper Lid Blepharoplasty

Section One

Preoperative Evaluation

11

Upper Eyelid Blepharoplasty: The Evaluation

Evan H. Black, John D. Siddens, Frank A. Nesi, Shoib Myint, and Geoffrey J. Gladstone

Understanding the patient's desires and expectations, whether functional, cosmetic, or both, is a critical element in eyelid surgery. The history and preoperative decision-making process is every bit as important as surgical technique.

1. The personalized interview of the patient by the surgeon is essential. During the visit, give patients a hand-held mirror so they can point out their concerns and how they want things changed.
2. Determine how and why the upper eyelids are bothering the patient. Find out what surgery they've had in the past. Are these cosmetic concerns or problems interfering with activities?
3. Obtain a detailed medical history, with particular attention to allopathic as well as homeopathic medications and supplements. Beware of drugs that interfere with platelet aggregation (aspirin, clopidogrel, ibuprofen) and the clotting cascade (heparin, warfarin).
4. Perform a complete ocular surface and adnexal exam, including visual acuity, slit lamp exam, basic secretor tear testing or tear meniscus inspection, regular visual fields, and then repeat with the eyelid skin taped up.
5. Watch out for warning signs during the exam: dry eye, corneal staining, poor Bell's phenomenon, or lagophthalmos.
6. Photos are critical. Get at least full face, downgaze, and side views. Close-up eye photos can be helpful, but with a modern digital camera these can be obtained from the full face photos.
7. Detailed measurements will differentiate ptosis, dermatochalasis, and brow ptosis. The upper margin reflex distance (MRD1) indicates the distance from the center of the pupil to the eyelid margin, which will indicate significant ptosis if 2.5 mm or less. The margin fold distance is the space between the lashes and the fold of upper eyelid skin, and gets smaller (or negative) with worsening dermatochalasis. See Figure 11.1.
8. Special attention must be given to the brow position. We cannot improve brow ptosis with a blepharoplasty procedure, and attempts to do so will cause complications. Be sure to look at the position of the lower border of *actual* brow skin ("plucked" or not); if significantly

below the superior orbital rim, this must be noted. The patient still may be a blepharoplasty candidate, but he or she must understand the limits of this procedure and possible need for future brow lift. Document this. See Figure 11.2.

9. Note that a unilateral brow elevation may indicate levator weakness on that side.

10. In a patient with a fullness above the supratarsal crease, check photos in youth as they may be seeking a look (hollowing) they never had.

11. Make sure to ask the patient to smile and note the wrinkling at the lateral canthi. They may think this will disappear with surgery, an effect that only botulinum toxin can achieve.

12. In addition to the unexpected surgical risks, discuss usual postoperative expectations with the patient. These include swelling and bruising, numbness of the eyelids and lashes, mild redness of the incision, and possible soreness.

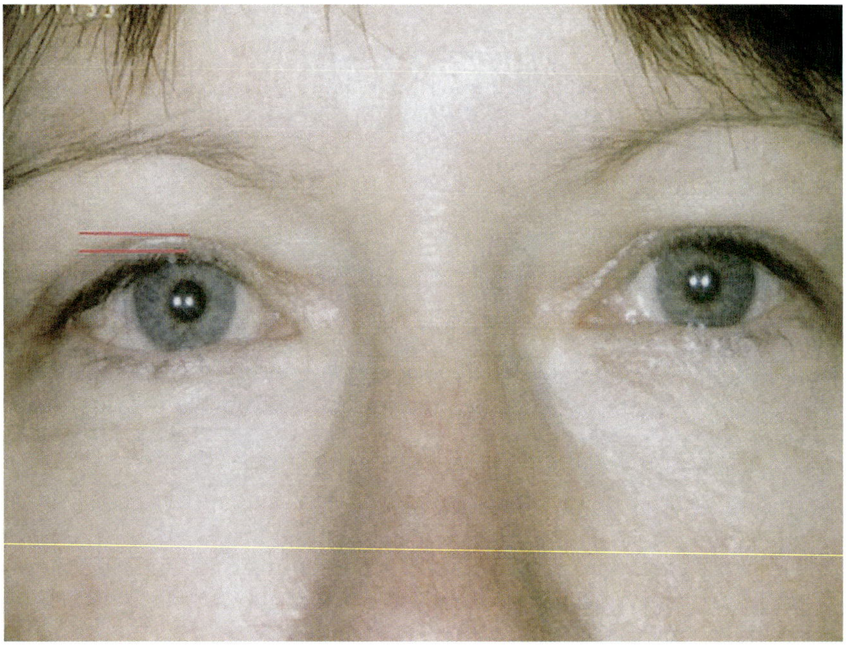

Figure 11.1. Margin fold distance.

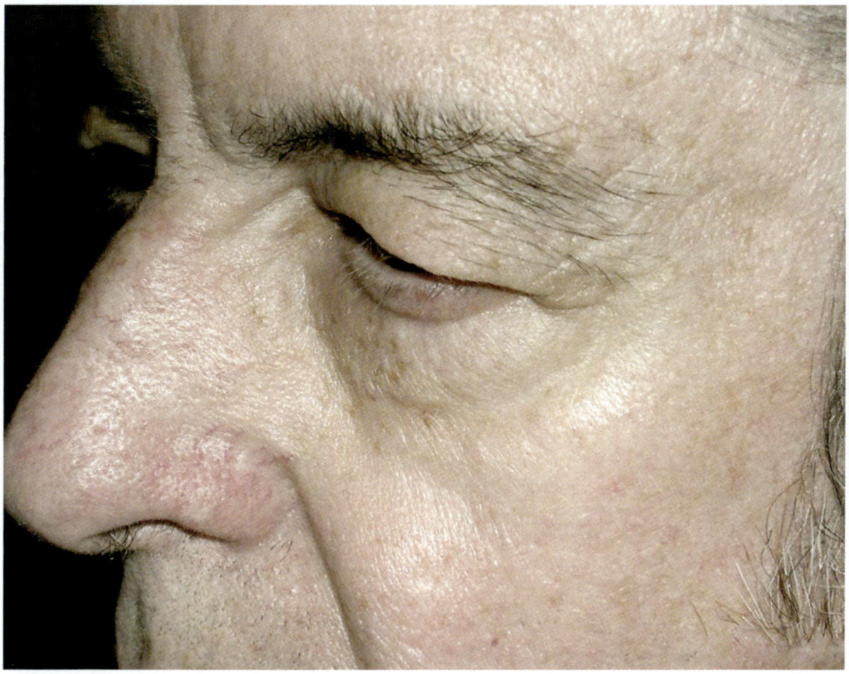

Figure 11.2. Brow ptosis.

12

Preoperative Examination Checklist for Upper Blepharoplasty

Philip L. Custer

When evaluating a patient for upper blepharoplasty, I go through the following anatomic checklist:

Brows: Brow ptosis contributes to the appearance of dermatochalasis and fullness of the superior sulcus. Brow elevation can be a compensatory response to eyelid ptosis or dermatochalasis. An elevated brow diminishes the appearance of dermatochalasis. Brow asymmetry may be congenital or related to the above factors. Brow hair may have been plucked, waxed, or shaved. The natural location of the brow can be identified by palpating the brow fat pad and noting the rather sharp transition between the thicker brow and thinner eyelid tissue.

Bony orbits: There is significant individual variation in orbital size. Orbital asymmetry can be present. A small orbit contributes to crowding and fullness of the superior sulcus, while patients with large orbits usually have naturally deep and hollow superior sulci. The eyelid crease is often lower in patients with smaller orbits.

Eyelid skin: The amount of redundant skin is graded for each upper eyelid. Note the position and quality of the upper eyelid crease. Webbing in the medial canthus may be related to anatomic variation or redundancy and poor fixation of the medial canthal-glabellar tissue. Blepharoplasty can accentuate medial canthal webs. While dependent edema occasionally develops within marked dermatochalasis, the presence of lid swelling warrants further evaluation for conditions such as thyroid disease. Eyelid inflammation (blepharitis) can be caused by allergy, mechanical trauma, and a variety of dermatologic conditions. Blepharitis should be treated before considering surgery.

Orbital fat: Fullness in the central or medial upper eyelid is usually related to prolapse of the orbital fat. The prominence of the fat pockets is graded prior to surgery.

Lacrimal glands: The primary lacrimal glands are located in the superior-lateral orbits. These glands occasionally become ptotic, contributing to fullness in the lateral upper lids.

Lid margin: While there is great variability, the natural position of the upper eyelid margins is usually about 2 mm below the corneal limbus when the patients looks in primary gaze. The lid margins are evaluated for symmetry, ptosis, or retraction. Further evaluation is needed if abnormalities are present. Review of old photographs is helpful in determining if changes are of recent onset. Blepharoplasty should not be used to surgically alter the position of the eyelid margin. The lower eyelid positions are also evaluated. Preexisting lower lid retraction or scleral show can predispose a patient to ocular dryness following upper lid surgery.

Ocular evaluation: Patients considering blepharoplasty should have an eye exam to determine if there are ocular conditions that could complicate surgery. The corneal surface and tear film are evaluated. A basal secretory rate (Schirmer's test performed with topical anesthesia) can be used to evaluate tear production. Patients undergoing recent refractive surgery may be at increased risk for developing post-blepharoplasty ocular irritation.

Visual fields: Visual fields should be performed with and without elevating the redundant eyelid tissue in patients desiring functional upper eyelid blepharoplasty. It is best to request prior determination of insurance coverage in such individuals.

Photographs: External photographs are obtained to document the preoperative findings. Informed consent: The risks of surgery are discussed and documented. It is reasonable to cover noticeable scarring, bleeding, infection, loss of vision, incomplete eyelid closure with ocular irritation, asymmetry, and need for additional treatment.

Preoperative instructions: While surgery can occasionally be safely performed on patients taking anticoagulants or platelet-inhibiting medications/supplements, these agents should ideally be withheld prior to blepharoplasty. Facial cosmetic products, jewelry, and contact lenses should not be worn the day of surgery. Patients with the following conditions may be at higher risk for complications following blepharoplasty or require specialized surgical techniques: unrealistic expectations, prior eyelid/facial surgery, dry eye symptoms, thyroid disease, prominent eyes, marked orbital asymmetry, significant coexisting medical problems.

13

Preoperative Evaluation and Documentation in Upper Blepharoplasty

Cat Nguyen Burkat

As with any procedure, upper eyelid blepharoplasty requires a thorough preoperative evaluation of the patient. Dermatochalasis may result in functional visual field obstruction or may create an aesthetically displeasing redundancy and fullness to the upper eyelids.

During the preoperative evaluation, any history of dry eyes and artificial tear use should be documented and addressed, as this will be exacerbated with eyelid surgery. Likewise, slit lamp examination of the corneal surface is important. Evaluation of the eyelids should include measurements of the margin-reflex distance (to look for concurrent eyelid ptosis), lagophthalmos, and eyelid skin as measured from the lash line to the thicker eyebrow skin. Documenting this in measured millimeters is a more precise and objective measurement, as opposed to a +1 to +4 scale that is difficult to compare between surgeons and residents. Degree of eyelid hooding over the margin in also documented, as well as the prominence of the nasal and preaponeurotic fat pads. Lateral eyelid fullness may suggest a prolapsed lacrimal gland that should be addressed during surgery (Figure 13.1), and eyebrow ptosis or eyebrow fat pad fullness should also be included in the management plan.

In Asian eyelids, any epicanthal fold should be documented and a careful discussion with the patient regarding the desired appearance of the eyelids should be undertaken. Having the patient bring in photos of others' eyelids, or magazine pictures, is helpful to determine the degree to which the patient wishes to retain the ethnic characteristic of his or her eyelids.

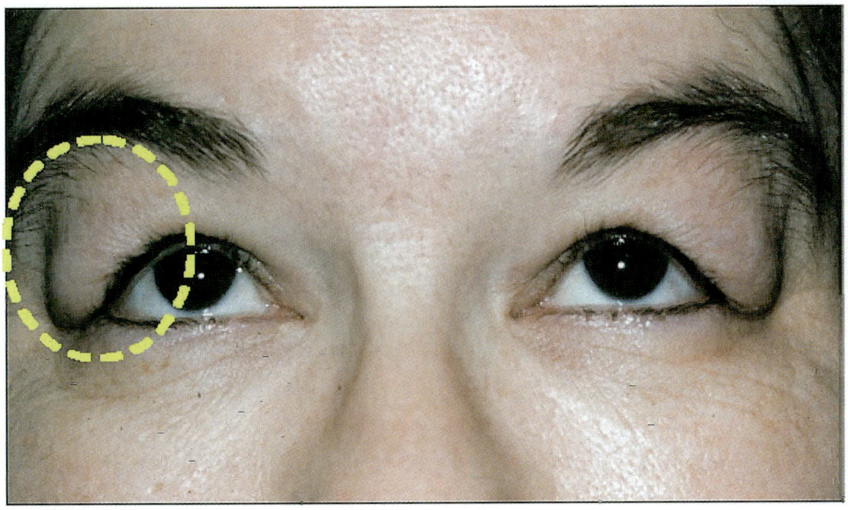

Figure 13.1. Lateral eyelid fullness may suggest a prolapsed lacrimal gland.

Section Two

Incision Planning

14

Marking Strategies for Upper Blepharoplasty

Guy G. Massry

Pinching skin to leave lids closed without redundancy of upper lid skin is the safest way to approach upper blepharoplasty. There may be a need for revision (especially temporally) on probably 20% of patients—especially in the cosmetic population, whose expectations are high (not so much in older patients in which insurance covers surgery and whose expectations are different). Leaving lash eversion and even up to 2 mm of incomplete closure is typically safe if orbicularis strength is good (check by forced eyelid closure and attempt to pry lids open) and other corneal protective mechanisms are intact (Bell's phenomenon, tear production, and corneal sensation).

Laterally one must balance skin excision with brow position and final outcome and discuss reasonable outcomes with patients preoperatively. More aggressive excision laterally is okay. It is very unlikely to develop corneal problems from excess temporal skin excision unless to the extreme. The brow tends to give and compensate for this. Unfortunately, the brow can become lowered, which can in itself cause a problem.

This is why, in patients who express a desire for more pretarsal show laterally, I often recommend browlift (not to elevate, but at least stabilize brow height). Elevating the temporal brow also shortens the lateral extent of the excision by reducing the pseudo-dermatochalasis components of the full temporal lid (by eliminating brow ptosis). In addition, postoperative sub-brow Botox injections (6U per side) are helpful during recovery.

Another helpful tip to prevent nasal webbing is to angle the incision up and medial slightly (mirror image of lateral incision). This tends to offset the vertical/horizontal disequilibrium that can occur and leads the development of webs.

Other hints:

- Wash off all skin prep before marking (especially Betadine) as it is harder to mark on skin with prep solution on it (especially when dry).
- Use a fine-tip marker. Thicker markers spread more, especially if lid gets wet from injection or if eyelid opens. This can lead to marks being millimeters off, which in the cosmetic population makes a difference.

- Mark, inject, and score (MIS). In my opinion this is critical. Many physicians mark before the prep and inject. After prepping I find the markings to be off (spread). I find MIS to be DOGMA. After prep (MIS), when both sides are scored, no matter what happens to the lid the incisions will be equal. The downside is less time for hemostasis from injection. This can be compensated for by waiting or doing lower lids (if scheduled).

I avoid muscle excision in most cases. There is enough lid thinning (anterior-posterior) by skin excision. I especially avoid this if orbicularis strength is not excellent in my preop evaluation. In addition, postop lagophthalmos can be divided into two types: (1) tethered—due to skin shortage or septal (or deep tissue) scar (adhesion); (2) paretic (I find most common)—due to weak orbicularis muscle. One can differentiate by what I call the tether test. Pull lashes down to close the eye—if tether present type 1 above is the case. This is rare compared to type 2. This is why I manipulate muscle as little as possible (the older the patient, the more prone to this). Lagophthalmos (especially nocturnal) can occur with adequate skin and is more likely to occur from orbicularis weakness. Avoid manipulating orbicularis as much as possible.

The best way to avoid hematoma is not to get one. When injecting, start temporal and hydrodissect skin from muscle. Bend needle to angle superiorly, keep tip up, and just under skin.

There are a percentage of patients that complain of misalignment of the relaxed skin tension lines of the lids after blepahroplasty. It is an arched incision—slight misalignment in patients with obvious vertical lines that can lead to this. It may also help to place two cardinal sutures (centrally and temporally) in the blepharoplasty incision. This turns a long arched incision into three small ellipsed ones and reduces the chance of webbing and skin misalignment.

I find that locking lateral sutures (a few) during the running suture is key. That is a dynamic area, and this prevents dehiscence. Another option is to run the suture and then place several interspaced interrupted sutures for tension and has the added benefit of everting the wound edges.

I have become less of a fan of brow fat sculpting in recent years. In some cases, I believe more in fat injections to elevate the ptotic brow fat pad.

15

Orbit Size and Lid Marking in Upper Blepharoplasty

Philip L. Custer

Prep and drape: Perform a full-face prep. Ensure the drape does not place traction on the lids or brows.

Marking incision: The inferior incision is placed in the location of the desired postoperative eyelid crease. Many patients have a well-defined, ideally positioned preoperative crease that can be used. Otherwise, the surgeon must determine the location for the desired crease. This location should be individualized, realizing that excessive high or low creases may have an abnormal appearance and can occasionally adversely affect eyelid function. A higher crease usually results in more visible pretarsal skin. General guidelines are:

	Higher crease	Lower crease
Larger bony orbit:	+	
Smaller bony orbit:		+
Females:	+	
Males:		+

This distance from the superior border of the lashes to the crease in the central lid is usually 9–10 mm in females and 8–9 mm males.

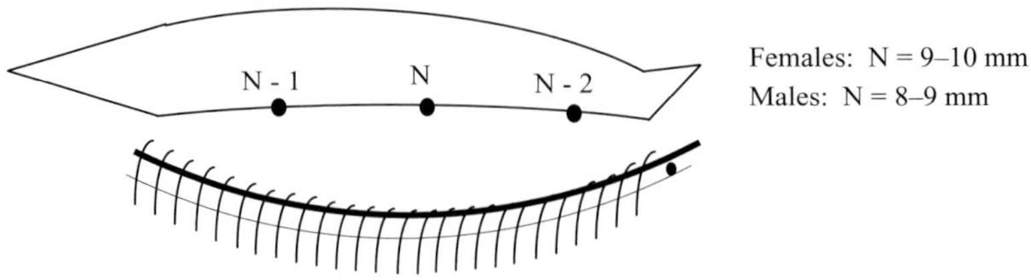

To minimize web formation, the medial and lateral extensions of the lower incision angle upward, starting before the lacrimal punctum medially and near the canthal angle laterally. With the patient gently closing his or her eyes, forceps are used to measure the amount of redundant skin across the lid, ensuring sufficient tissue is left in place to allow full eyelid closure. More conservative skin excision is indicated in patients with dry eyes or at risk for lagophthalmos. The two sides are examined for symmetry. Asymmetric skin excision may be needed in patients with uneven skin redundancy or orbital asymmetry.

It may be necessary to incorporate a medial "M-plasty" in patients with marked excess skin or preexisting epicanthal folds.

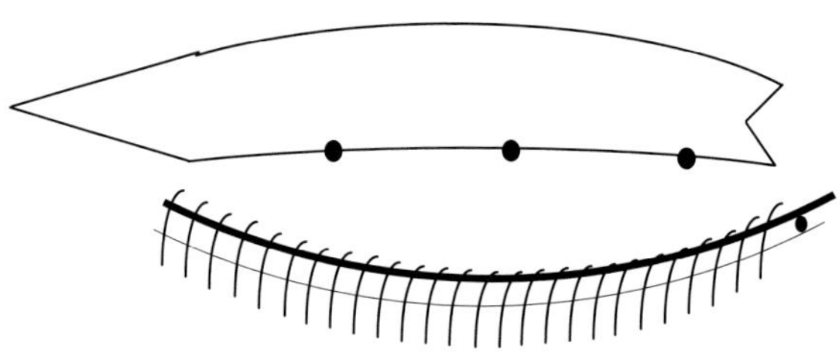

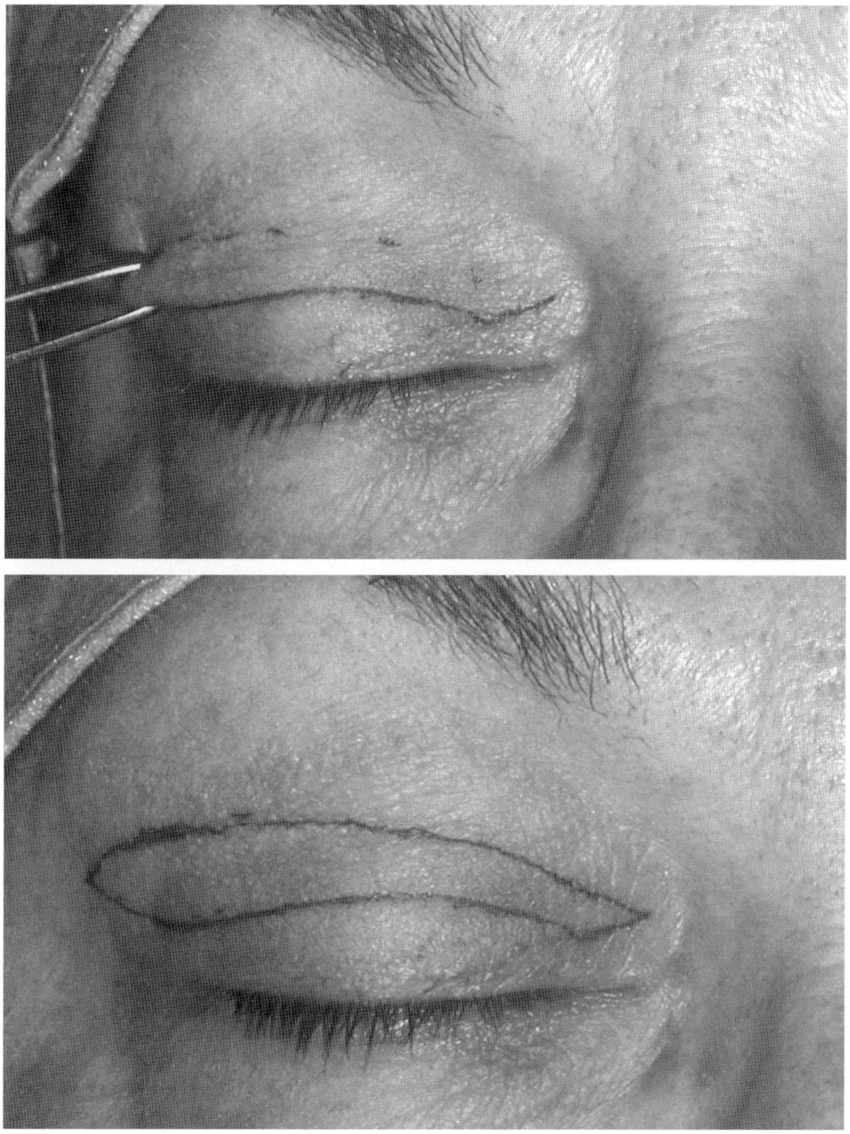

A

B

Figure 15.1. Incision mark for upper blepharosplasty.

16

Incisional Guidelines When Marking the Skin in Upper Eyelid Blepharoplasty

Sheri L. DeMartelaere, Todd R. Shepler, Sean M. Blaydon, Russell W. Neuhaus, and John W. Shore

For those patients without a discernable lid crease (Figure 16.1), the following measurements can provide a good incisional guideline:

- 7–9 mm above the mid-eyelid margin for men and 8–10 mm for women
- 6 mm above the medial eyelid margin at the level of the punctum
- 6–8 mm above the lateral eyelid margin at the level of the lateral canthus
- Lateral eyelid crease incision then swings upwards at the lateral canthus to end 15–18 mm from the lateral canthus at a 45° angle

An axiom that is useful for those starting out: always leave behind at least 2 cm of skin between the lash margin and lower eyebrow hairs and you should never have difficulty with postoperative lagophthalmos. This means that the upper limit of skin excision should leave 10–15 mm of skin between the inferior brow and upper skin incision. This limit can be marked at the beginning of the case as a reminder.

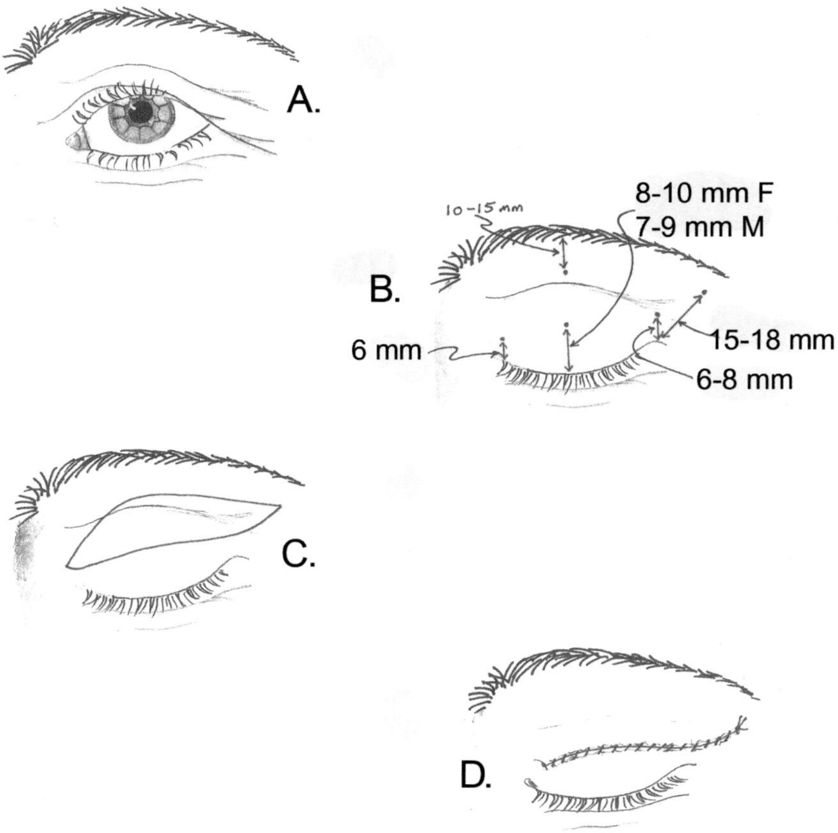

Figure 16.1. Artist's sketch depicting incision guidelines for upper eyelid blepharoplasty. (A) Preoperative sketch of upper eyelid dermatochalasis. (B) Castrovierjo calipers are used to measure the eyelid. (C) Planned incision. (D) Skin excision closed with running suture.

17

Marking the Proposed Upper Eyelid Crease: Determining the Safe Amount of Skin Removal—The Pinch Technique

Jemshed A. Khan

The success of the upper belpharoplasty operation rests on the foundation of perfectly symmetrical skin markings. Any asymmetry in this initial step will carry forward in the operation and adversely affect the final outcome.

With the patient in the supine position, determine the amount of skin removal using the pinch technique (Figures 17.1–17.3). Be certain that the lids can passively close while pinching. This should prevent postoperative lagophthalmos due to excessive skin removal.

The medial extent of removal is superior to the punctum but should be moved laterally when there is a tendency to medial canthal webbing. The tendency toward nasal webbing may be determined preoperatively by the web test: gently pinch the lateral walls of the nasal bridge and tug inferiorly. Observe the medial canthal area for webbing during this maneuver to judge the pateint's tendency toward webbing. The lateral extent of removal is often determined by hooding and may be limited by the lateral orbital rim. Ink the margins for resection and then remeasure with calipers after marking to ensure perfect symmetry.

Reprinted with permission from: Chen WPD, Khan JA, McCord, Jr, CD. Color Atlas of Cosmetic Oculofacial Sugery. Philadelphia: Butterworth Heinemann/ Elsevier, 2004.

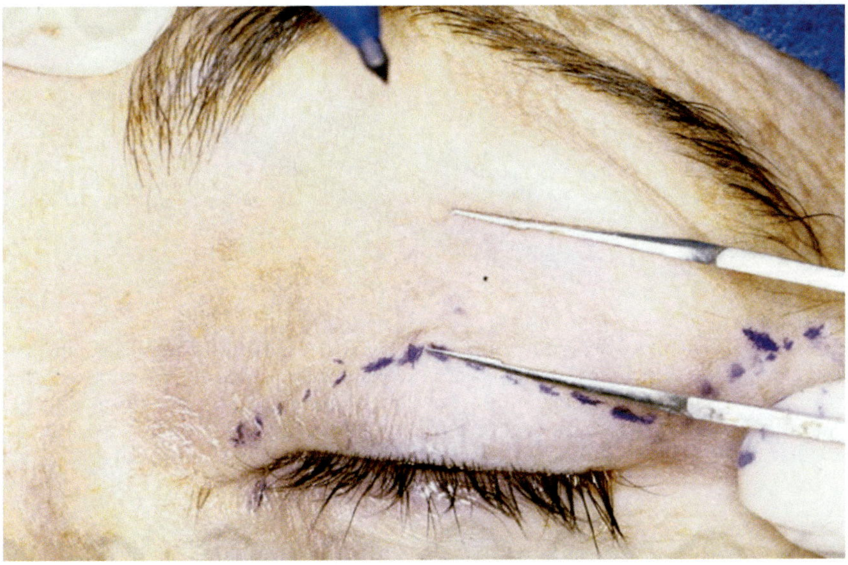

Figure 17.1. Pinch technique: the inferior jaw of the forceps engages the inferior skin mark.

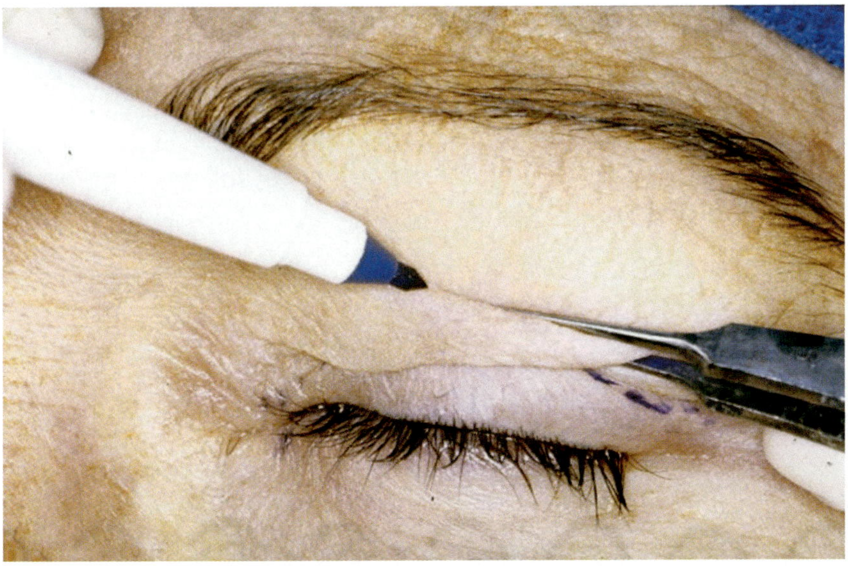

Figure 17.2. Redundant skin is gathered between the forceps jaws. Care is taken that no lagophthalmos is induced and the superior resection margin is inked.

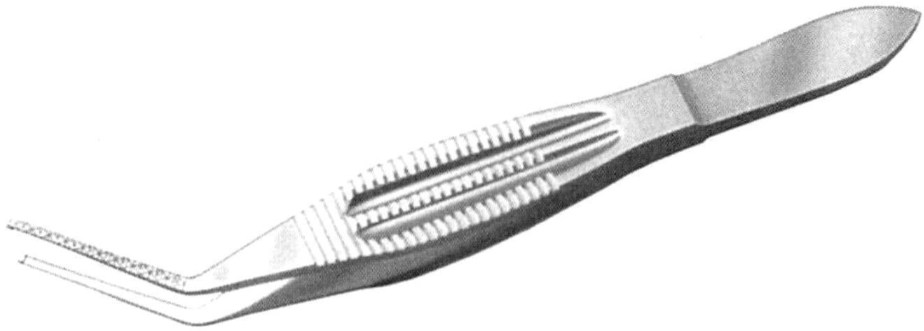

Figure 17.3. Specially designed ambidextrous "Khan Ink and Pinch" forceps for blepharoplasty skin marking. Note square atruamatic jaws are offset from the foceps shafts to allow gathering of redundant skin. Minute tip serrations engage the inferior crease. Calibrated millimeter markings help ensure symmetry. (Courtesy Storz® Instruments/Bausch and Lomb Inc, San Dimas, CA.)

18

Preoperative Measurements in Upper Blepharoplasty: Patient Selection

Jemshed A. Khan

- When examining the patient preoperatively, special attention should be paid to the brows.
- The MRD obtained with eyebrows manually raised (refered to as MRDb) is highly predictive of the postblepharoplasty MRD.
- While the brows are manually raised, the superior sulcus is examined for evidence of herniating nasal and preaponeurotic fat pads and to search for lacrimal gland prolapse.
- Ballottement the globe while examining the superior sulcus helps determine which fat pads should be resected. Any preexisting eyebrow ptosis, eyelid ptosis, or nasal webbing should be both documented and emphasized to the patient.
- Finally, the extent of lateral hooding and retro-orbicularis oculi fat (ROOF) should be noted.
- Examine for lagophthalmos by having the patient passively close his or her eyelids as if sleeping.

Reprinted with permission from: Chen WPD, Khan JA, McCord, Jr, CD. Color Atlas of Cosmetic Oculofacial Sugery. Philadelphia: Butterworth Heinemann/ Elsevier, 2004.

19

Keys to Success When Marking the Skin in Upper Blepharoplasty

John R. Burroughs and Richard L. Anderson

- There are few procedures in oculofacial plastic surgery more gratifying to the surgeon and patient than upper blepharoplasty. Keys to success are a strong patient–physician relationship and making certain that the desired goals are also realistic expectations.
- We avoid removing upper eyelid skin that would leave less than 20–22 mm between the eyelid margin and the brow cilia.
- Patients should marked in an upright position.
- We wipe the skin with alcohol to remove oils prior to marking to ensure the surgical markings will remain after patient prepping.
- We use the extra-fine point skin marker by Scanlan™ (1-800-328-9458) as it has an ultra-fine tip and allows extremely precise marking (Figure 19.1). The white cap on the bottom of the marker is approximately 10 mm in length and readily serves as a quick way to estimate the placement of the incision markings (Figure 19.2)
- We advise against placing the lower skin incision any lower than 9–10 mm in most eyelids unless the natural crease is lower. Simply marking the patient's natural eyelid crease can be quite variable, and in acquired ptosis patients may be remarkably higher than normal. Symmetry in the lid crease markings is key in upper blepharoplasty.
- We then mark the upper incision in the sitting upright position by having the patient gaze straight ahead to help determine the upper extent of the upper blepharoplasty incision.
- The bottom white portion of the of the Scanlan marker (Figure 19.2) is used to quickly check that at least 10 mm of eyelid skin remains above and below the marked areas for skin removal.

It is critical to maintain symmetry in the height, depth, and fold of the eyelid crease, which is paramount in the success of the upper blepharoplasty.

We avoid medial webbing by drawing a gentle upturn to the medial incision markings. Laterally we extend the markings to approximately 5 mm above the lateral canthus, then upturn to hide the lateral incision and to avoid elevation of the temporal eyelid crease (Figure 19.3).

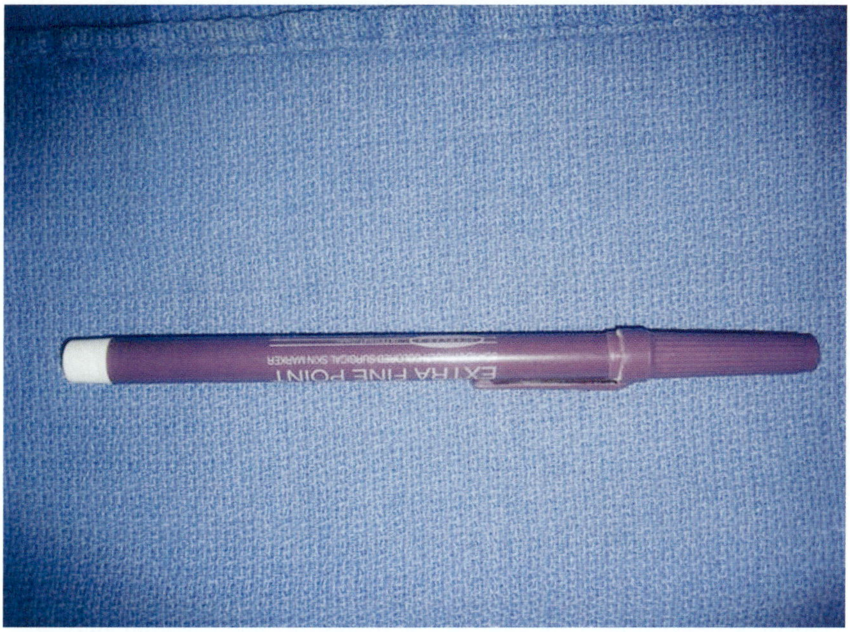

Figure 19.1. Scanlan^{TM} marking pen with white end-cap that is approximately 10 mm in length.

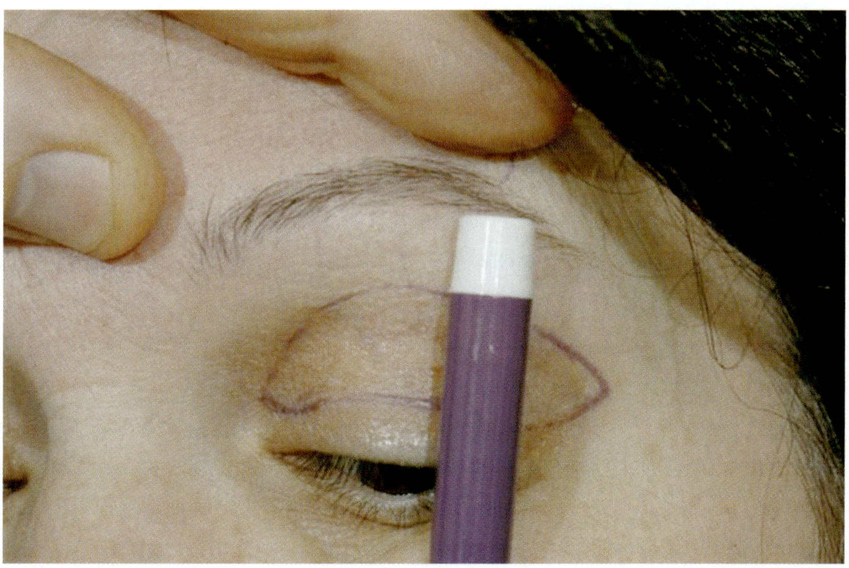

Figure 19.2. Blepharoplasty skin marking showing gentle medial and lateral upturn. White end-cap showing at least 10 mm of skin between upper marking and browcili.

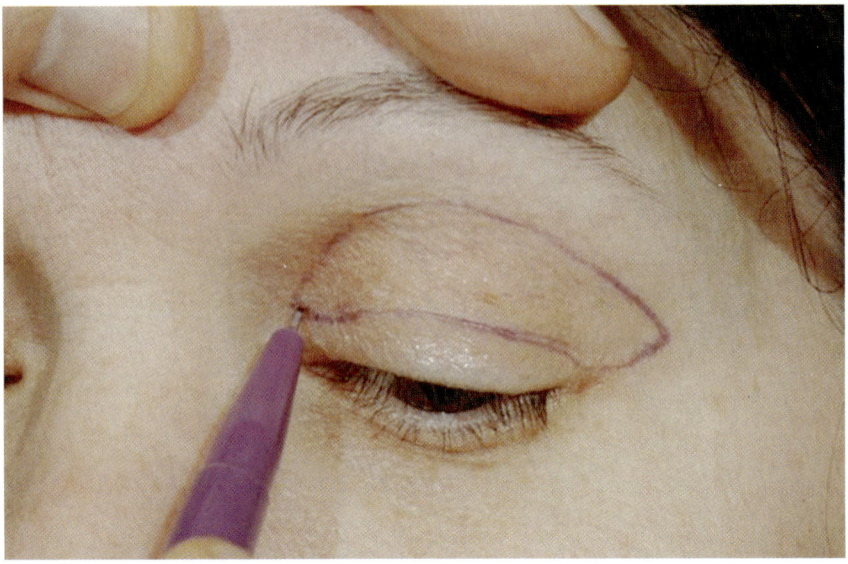

Figure 19.3. Gentle medial upturn to avoid medial webbing andmarking within 5 mm of lateral canthus. Lateral upturn helps hide the incision temporally.

20

Skin Marking in Upper Blepharoplasty—Avoiding Pitfalls

Cat Nguyen Burkat

At surgery, the skin marking is probably one of the most important steps and therefore warrants careful attention to detail. The placement of the skin incision is crucial to the perceived success of the surgery postoperatively as the eyelid crease is the most distinguishing feature of the upper lid. I prefer to mark the incisions with a fine-tip marking pen prior to injection of local anesthetic to avoid distortion of the tissues from the anesthetic. The eyelid crease heights are first measured and compared on both upper eyelids. If they are symmetric and appropriate for gender (8–11 mm for women, 6–8 mm for men), the creases are marked with the pen (Figure 20.1). Occasionally, the crease heights are asymmetric, contain double lines, or are discontinuous. Therefore, careful comparison between the two sides will help guide the proper placement. In addition, if involutional ptosis is also present, the eyelid crease will be anatomically elevated up to height of 15–20 mm (due to dehiscence of the anterior fibers of the levator aponeurosis that attach to dermis and skin at the level of the lid crease). Placement of the incision at these elevated crease levels would result in a suboptimal and unnatural appearance to the eyelids.

Gender and ethnic considerations are also incorporated into placement of the skin marking, with the crease incision rounder and more arched in women, as opposed to a flatter and lower crease incision in men. In Asian eyelids, the medial aspects of the flap markings should blend into the epicanthal fold. In addition, the height of the eyelid crease in Asians will be much lower at 4–6 mm. Placing the incision at the normal 8- to 11-mm height would result in a westernized Caucasian eyelid that would be unfavorable to the Asian patient.

In general, the upper eyelid skin should measure 19–20 mm from eyelid margin to the transition to eyebrow skin. This measurement eliminates the risk of postoperative lagophthalmos from aggressive tissue excision (Figure 20.2). In addition, it is a useful tool for teaching residents in training. Therefore, the height of the eyelid crease is subtracted from a total of 20 mm (Figure 20.3). This amount is then measured from the inferior edge of brow skin, which will thus represent the superior border of the skin flap to be removed (Figure 20.3). This is measured at the central lid first and then medially. Many times surgeons tend to excise too much skin medially and cause medial lagophthalmos or webbing (Figure 20.4). Laterally, an extra 1–2 mm may be removed as there is usually some degree of lateral eyebrow ptosis. Care should be taken to avoid confusing the true junction of the inferior brow (where the thin eyelid skin transitions to thicker, larger porous brow skin with a different color) in women who pluck their eyebrows to a higher height (Figure 20.5). Measuring the upper incision to the plucked eyebrow level would thus result in erroneous excess skin removal.

The pinch technique is then performed to confirm that an adequate 19–20 mm of skin is preserved, done by pinching together the skin between the inferior and superior markings and measuring the remaining skin from the eyelid margin to the brow skin. If the skin pinch results in a tightness to the thin eyelid skin, vertical striae to the skin, or retraction or eversion of the eyelid margin, too much skin is being excised (Figure 20.6).

Other important pearls are keeping the medial extent of the skin marking no further medial than the upper punctum. Incisions that extend medial to the punctum increase the risk of webbing in the nasal eyelid region (Figure 20.4). In the event that there still remains an excess of skin medially, a Burow's triangle is sometimes helpful while still avoiding medial webbing.

The lateral extent of the skin marking should also be measured from the lateral canthal angle with a caliper. This ensures that the incisions extend for the same length bilaterally, which is often noticeable to the patient. In addition, the lateral extent should not extend into the thicker temporal skin.

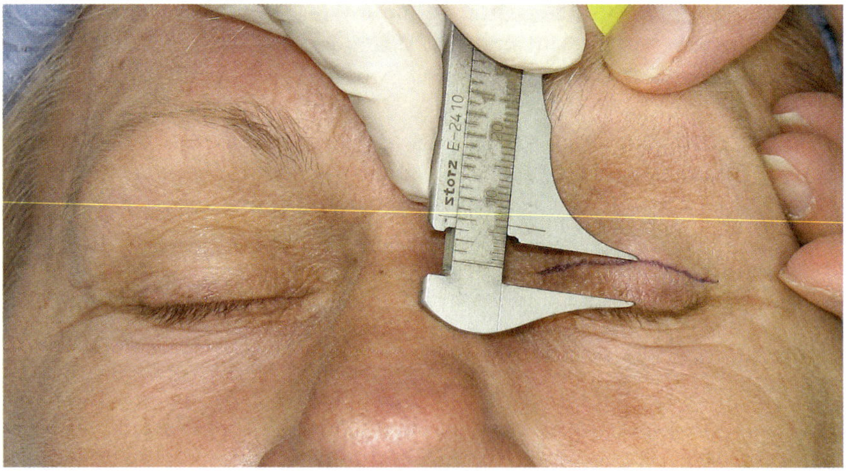

Figure 20.1. Measuring and marking the eyelidcrease incision from the eyelid margin.

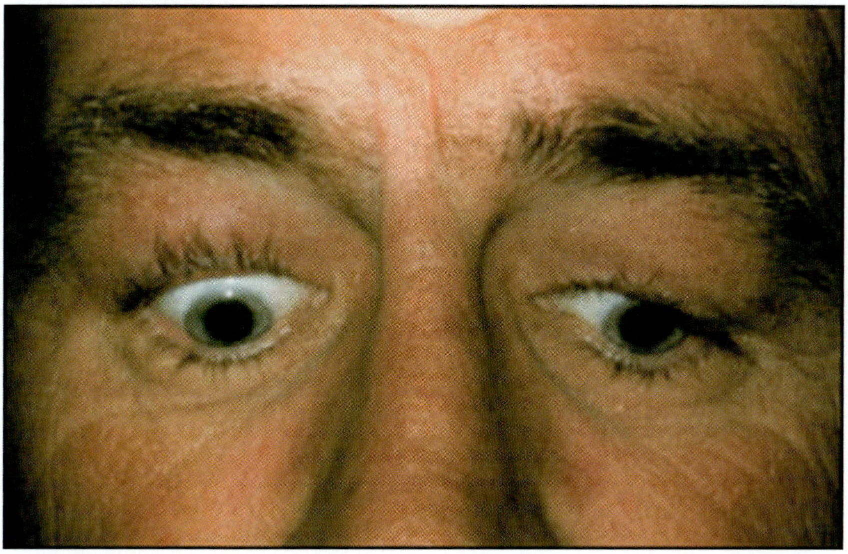

Figure 20.2. Postoperative lagophthalmos following aggressive skin incision.

A

B

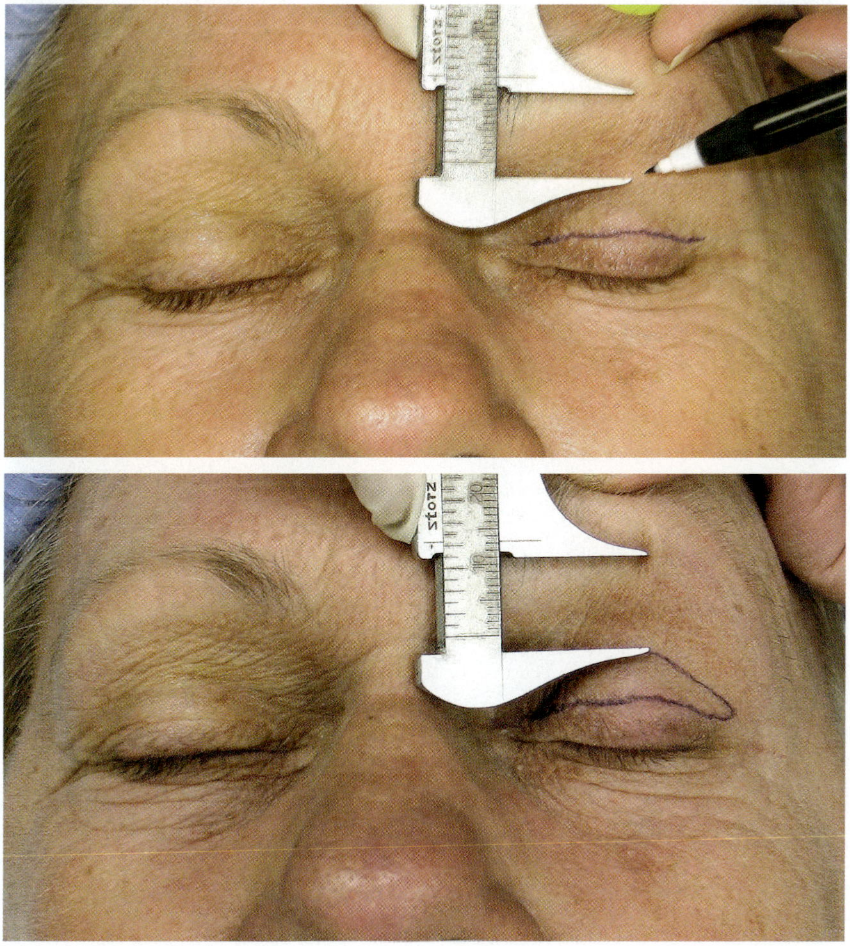

Figure 20.3. Marking the superior incision from the thick eyebrow skin.

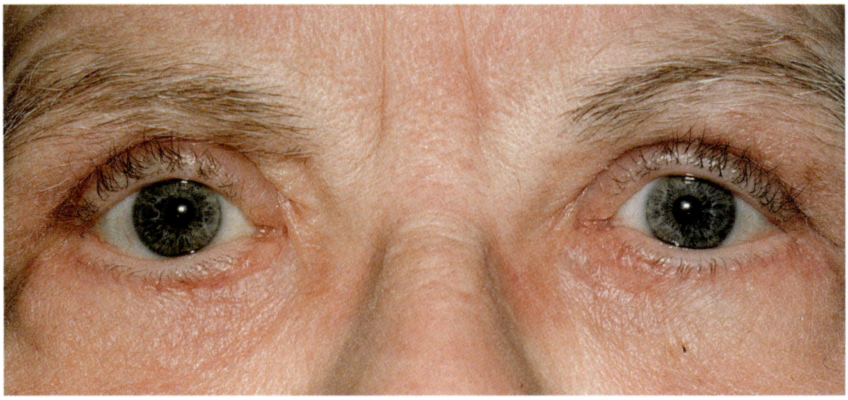

Figure 20.4. Webbing of skin medially due to extension of incision past the superior punctum.

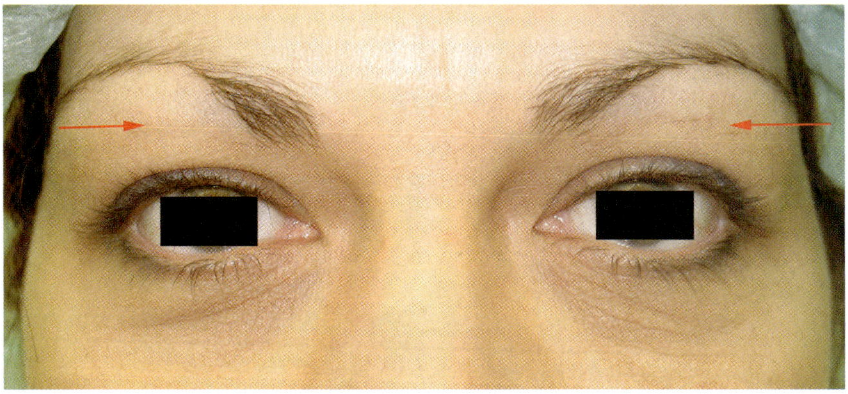

Figure 20.5. Arrows demarcate the transition from thin eyelid skin to thick eyebrow skin, which may be considerably below the level of plucked eyebrows.

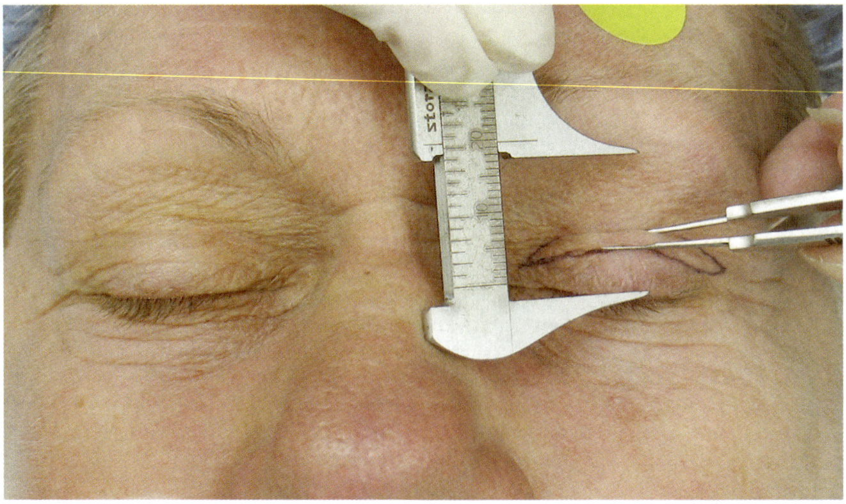

Figure 20.6. The pinch technique confirms that 20 mm of skin has been retained.

Section Three

Upper Blepharoplasty Procedure Pearls

21

Upper Blepharoplasty: Pearls for the Procedure

Evan H. Black, John D. Siddens, Frank A. Nesi,
Shoib Myint, and Geoffrey J. Gladstone

1. Meticulous marking is critical. We recommend marking prior to injection. A fine-tip marker is preferred, as the larger markers smear and do not allow the precision necessary for eyelid surgery.
2. The supratarsal lid crease should be marked from punctum to lateral canthus. If the patient's natural creases are appropriate and symmetrical, they can be used. Otherwise adjustments should be made.
3. The pinch technique will determine how *little* skin can be excised to achieve optimum results. Be careful to make the endpoint the eversion of lashes. This part is critical to prevent lagophthalmos. Care is taken not to remove sub-brow skin to prevent postoperative brow ptosis. Less is more with skin removal.
4. The lid crease marking should slope gently upward medial to the punctum and lateral to the lateral canthus. Avoid aggressive medial skin excision or going too close to the lid margin medially, as this can cause webbing.
5. To achieve adequate hemostasis, 2% lidocaine with 1:100,000 epinephrine mixed with 0.5% marcaine with 1:200,000 epinephrine is used. Hyaluronidase can be used in the mixture to help dispurse the anesthetic.
6. When incising the skin–muscle complex, be careful not to damage the levator complex. This can result in ptosis. Orbital fat is a good landmark as it lies anterior to the levator.
7. Prominent lacrimal gland tissue may need to be tucked to create an aesthetically pleasing appearance to the lateral eyelid.
8. With fat removal, being conservative is better. A subjective preoperative grading system should be implemented to prevent under correction or overcorrection of the orbital fat. Prominent medial fat pads should be reduced.
9. Excessive cautery medially can damage the trochlear region, resulting in diplopia. One should be meticulous with hemostasis, however, to avoid the rare complication of orbital hemorrhage. Use of handheld or bipolar cautery is useful.
10. Lid crease fixation suture can be used to enhance the appearance of the crease, especially in females or when less skin is taken.

11. The chance of milia, granuloma, or epithelial suture cysts can be reduced by using subcuticular closure with a nonreactive permanent suture such as 6-0 polypropylene. If an absorbable suture is used, the remaining sutures should be removed at about 7 days.

22

Fat Excision in Upper Blepharoplasty

Sheri L. DeMartelaere, Todd R. Shepler, Sean M. Blaydon, Russell W. Neuhaus, and John W. Shore

The nasal fat pocket can sometimes be difficult to access, is more vascularized, and is more innervated than the rest of the preaponeurotic fat. Additional local anesthetic injected within the fat pocket during excision will improve patient comfort. A small Desmarres retractor can be used to retract the skin nasally and better expose the nasal fat. The nasal orbital septum is carefully opened and the nasal fat pocket exposed. While grasping the fat with forceps, the surrounding tissue is pushed posteriorly using cotton-tipped applicators. The nasal fat can then be carefully excised with small snips of Wescott scissors or using pin-point monopolar cautery. Hemostasis should be achieved before the fat retracts back into the orbit.

In elderly patients, beware of the prolapsed superior ophthalmic vein presenting nasally within the preaponeurotic fat. Inadvertent disruption of this vein can cause significant hemorrhage, sometimes requiring suture ligation and placement of an orbital drain to manage. If a prominent vein is found medially on one side, expect to find it on the opposite side.

It is important not to remove too much fat, particularly in men. Consideration should be given to excising a minimum of fat out temporarily in order to avoid skeletonizing the orbital rim.

23

Mobilizing and Excising the Nasal Fat Pad in Upper Blepharoplasty

Jemshed A. Khan

After the initial incision and removal of skin and muscle, bluntly spread the fascia over the nasal fat pad with a hemostat. Ballottement the globe will prolapse the fat pad forward. Make an "X"-shaped incision over the nasal fat pad, deepening the incision until the fat prolapses. Grasp the protruding knuckle of fat with forceps and use a cotton-tip applicator to bluntly strip away tissues retaining the nasal fat pad. Supplemental local anesthesia injection is usually required at the base of the nasal fat pad. The fat pad may be excised across a closed hemostat or divided using a laser against a backstop. Adequate hemostasis is important because of the caliber of vessels associated with the fat pocket.

Reprinted with permission from: Chen WPD, Khan JA, McCord, Jr, CD. Color Atlas of Cosmetic Oculofacial Sugery. Philadelphia: Butterworth Heinemann/ Elsevier, 2004.

24

Tissue Removal Considerations in Blepharoplasty Surgery

Rona Z. Silkiss

When deciding how much tissue to remove in cosmetic upper blepharoplasty, it is important to remember a few critical mantras:

1. It is not the tissue that you remove, but what you leave behind that counts. As we are all asymmetric, measure not what you remove, but the residual eyelid tissue for symmetry.
2. Function trumps form every time. Blepharoplasty is not a procedure designed to achieve maximum tautness of the lids. This in fact is an aging change. It is critical to ensure that the patient can close their eyes completely on the OR table. It is not recommended that the patient have residual lagophthalmos. If the patient has lagophthalmos in the OR, he or she certainly may have lagophthalmos in the office the next day. This situation does not improve spontaneously. Additionally, it is important to leave the orbicularis. This is not a structure that becomes redundant with age. The orbicularis is important to ensure adequate eyelid closure, especially in a population at risk for dry eye.
3. Blepharoplasty is not a procedure designed to achieve maximum skeletonization or excavation of the eyelids. Fat is the lubrication of the eyelid. A cushion of fat is a sign of "youthfulness," ensures adequate levator function, and decreases the possibility of postoperative scarring. Overexcision of fat can overly hollow the eyelids, leading to a "lost in time," obviously surgical appearance.

25

Fewer Hematomas in Upper Blepharoplasty

Martin H. Devoto

The following text and photos illustrate how I perform upper blepharoplasty surgery. The settings are specific to the ERBE ICC 80 unit and may not be directly transferable to another brand of electrosurgery unit.

1. Carefully adjust monopolar cutting cautery settings for each step ("Effect 2" setting used throughout).
2. Use a fine needle tip, such as a Colorado® needle or equivalent clone.
3. Continuously ice the side you are not working on (Figure 25.1)
4. Skin incision cutting mode 7. Incise gently and smoothly to avoid excess heat (Figure 25.2).
5. Skin–muscle flap excision, coagulation mode 10 (Figure 25.3).
6. ROOF fat sculpting, coagulation mode 15 (Figure 25.4).
7. Hemostats are used to hold gauze that secures ice over each eye (Figure 25.5). This prevents ice from falling. Only the lower hemostat is moved to switch eyes.
8. Use of a tapaered needle prevents orbicularis bleeding with closure (Figure 25.6).
9. Early postoperative photos (Figure 25.7).

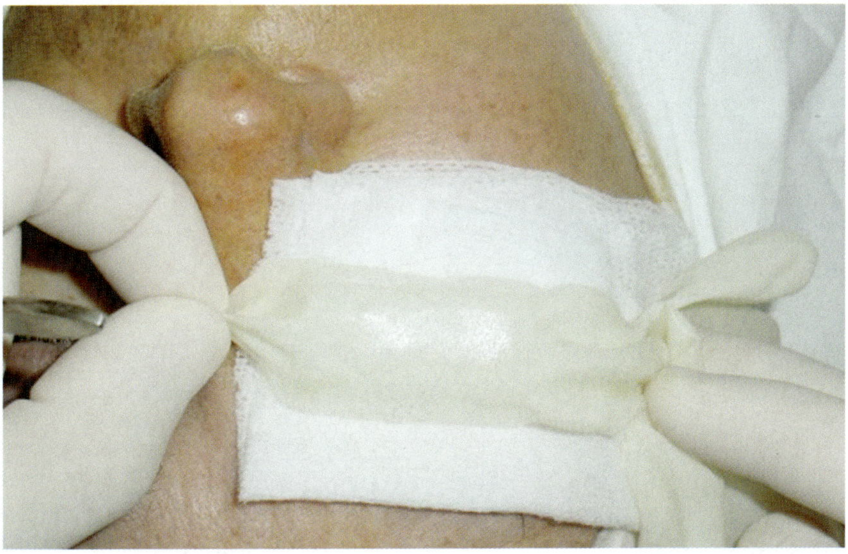

Figure 25.1.

A

B

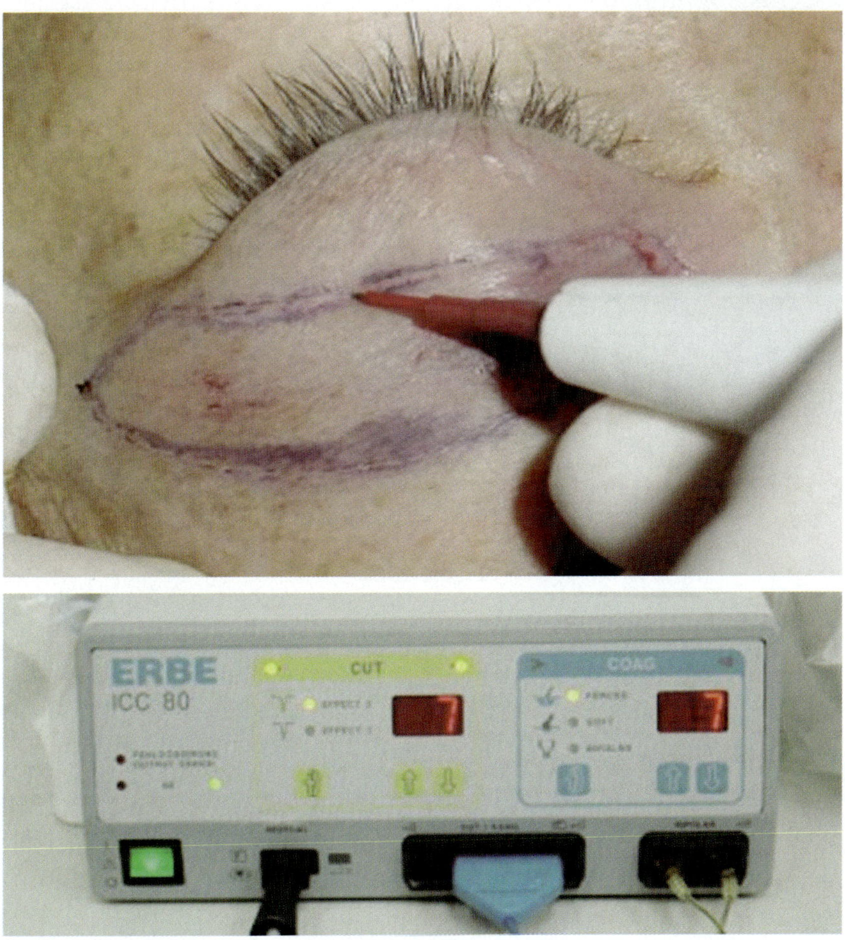

Figure 25.2.

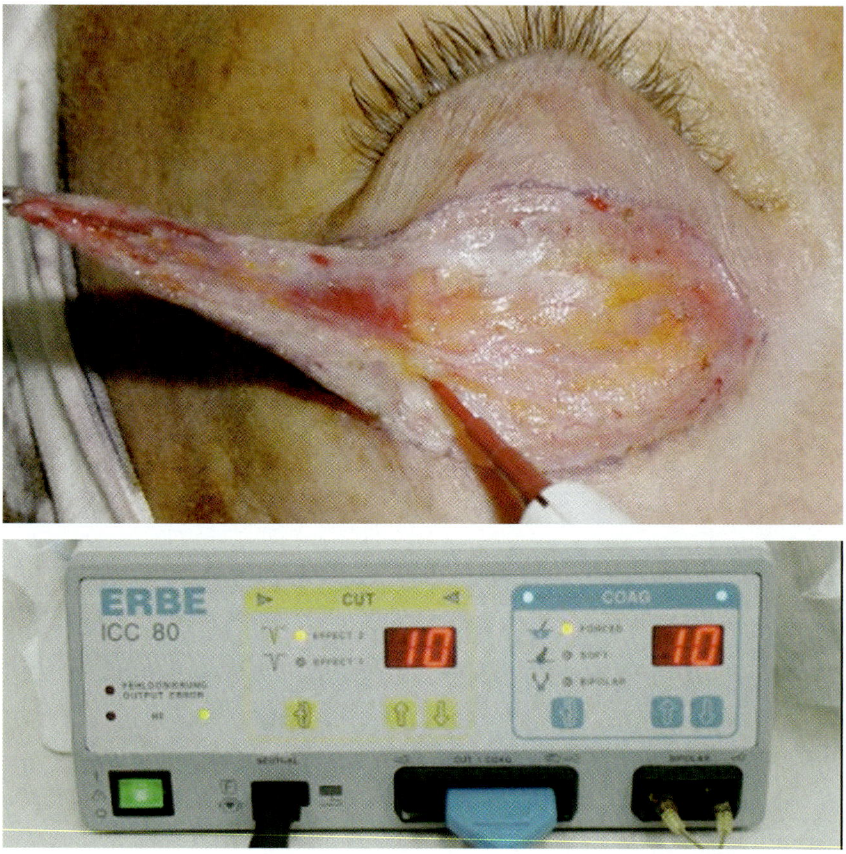

A

B

Figure 25.3.

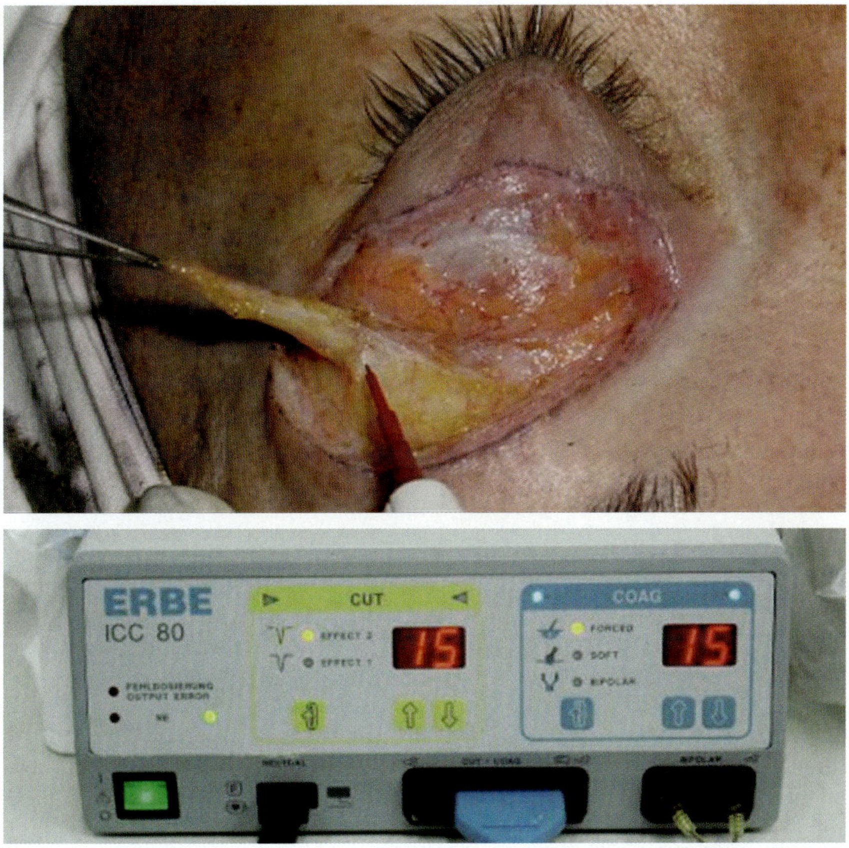

A

B

Figure 25.4.

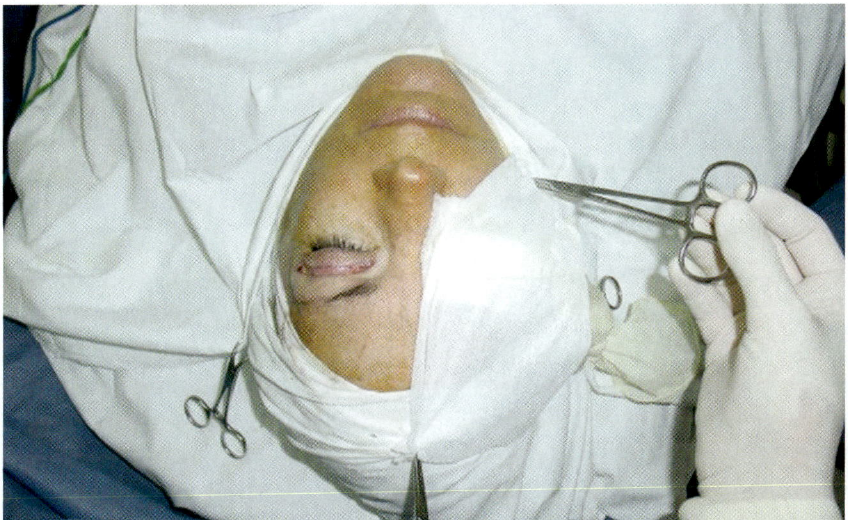

Figure 25.5.

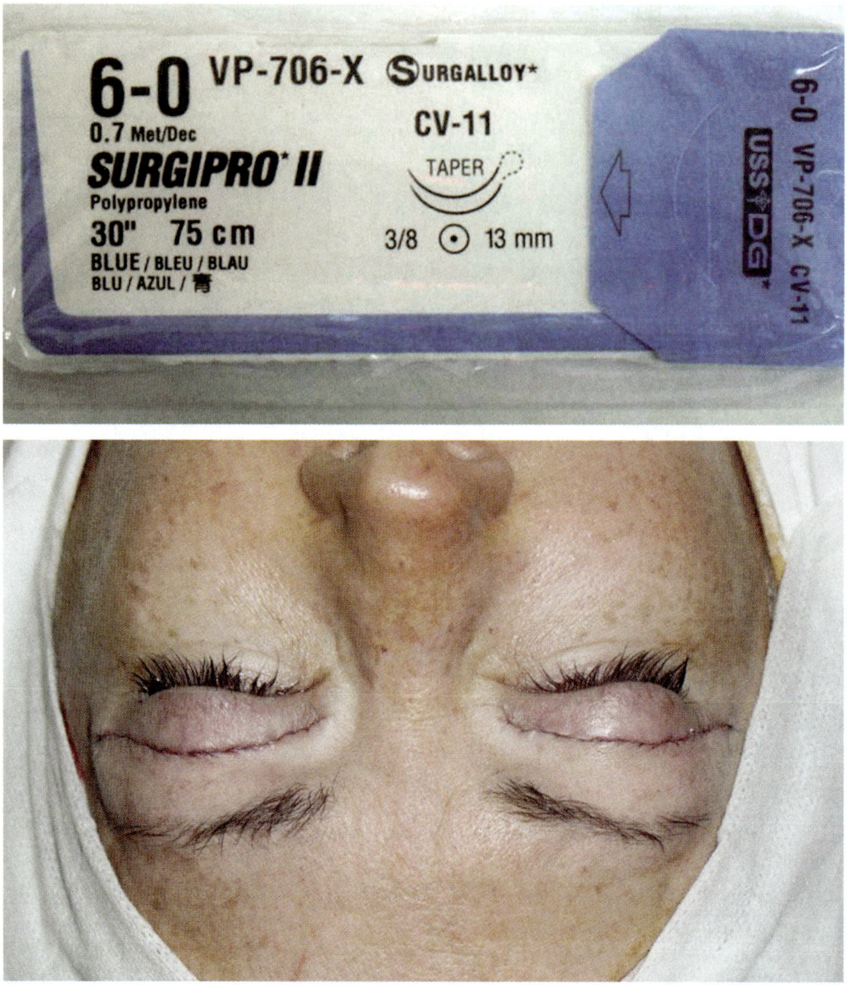

A

B

Figure 25.6.

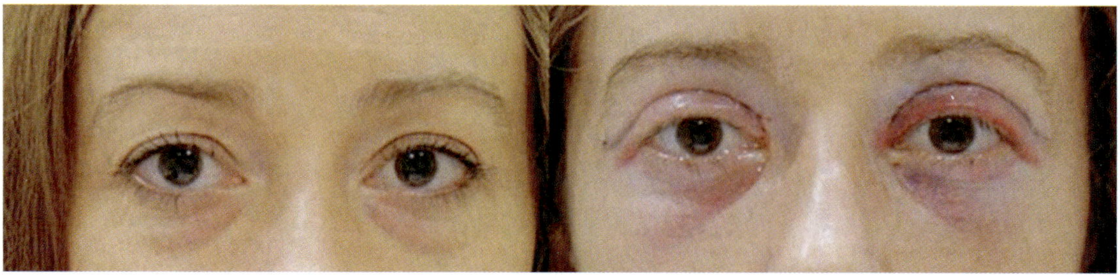

Figure 25.7.

26

Blepharoplasty Incisional Modalities: 4.0 Radiowave Surgery vs. CO_2 Laser

Joseph Niamtu, III

Many modalities have been used for blepharoplasty incision, including scalpel, scissors, cautery, laser, and electrosurgery and radiowave surgery. Incision with hemostasis has many advantages in the extremely vascular periorbital tissues. Bleeding in the surgical field presents many problems for the surgeon and the patient. Poor visualization is a negative thing in any procedure. Increased bleeding can translate into increased postoperative swelling, bruising, and pain and prolongs healing. Using a bloodless incisional modality mitigates all of the above for the patient and hastens the procedure for the surgeon.

Radiowave surgery should not be confused with electrosurgery as vast differences exist.[1–3] Standard electrosurgery was invented in 1928 and has changed little since. It operates at lower frequencies than radiowave surgery (about 1 million cycles per second), and the electrode tip provides the resistance for the circuit. This means that the electrode becomes heated and transfers this heat to the lateral tissues. This increased heat causes lateral tissue damage up to 650 μm. This lateral tissue damage also translates into increased pain and swelling, delays healing, and produces a more significant scar.

Modern radiowave surgery is a patented technology (Ellman International, Oceanside, NY) that operates at 4.0 MHz. Multiple studies have shown this technology to have as little as 20 μm of lateral tissue damage, which is commensurate with histologic studies of scalpel incision.[4–6] 4.0 MHz radiowave surgery can produce a bloodless incision with minimal lateral tissue damage. These attributes indicate its use in blepharoplasty surgery.

The CO_2 laser operates at a wavelength of 10,600 nm and has an affinity for water. The skin is abundant with this target chromophore, and at a specified fluence the tissue is vaporized. Although CO_2 laser produces a bloodless incision, it can generate lateral thermal damage up to 500 μm. The eyelids, being very forgiving, can tolerate this without abnormal scarring, but other facial incisions are not generally made with the CO_2 laser.

Study

Thirty consecutive cosmetic blepharoplasty patients were treated by the author using 4.0 MHz radiowave surgery (Ellman International, Oceanside, NY) on one lid and a 0.2-mm CO_2 handpiece at 8 watts (Lumenis Inc., Santa Clara, CA) on the other lid. Routine cosmetic blepharoplasty was performed by removing a predetermined skin ellipse, a 5-mm band of orbicularis oculi muscle, and reduction and recontouring of both upper periorbital fat pads. All incisions were closed with a running 6-0 nylon suture, which was removed a 5 days postop, and all patients were instructed in the same wound care.

Results

Of the 30 patients in the study, 23 presented for 1 year followed with digital photography. Digital photos were printed on high-quality paper, and the scars (patients eyes closed, brows raised) were evaluated by blind observers. The observers were experienced blepharoplasty surgeons and included a plastic surgeon, a facial plastic surgeon, an oculoplastic surgeon, an oral and maxillofacial surgeon, and a dermatologist. Observers were asked to score which eyelid scar was aesthetically superior or if they were both the same. Interestingly, 37% of the observers rated the radiowave surgery side as most aesthetic, 37% rated the CO_2 laser side as most aesthetic, and 26% scored both sides as equal. Statistically there was no significant difference between the sides; therefore, in this study both modalities produced equally pleasing scars as rated by experienced observers.

Both 4.0 MHz radiowave and CO_2 laser produce a bloodless incision with an aesthetic scar. Clinical advantages existing for the 4.0 MHz include affordability, portability, the ability to use in many other surgical applications, and the broad availability of customized electrode tips to suit hundreds of situations in multiple specialties. Advantages of the CO_2 laser include the ability to resurface facial eyelids and skin with a single modality.

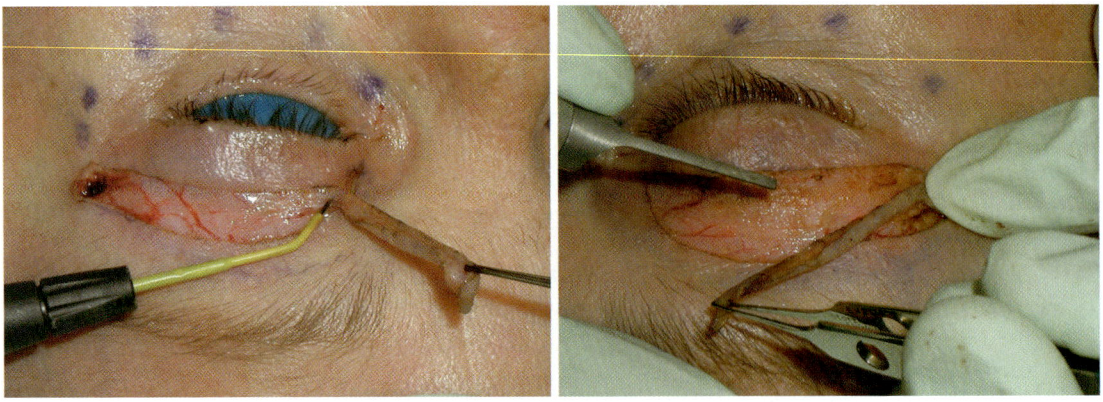

Figure 26.1. Both radiowave and CO_2 laser provide simultaneous incision and hemostasis for cosmetic blepharoplasty surgery.

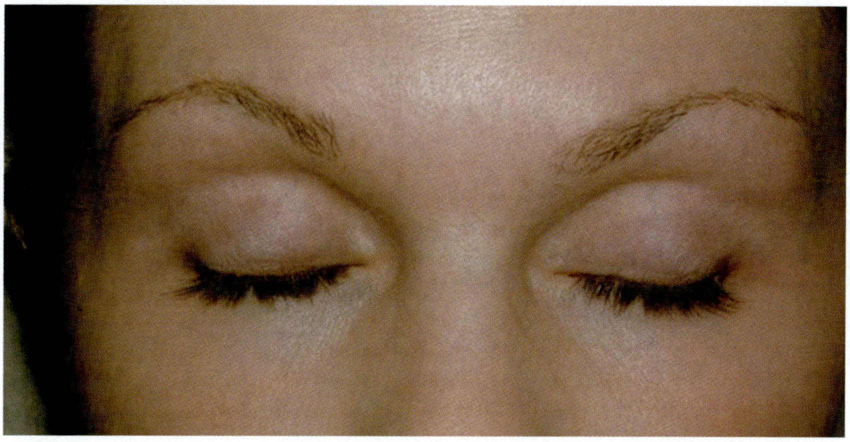

Figure 26.2. A case from the study where both radiowave surgery and CO_2 laser produced excellent postblepharoplasty scars. This patient's left upper eyelid was treated with 4.0 MHz radiowave surgery and the her right upper lid was treated with CO_2 laser.

References

1. Niamtu J. 4.0 MHz Radiowave surgery in cosmetic surgery. Australas J Cosmet Surg 2005;1(1):52–59.
2. Niamtu J III. Cosmetic Blephaoplasty. Atlas of Oral Maxillofacial Surg Clin N Am 2004;12:91–130.
3. Bosniak S, Cantisano-Zilkha. Radio-surgery: a 24 year history of scarless mole removal. Oculoplastic Orbital Reconstr Surg 2001;4(22):109–112.
4. Bridenstine JB. Use of ultra-high frequency electrosurgery (radiosurgery) for cosmetic surgical procedures. Dermatol Surg 1998;24:397–400.
5. Kalwarf KL, Kreici FR, Edison AR, Reinhardt RA. Lateral heat production secondary to electrosurgical incisions. Oral Surg Oral Med Oral Pathol 1983;55(4):344–348.
6. Olivar AC, Parouhar FA, Gillies CA, Servanski DR. Transmission electron microscopy: Evaluation of damage in human oviducts caused by different surgical instruments. Ann Clin Lab Sci 1999;29:281–285.

27

Fat Preservation and Other Tips for Upper Blepharoplasty

Cat Nguyen Burkat

I prefer using the Ellman radiofrequency unit with a microdissection tip or the monopolar unit with a Colorado tip to incise the skin, as these afford simultaneous cutting and excellent hemostasis. The skin and orbicularis muscle are removed as single flaps generally, although a skin flap alone could be removed if there is preoperative concern for poor eyelid closure function. Next, the fat pads are addressed if prominent on the preoperative evaluation (Figure 27.1). In general, limited fat removal should be performed in order to avoid the appearance of a hollow superior sulcus. The trend in upper eyelid blepharoplasty has shifted to preservation, repositioning, or filling of the upper lid fat, rather than aggressive removal. If debulking is indicated, the fat should be conservatively removed over a curved hemostat in order to avoid orbital hemorrhage. Medial fat pad removal should bear in mind the location of the trochlea and superior oblique tendon, as well as the numerous fibrous attachments of these structures to the orbital fat. Generally, the orbital fat pads can be thermally sculpted with the Ellman roundball tip or the Colorado tip over an intact orbital septum, which limits the risk of hemorrhage or injury to adjacent structures, as well as requires much less operative time.

In the lateral upper eyelid, a prolapsed lacrimal gland may be found in up to 10–15% of young patients undergoing blepharoplasty (Figure 27.2). The lacrimal gland will exhibit a characteristic pink color, with a lobulated shape. Failure to recognize this during surgery may lead to inadvertent lacrimal lobectomy and possible postoperative hemorrhage or dry eye. On the other hand, if left uncorrected, this may result in eyelid asymmetry, persistent lateral fullness, and therefore, poor cosmesis. The lacrimal gland, if prolapsed, should be resuspended under the superolateral orbit with several interrupted sutures.

Any additional eyelid or eyebrow procedures may also be performed through the blepharoplasty incision: these include external levator repair, internal browpexy with or without implants, ectropion repair, and/or weakening of glabellar musculature (Figure 27.3).

Meticulous layered closure is performed using 7.0 Vicryl to close the orbicularis muscle at three to four sites, followed by 6-0 fast-absorbing plain gut suture to approximate the skin edges in a running fashion, taking care to evert the skin edges. Although some surgeons prefer nonabsorbable prolene or nylon suture, patients greatly appreciate the absorbable aspect, and this also saves time in the clinic without compromising the final appearance to the incisions. Closure is performed from medial to lateral, as any dog-ear deformity, if present, is better addressed and camouflaged laterally. In Asian eyelids, closure of the orbicularis muscle layer should incorporate the levator aponeurosis at several sites to recreate a defined eyelid crease, and the incision should blend nicely into the medial epicanthal fold.

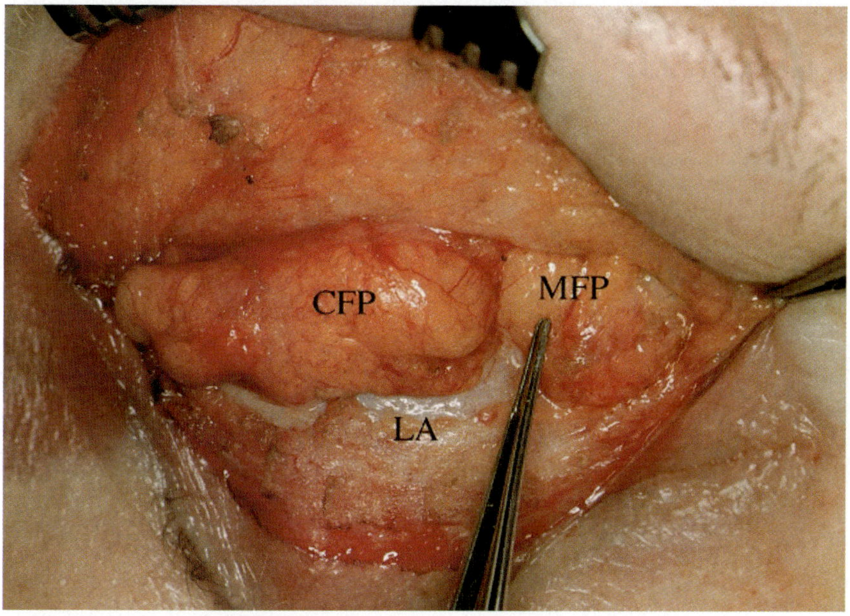

Figure 27.1. Introperative view of upper eyelid fat pads posterior to the orbital septum. The levator aponeurosis lies posterior to the orbital fat pads. MFP, medial fat pad; CFP, central fat pad; LV, levator aponeurosis.

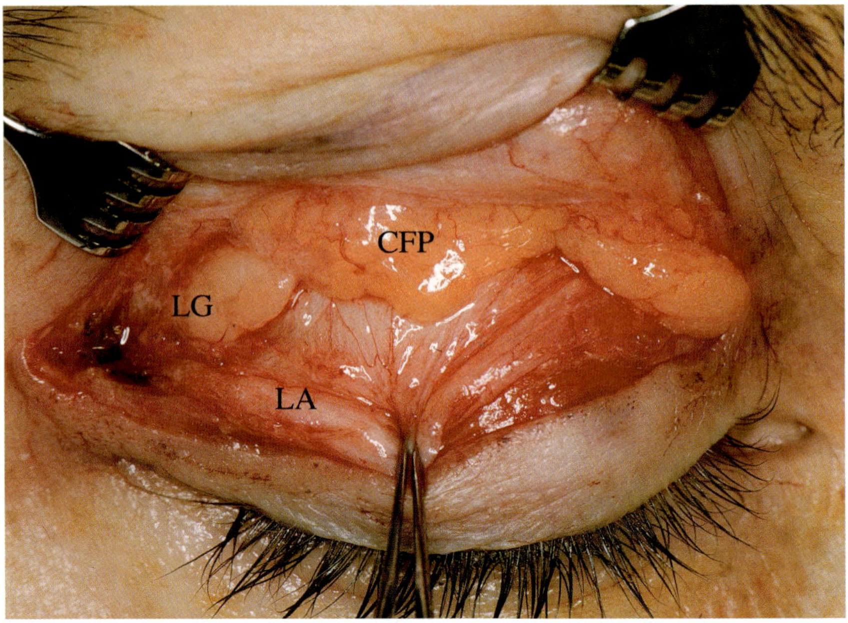

Figure 27.2. A prolapsed lacrimal gland may be seen lateral to the central fat pad and should not be mistaken for fat and inadvertently excised. LB, lacrimal gland; CFP, central fat pad; LV, levator aponeurosis.

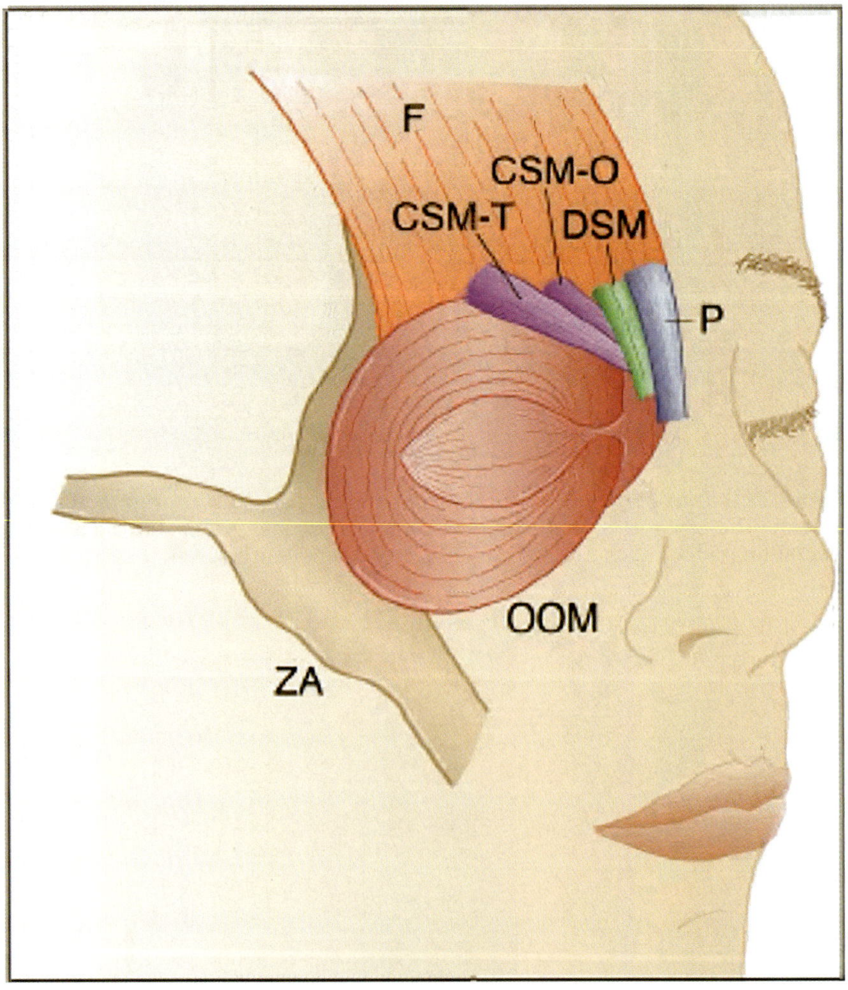

Figure 27.3. The medial eyebrow depressors may be weakened or excised through the medial aspect of the blepharoplasty incision. CSM-O, corrugator supercilii muscle oblique head; CSM-T, corrugator supercilii muscle transverse head; SM, depressor supercilii muscle; F, frontalis; P, procerus muscle; ZA, zygomatic arch; OOM, orbigularis oculi muscle.

28

Asian Blepharoplasty

Samuel M. Lam

Asian blepharoplasty is a distinct challenge for the Western surgeon who may not have frequent encounters with the Asian patient and thereby may lack the technical knowledge of how to perform the procedure as well as cultural sensitivity in approaching the Asian patient. There are as many different styles of creating a supratarsal crease in the Asian patient as there are practicing surgeons who undertake this procedure. I will discuss the personal strategy that I have developed and the accompanying pearls and pitfalls that I have encountered along the way.

All of the methods can be more broadly classified as one of three major types: suture, partial or limited incision, and full incision. For younger patients, I have come to rely on the partial-incision method that employs a simple 1.5-cm incision in the central aspect of the upper eyelid (Figure 28.1). However, when I encounter patients who have some incipient or pronounced dermatochalasis, I prefer to use the full-incision method, which permits some removal of redundant skin (Figure 28.2). Due to the ephemeral nature of the suture method with the potential for fold loss over time, I do not use this method.

The partial incision method developed by Young-Kyoon Kim is a reliable and expedient method to create a supratarsal crease in the younger patient.* The abbreviated incision permits a relatively shorter recovery time with a result that can look socially acceptable occasionally after 1 week , but more often after 1 month, can look very good by 3 months, and at the desired endpoint by the 7th to 8th month. However, what I have learned from Dr. Kim is the very important lesson to use only permanent sutures—so-called internal fixation sutures—to fixate the levator to the skin.

Also, each suture must not only bite the levator and skin edge, but also pass through approximately a half to a full millimeter of the epidermis to engender a foreign body reaction and thereby establish greater permanence of the fold.

---

*The surgical methods described in this chapter are recounted in stepwise fashion in my book, *Cosmetic Surgery of the Asian Face* (2nd ed.), Thieme Medical Publishers, Inc., New York, 2005.

When I first started performing the partial-incision method, a high percentage of my patients lost their fold principally due to my not adhering to this admonition. The major limitation of this technique is the potential for fold loss due to the short distance of levator-skin fixation. Besides the above caveats, the surgeon should also not remove any fixation sutures that become exposed until at least 3 months have transpired to ensure that a durable scar has developed.

Fortunately, the short incision of this technique permits an easier revision procedure, if needed, which is always difficult no matter what technique is pursued.

Caution: Never undertake revision surgery in only one eyelid, as the edema that results on one side alone makes discernment of symmetry elusive. If asymmetry persists by the second week, the surgeon should elect to undertake revision surgery when the scar has not matured, facilitating a far easier, faster, and safer revision procedure.

For patients who manifest dermatochalasis, I prefer the full-incision method of Dr. John A. McCurdy, Jr., in Hawaii, to remove some of this extra skin. This method will result in a longer convalescence that may look unnatural for even several months. Unfortunately, most patients who undergo a full incision in my office are older and are less tolerant of having a longer period of looking unnatural. It is also harder to perform a revision surgery when the full-incision method is used. In the partial-incision method, a revision procedure can be undertaken by extending the incision to the full length and then working down to the levator in virgin territory to avoid injury to this muscle. This luxury is not possible with the full-incision method. In revision surgery after a full-incision double-eyelid procedure, one should stay more superiorly and use the nondominant hand to apply pressure to the eyelid/globe so as to elicit herniation or propulsion of the preaponeurotic fat, which is the safety landmark from injury of the levator.

The old term "westernization" of the Asian eyelid is quite outdated for many reasons. First and foremost, many Asians do not desire to look Caucasian per se but to look more like the paragons of beauty from their own culture. Large creases with hollow upper eyelids simply never look good on Asians but render them looking very strange and unnatural. In fact, I often do not remove any fat from the upper eyelid in the Asian, especially if there already is a paucity of preaponeurotic fat to begin with.

I have devised a classification of the aging Asian eyelid that may be helpful for surgeons who would like to understand when and how to apply judgment for Asian blepharoplasty in the aging Asian eyelid and even for those who simply would like to know if they could proceed without having to create a crease. This classification scheme divides the aging Asian eyelid into three categories:

1. Aging Asian eyelids with a natural crease
2. Aging Asian eyelids without a crease
3. Aging Asian eyelids with a man-made crease

The first category, aging Asian eyelids with a natural crease, seems intuitively straightforward. If there is a crease present, then the surgeon should assume that a standard blepharoplasty could be undertaken without concern of levator fixation, symmetry, etc. However, there are some subtle but important considerations. First, what constitutes a crease in some Asian eyelids may be far less than what is traditionally encountered in the Caucasian upper eyelid. The crease may be as small as 1–2 mm and only partially visible or only established on one side. If this is the case, the surgeon should really deem this rudimentary crease as no crease at all and treat the patient accordingly. The surgeon should also be wary with indiscriminate removal of skin in these very low creases as the levator that lies in close apposition to the skin at this inferior level can be damaged if the skin incision is cut too deeply. For the patient with a standard Occidental-like natural crease, the surgeon should still be cautious because Asians are very sensitive about the position of their lid fold. Caucasians tend not to care if they show more lid crease or less. If the surgeon removes a substantial amount of skin from above the crease, as would be performed during a standard blepharoplasty, the crease can be overly elevated in position and deemed unnatural. Any crease elevation in fact may be considered unacceptable. Accordingly, the surgeon should have a detailed discussion with the patient about this likelihood. Always err on the side of conservative skin removal for this reason.

The patient that has a surgically fabricated supratarsal crease probably had it constructed when he or she was much younger during an era when westernization procedures were popularized. Therefore, the initial crease could have been excessively high and with time either become much smaller or altogether disappeared due to brow ptosis, fat absorption, and dermatochalasis. The surgeon should inspect the original crease height by lifting upward on the overlying skin to evaluate whether it is very high. If so, the surgeon is advised to warn the patient that removal of skin during a standard blepharoplasty could result in re-creation of that very high lid fold that may be unacceptable to the patient. In general, it is almost impossible to lower a crease that has already been made too high. It is also quite difficult to fill in using fat grafting a completely vacuous eyelid either due to aging, prior surgery, or both owing to the prolonged recovery time and risk of morbidity associated with possible lumpiness in the thinner skin when putting that much fat in the upper eyelid. Furthermore, the surgeon can potentially lose the fold during a conventional blepharoplasty if a suture technique was undertaken since the tenacity of this created fold is very weak.

Finally, a patient with aging Asian eyelids without a discernible crease can be approached using a standard full-incision double-eyelid blepharoplasty technique. If the surgeon tries to remove simply skin in a premeasured marked line in the upper eyelid skin without taking some preaponeurotic fat with it, the fullness of the Asian eyelid due to the low position of the levator insertion or lack of insertion altogether must be addressed. However, removal of preaponeurotic fat along with skin without addressing the levator fixation may lead to a problem with variable crease formation due to random adhesion of the postseptal tissue to the skin. Besides these problems, Asian double-eyelid blepharoplasty also carries with it some additional issues. First, creation of a supratarsal fold at a later age in life may alter an individual's self-perceived identity, a condition more prevalently suffered by the male. Preoperative counseling about this matter should be incorporated to minimize this outcome. Also, even 1–2 mm of lid edema that can persist for months may be deemed unacceptable, especially in men, who have a harder time adjusting to changes and recovery and who do not normally wear any mascara to camouflage the swelling. I tend to ask if the patient associates more with Asians or Caucasians simply because Asians know about this procedure and would recognize the postoperative stigma, whereas Caucasians and other minorities would most likely not know anything was done since they are not very sensitive about lid crease height and have never heard about a double-eyelid procedure.

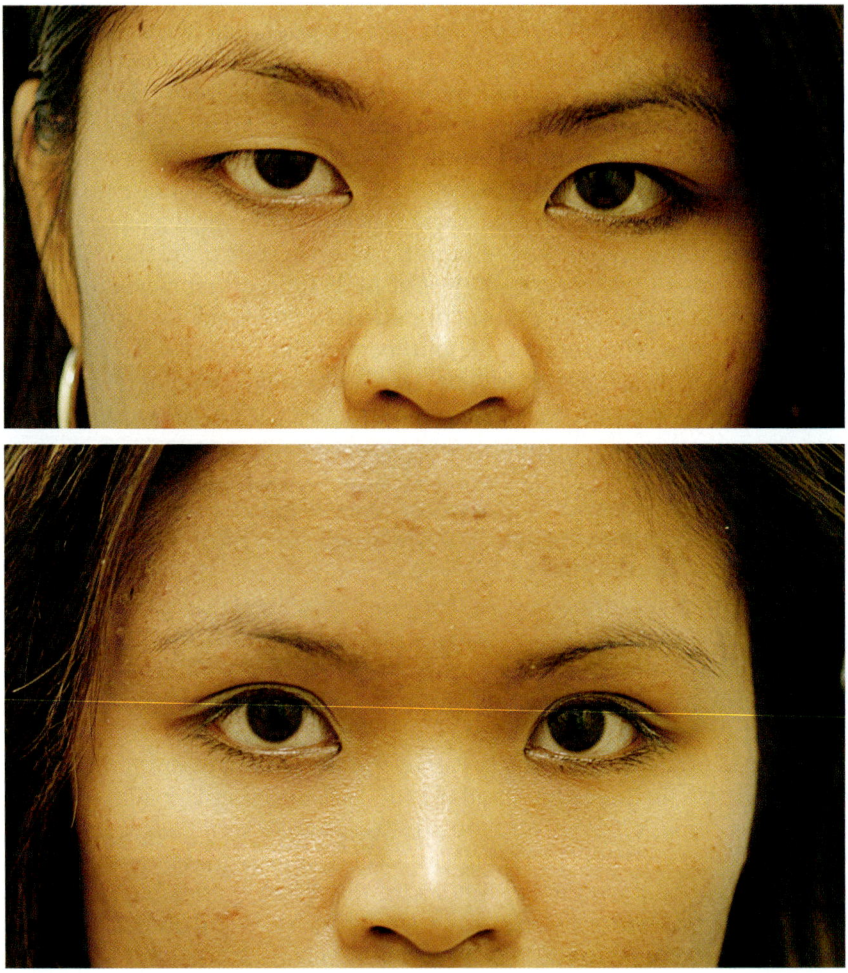

A

B

Figure 28.1. This 24-year-old Chinese woman underwent a partial-incision double eyelid blepharoplasty and shows a favorable aesthetic result 3 months postoperatively. Of note, she started with asymmetric lid creases and therefore asymmetric palpebral fissures, which was corrected by a symmetric double-eyelid blepharoplasty.

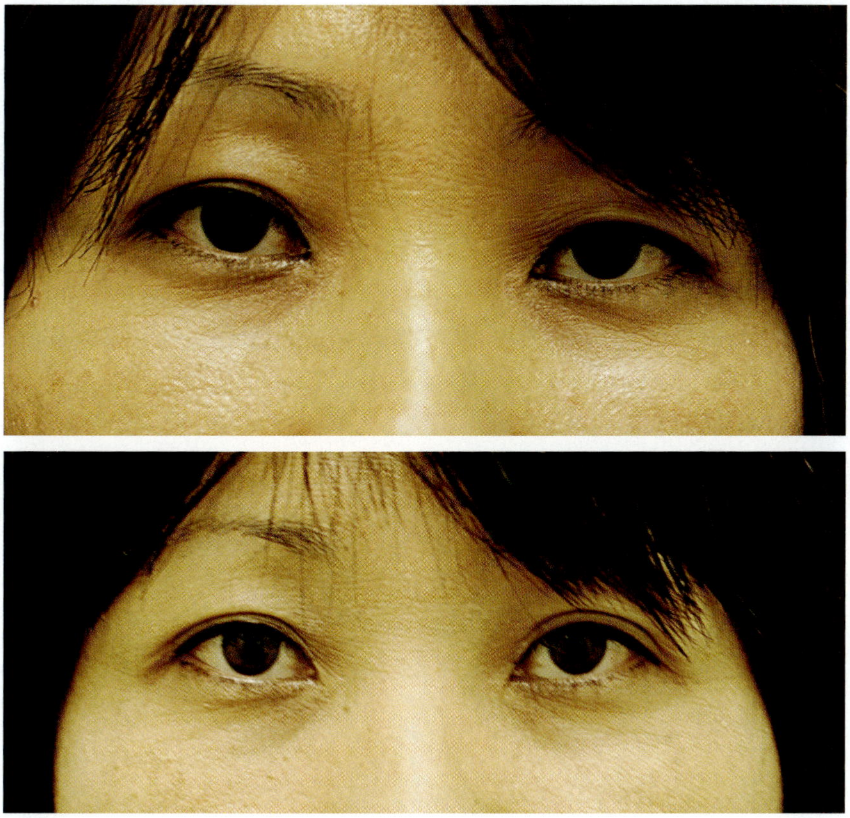

A

B

Figure 28.2. This 39-year-old Japanese woman underwent a full-incision double-eyelid blepharoplasty and is shown 7 months postoperatively. Of note, she has asymmetric creases preoperatively that have been rectified by symmetric crease fixation.

Section Four

Adjunctive Procedures in Upper Blepharoplasty

29

Internal Brow Elevation with Corrugator Removal

John R. Burroughs and Richard L. Anderson

To yield optimal results, we strongly encourage our patients to undergo adjunctive transblepharoplasty procedures to the standard upper blepharoplasty.

Our most common adjunctive procedure is internal brow elevation, which we suggest to any patient who has less than 10 mm of skin between the upper eyelid crease and the inferior brow cilia and is not interested in more aggressive brow elevation. It is ideal for heavy ptotic brow fat pads.

This procedure involves the sculpting of the brow fat pads and release of the orbital ligament for both upper eyelids. The orbital ligament is the confluence of the anterior leaf of the deep galea and the superficial temporalis fascia (Figure 29.1). Grasping this structure with forceps ensures the proper area to transect as it tethers the eyebrow until it is released. It should be transected at its most inferior extent between the lateral canthal tendon and the zygomaticofrontal suture (Figure 29.2). Stevens scissors are then used to open the anterior leaf of the deep galea and release it from the periosteal attachments along the superolateral orbit. During this release the scissors should be kept at least 1 cm above the superior orbital rim to avoid transection of the supraorbital, supratrochlear, and lacrimal vessels. Oversculpting of the brow fat pads should be avoided to reduce the risk of a pronounced bony appearance postoperatively. The underyling orbicularis superior to the upper blepharoplasty incision and the posterior leaf of the deep galea and underlying periosteum must be left intact to avoid postoperative dimpling and adhesion sites.

Corrugator removal is suggested while performing internal brow elevation in patients with aggressive glabellar furrowing or medial brow ptosis.

The corrugator muscle capsule becomes exposed upon release of the anterior leaf of the posterior galea overlying the superomedial aspect of the wound. The oblique fibers of the corrugators may then be meticulously excised (Figure 29.3). Aggressively elevating the corrugator muscles during piecemeal removal away from the deeper tissues minimizes the risk of damage to the underlying neurovascular structures. Dissection further medially and inferiorly exposes the depressor supercilii, which should be extirpated and/or transected to optimize the medial eyebrow elevation (Figure 29.4). The glabellar folds are then undermined to weaken the attachments to the skin, which will lessen their appearance postoperatively. The procerus muscles may also be bluntly weakened during this undermining, but one must be careful to avoid bleeding distant from the operative site that would be difficult to cauterize (Figure 29.5). Botox® can provide a temporary stronger weakening, but we find approximately a 50–60% improvement through this surgical approach. The requirement for postoperative Botox® injections, if needed, is lessened.

For patients with more severe forms of brow ptosis, we recommend an endoscopic forehead lift, but have found a very high acceptance rate with internal brow elevation in patients presenting for upper blepharoplasty

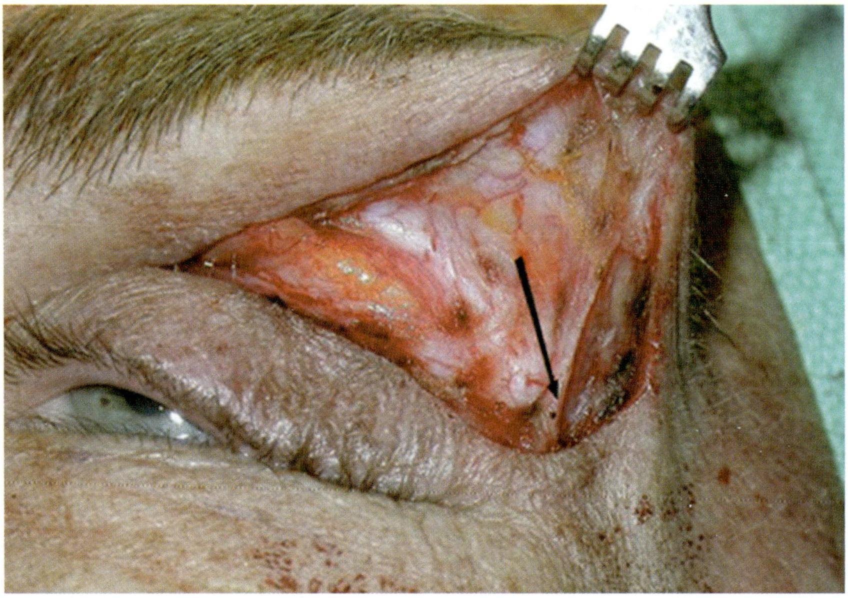

Figure 29.1. Intraoperative photograph of the confluence of the orbital ligament and the anterior leaf of the deep galea. Note the dense attachment at the lateral orbital rim. Arrow is pointing to the orbital ligament.

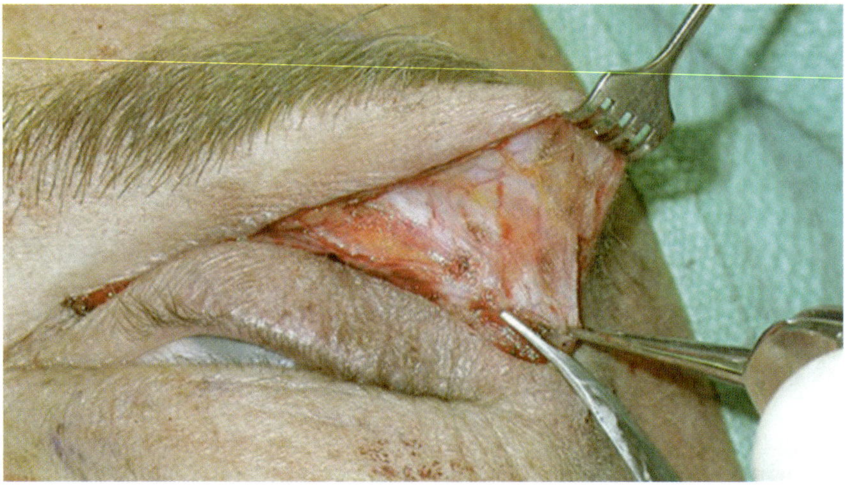

Figure 29.2. Intraoperative photograph of surgeon grasping the orbital ligament with forceps and the anterior leaf of the deep galea demonstrating its firm attachment to the lateral orbital rim. The brow fat pad lies directly beneath this tissue.

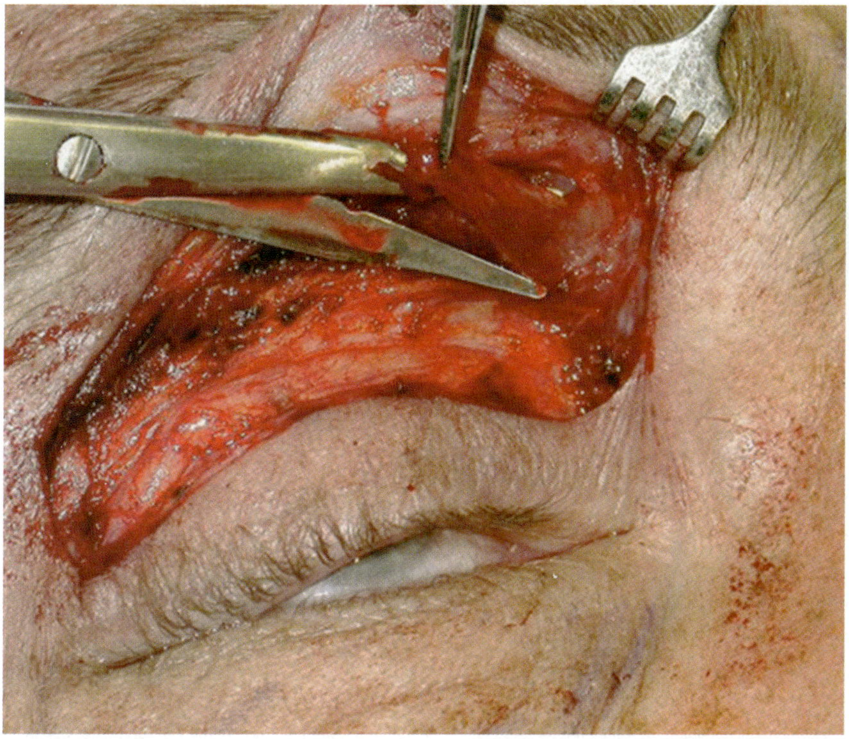

Figure 29.3. Corrugator supercilli muscle shown in the forceps during removal.

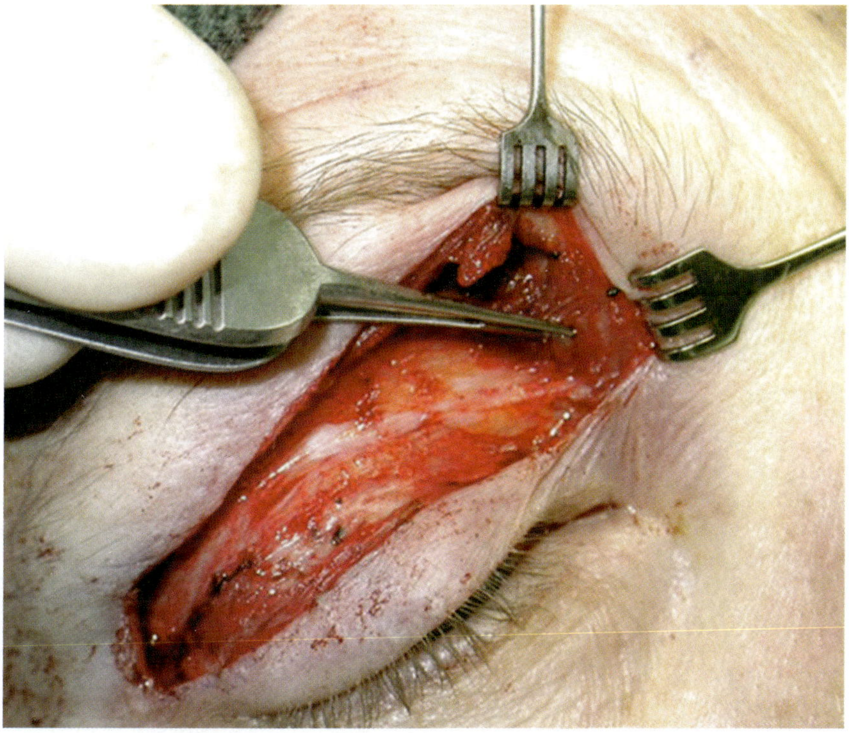

Figure 29.4. Depressor supercilli muscle shown in forceps during removal.

A

B

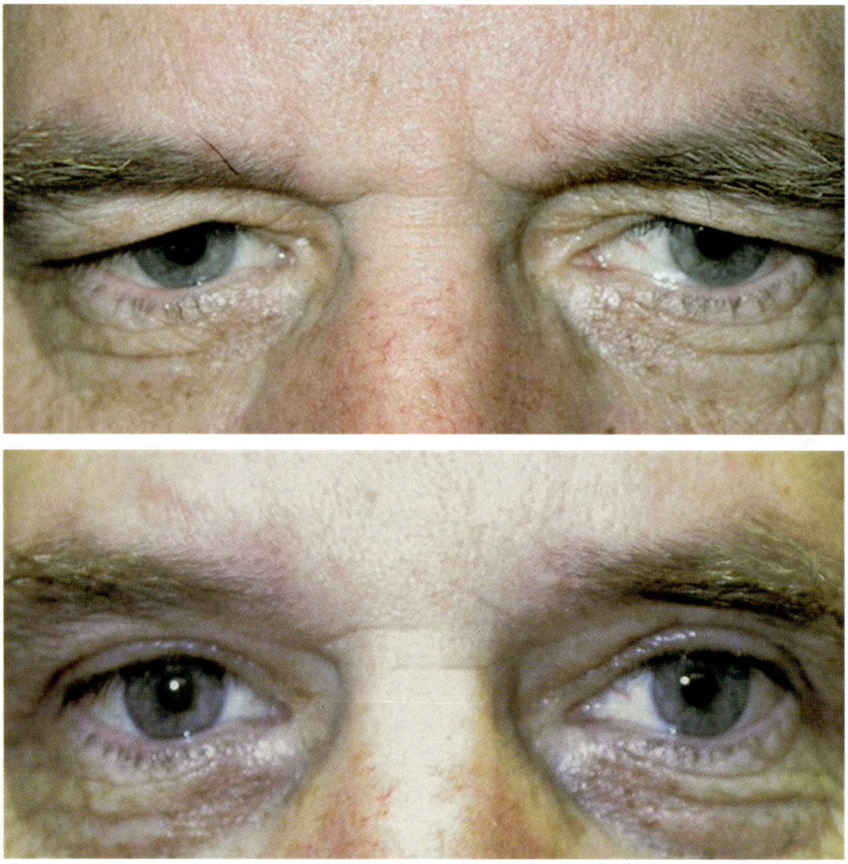

Figure 29.5. (A) Preoperative photograph showing marked blepharoptosis, bulky brow fat pads, and brow ptosis on both sides. (B) Excellent postoperative result seen after internal brow elevation, corrugator removal, and upper blepharoplasty.

30

Excision of ROOF During Upper Blepharoplasty

Jemshed A. Khan

During upper blepharoplasty, it may be necessary to excise the retro-orbicularis oculi fat (ROOF). This is usually helpful in patients with thick redundant tissues obscuring the lateral half of the orbital rim.

To excise ROOF, grasp the orbicularis of the upper wound edge. Trim the orbicularis and underlying ROOF flush with the skin edge, and then reflect the ROOF from the deep connective tissue overlying the orbital rim. Care should be taken not to expose bare periosteum because the skin may become adherent after surgery. Cauterize any bleeders. Proceed with the blepharoplasty in the usual fashion.

Reprinted with permission from: Chen WPD, Khan JA, McCord, Jr, CD. Color Atlas of Cosmetic Oculofacial Sugery. Philadelphia: Butterworth Heinemann/ Elsevier, 2004.

31

Addressing the Brow During Upper Blepharoplasty

Philip L. Custer

Internal Browlift

The central-lateral brow can be slightly elevated via the blepharoplasty incision. This technique often does not produce a dramatic change and should only be considered in patients requiring mild elevation or who are not candidates for alternative methods of browlift.

The lateral brow is manually elevated to the desired position during the skin excision–marking process. The brow dissection is performed after completing the skin, orbicularis muscle, and fat excision. The orbital septum is divided near the superior orbital rim and the periosteum is exposed. The soft tissue of the brow and forehead are elevated off of the periosteum superiorly for at least 2 cm. The dissection is performed lateral to the supraorbital notch to avoid trauma to the supraorbital neurovascular structures. The deep soft tissue of the brow is then sutured to the periosteum with several 5-0 Prolene sutures. The brow is examined to ensure there is an appropriate contour and position. The blepharoplasty is then completed.

Alternatively, the brow position may be maintained with an absorbable fixation device. The soft tissue of the lateral brow and inferior forehead are elevated in a subperiosteal plane, and the fixation device is inserted into a hole drilled above the superior orbital rim.

Thinning of Brow Fat Pad

Patients with low, full brows or small bony orbits may benefit from thinning of the retro-orbicularis oculi fat pad (ROOF). This procedure is performed before closing the blepharoplasty incision. The combined skin-orbicularis muscle is elevated as a flap off of the ROOF across the lateral aspect of the lid. The hair follicles of the brow are easily avoided, since the dissection is isolated to the tissue below the hair-bearing skin.

A portion of the ROOF is then excised off of the underlying orbital septum, improving the contour of the sulcus. It is important to leave the septum and some fat in place to avoid "skeletonizing" the orbital rim or adhesions between the orbicularis and deeper eyelid structures. The blepharoplasty wound is then closed. Patients often develop more swelling and ecchymosis after ROOF excision. They may also report hypesthesia of the upper lid, a finding that is often transient.

32

Transblepharoplasty Incision Lower Lid Canthopexy

John R. Burroughs and Richard L. Anderson

Many patients benefit from addressing lower eyelid lateral dystopia, the "sad" age-related downward slant. Lateral canthopexy is performed on most of our cosmetic patients when they undergo upper blepharoplasty. We prefer a 5-0 vicryl or PDS on a P-2 needle to suture the inferior crus of the lateral canthal tendon to the orbital rim more superiorly (Figure 32.1). This helps provide a pleasing upturn to the lateral lower eyelid, yielding a more almond shape that is aesthetically pleasing.

Through the lateral portion of the upper blepharoplasty incision, one can elevate the suborbicularis oculi fat (SOOF) pads and cheek. Closed Stevens scissors are used to undermine the lower eyelid tissues laterally to gain access to the SOOF. The temporal tissues can be sutured with a 5-0 or 4-0 vicryl on a P-2 needle more superiorly to the temporalis fascia to elevate the SOOF and cheek. One must not overelevate the SOOF pads or this will cause a large area of dimpling above the blepharoplasty incision once it is closed. Furthermore, dimpling of the skin can be avoided by not incorporating superficial skin tissue during the suturing of the temporal tissues. This provides a nice lift to the lower lateral eyelid and a subtle elevation of the midface. Our preferred treatment for nasolabial folds, however, remains injection of fillers, more aggressive midface lift, and/or facelift.

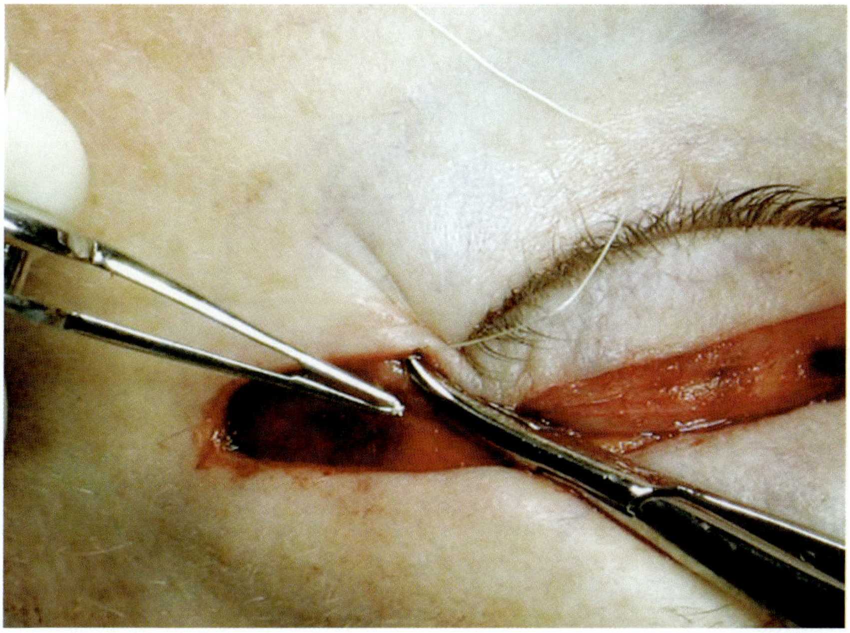

Figure 32.1. P-2 needle engaging periosteum inside lateral orbital rim after it has been placed through the inferior crus of the lateral canthal tendon (view, left side from above).

33

Lower Lid Canthopexy Through Upper Lid Incision

Guy Ben Simon and John D. McCann

Some surgeons routinely perform canthopexy in lower eyelid blepharoplasty. This can be done through a lower or upper eyelid. It eliminates unnecessary skin resection and is believed to restore tone and youthful contour.[1]

Through an incision in the upper eyelid crease,[2] dissection is extended inferiorly to the level of the lateral orbital rim, leaving the periosteum intact. This stage of dissection can facilitate lateral fad pad resection if this was not fully addressed during lower blepharoplasty. The inferior limb of the lateral canthal tendon can be cut with scissors under visual inspection. A double-armed suture on a semicircular needle is placed 2 mm above Whitnall's tubercle inside the orbital rim. The suture then travels through the orbital rim periosteum and emerges in half-buried horizontal mattress fashion through the inferior canthal tendon. Additional sutures can be used to tighten the orbicularis muscle to the superficial orbital rim. Alternatively, lateral canthal resuspension can be performed using the lateral canthal strip procedure described by Anderson and Gordy.[3]

References

1. Flowers R. Canthopexy as a routine blepharoplasty component. Clin Plast Surg 1993;20:351.
2. Jelks G, Glat PM, Jelks EB, Longaker MT. The inferior retinacular lateral canthoplasty: a new technique. Plast Reconstr Surg 1997;100:1262.
3. Anderson RL, Gordy DD. The tarsal strip procedure. Arch Ophthalmol 1979;97:2192–2196.

Section Five

Wound Closure and Postoperative Care

34

Avoiding Dog Ears During Upper Blepharoplasty Closure

Peter S. Levin

The medial and lateral "dog ears" that may form at the ends of upper blepharoplasty can be minimized by equalizing tension across the upper eyelid incision. One way to do this is to place the medial and lateral ends of the incision on horizontal stretch. Maintaining tension across the wound produces excellent alignment of skin edges and prevents "surprise" dog ears at the ends of the incision. Careful placement of a fine hemostat (medially) and a single skin hook (laterally) enables closure of the upper blepharoplasty incision, often without the need for a surgical assistant.

Surgical Technique

After upper blepharoplasty is performed, the extreme medial aspect of the wound is closed and tied with a 6-0 polypropylene or other suture. A long suture tail is left and is secured with a fine hemostat. The hemostat is then held across the nose by the surgical assistant, or it is draped over the nose by the surgeon. At the lateral aspect of the incision, a single skin hook is placed which is either held by the surgical assistant or allowed to hang freely (Figure 34.1). The directions in which the medial hemostat and lateral hook pull are checked to equalize tension across the wound. The incision is closed with running 6-0 polypropylene. Halfway through the closure, the tension placed medially is no longer required and the hemostat is released. The closure is completed without lateral dog ear formation.

Dog ears are almost always avoided laterally with this technique. However, medially a dog ear is inevitable if the upper and lower incisions meet at a relatively acute angle, as is common with aggressive excisions in this area. In the medial area, the relative surplus of superior eyelid skin relative to inferior skin relative is apparent when the initial prolene suture is placed on medial stretch. Options for dealing with excess superior skin—which leads to a dog ear—include "w-plasty" or medial extension of the incision. Once the medial dog ear is addressed, the technique described above can be used for the remainder of the closure.

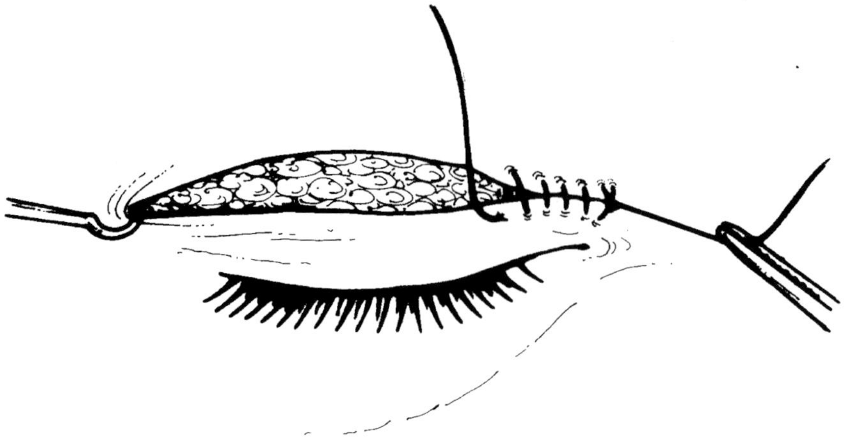

A

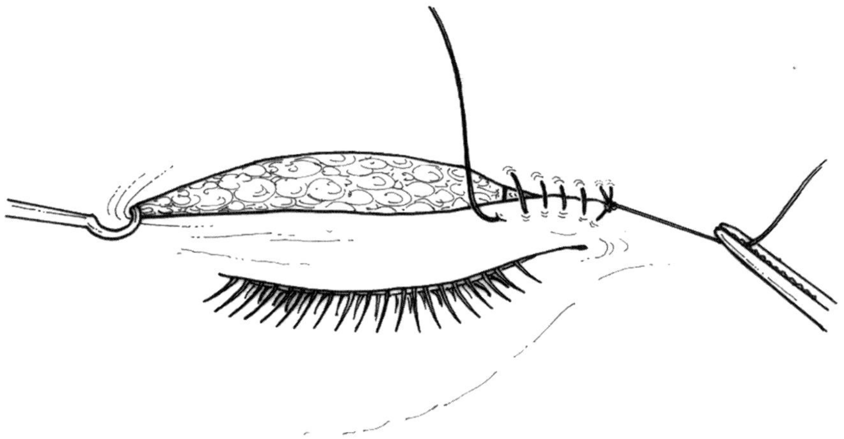

B

Figure 34.1. A hemostat is placed on the tail of the running suture to place medial traction on the incision. A single skin hook placed at the lateral aspect of the incision provides lateral traction on the incision.

35

Crease Formation in Upper Blepharoplasty

Philip L. Custer

Crease formation: A soft, subtle crease can be formed by suturing the edge of the pretarsal orbicularis muscle to the levator aponeurosis with three 7-0 Vicryl sutures. Inspect the lid position and contour after placing these sutures to ensure the natural lid position has not been altered.

Wound closure: Place one or two buried 7-0 Vicryl sutures to close the orbicularis muscle lateral to the canthus. Several interrupted 7-0 Prolene sutures are placed in the medial lid incision. The remaining wound is closed with a running 7-0 Prolene. A more defined crease can be achieved by incorporating the aponeurosis in the skin closure sutures.

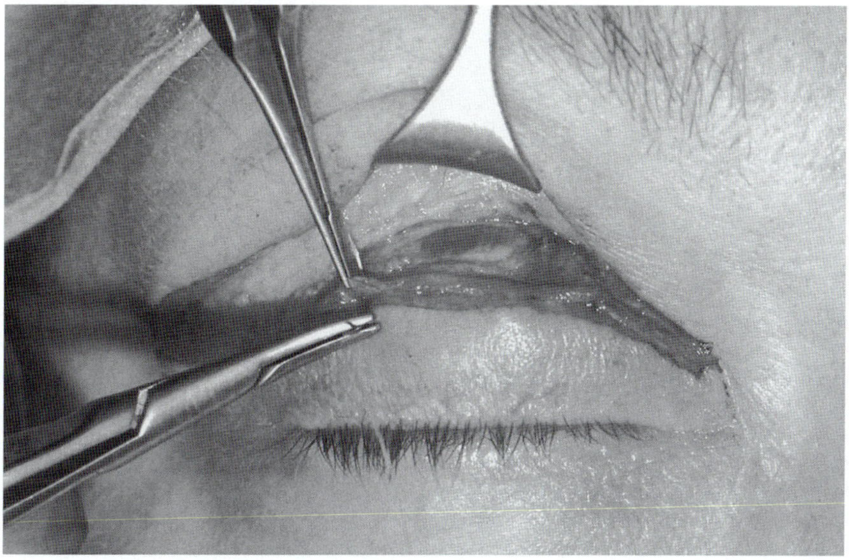

Figure 35.1. Creation of a suble eyelid crease.

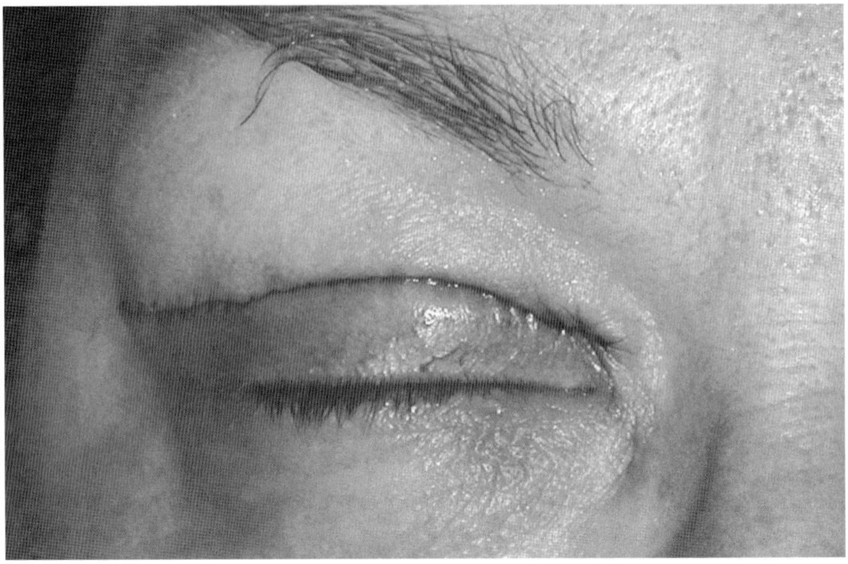

Figure 35.2. Upper blepharoplasty wound closure.

36

Use of Tissue Adhesive for Oculoplastic Incision Closure

Charles B. Slonim

Cyanoacrylate adhesives, such as Dermabond® are options for ocuplastic wound closure. The applicator provided by the manufacturer does not work for these sorts of wounds, and the tips below will allow the use of these products.

1. The skin edges must be absolutely dry and free of debris, dried blood, and dried betadine.
2. The assistant pushes slightly gapped wound edges together during the application. A good subcutaneous layer (closure) is necessary for the skin edges to rest on (e.g., DCR and orbitotomy incisions).
3. The Dermabond vial is crushed, and its contents are squeezed out into a disposable plastic container (e.g., lid of the specimen container). The applicator tip contains a chemical initiator that the adhesive needs to pass through. Tilt the lid so that all the adhesive runs to an edge or groove of the container.
4. Draw the adhesive up with the 26- or 27-gauge needle already attached to a tuberculin syringe.
5. Invert the syringe (needle pointing up) and draw the entire adhesive down to the plunger.
6. Evacuate all except 0.05 mL of the air just up to the needle hub. There will be about 0.5 cc of adhesive in the syringe.
7. Change to a 30-gauge needle and turn the syringe so the needle points downward. The 0.5 cc of air is now between the plunger and the dermabond.
8. Gently push the adhesive so that a micro-droplet just appears at the bore of the needle tip.
9. Place the first droplet in the middle of the wound. The liquid adhesive will run a few millimeters in either direction along the wound edges.
10. Continue to divide the wound in halves and place droplets along the rest of the wound.
11. After the first layer has had a chance to polymerize (i.e., dry), place a second layer on top of it.
12. Keep the wound dry. Iced soaks need to be done over a dry cloth or gauze to prevent the wound from getting "soggy" wet.

37

Avoiding or Minimizing Postoperative Swelling

John R. Burroughs and Richard L. Anderson

Potential causes of increased postoperative swelling include rough tissue handling, excessive cauterization, and lymphatic disruption. Other contributing factors are poor patient compliance with cool compresses, head elevation, and rest. Progressive postoperative periorbital and orbital inflammation is usually considered to be infectious or toxoallergic in etiology. Clinical onset, signs, symptoms, and response to empiric therapy often help distinguish the diagnosis.

More common causes of postoperative swelling as outlined earlier include surgical issues (e.g., surgical disruption of lymphatics, poor wound handling, and excessive cautery); an adverse reaction to topical or oral agents; and infections.

Intraoperatively, we place the patient's head at a slight elevation (reverse trendelenburg) and when switching from one side to the other will cover the operative site with a cool, dampened gauze until returning to this side, which minimizes bleeding and reduces swelling.

We utilize a nonstick-type bipolar cautery (Stryker SILVERGlide™ 800-253-3210), which provides quicker and more precise method of controlling bleeding. Immediately following surgery, we place ice compresses (e.g., bag of frozen peas) over the eyes.

We encourage constant ice compresses for the first 24 hours while awake, and at least every few hours for 20-minute intervals for another 24–48 hours. Between 48 and 72 hours, we instruct patients to switch to warm compresses. Patients should be warned to not microwave a wet towel, as this can lead to burns of the skin, especially while the sensory perception is reduced in the early postoperative period. Instead, we advise patients to use hand towels soaked with warm tap water or an electric heat pad, as this is much safer. Patients are also advised to sleep with their heads elevated for the first several days following surgery.

Reactions to topical agents can take several days to a week before becoming apparent. Neomycin-associated dermatitis can take up to a week, but some topical induced reactions can occur much quicker. Early infections commonly present with erythema, swelling, and pain before any puruluent wound discharge develops. Therefore, a high index of suspicion for an infection should be present when swelling progressively worsens after the first 48 hours postoperatively.

We have found that patients with seasonal allergy-related eye complaints, thyroid eye disease, and preoperative edema will generally swell more profusely, and often we will treat with a Medrol dose pack immediately following surgery. We point out in preoperative photographs any patients with even mild festoons that this will likely worsen for several months following their surgery. We also routinely recommend vitamin C and Arnica Montana to our patients undergoing multiple periocular procedures to lessen bruising and speed resolution. Currently, our preferred arnica montana formulation is SinEcch (888-746-3224), which has an easy dosing schedule and empirically in our practice seems to reduce both the severity and the duration of bruising and swelling. Our aestheticians utilizing lymphatic massage (synergy) treatments help postoperative edema, and some topicals, including Preparation H, often help reduce longstanding eyelid edema and festoons.

38

Management of Postblepharoplasty Dry Eye

Morris E. Hartstein

Postblepharoplasty dry eye can range from being a mild inconvenience to having catastrophic consequences. As with most complications, the best management strategy is to avoid it in the first place. Here are some general guidelines and tips.

A thorough eye history and exam should be performed on all prospective blepharoplasty patients, paying specific attention to the following:

- Do patients currently use artificial tears?
- Do their eyes burn; do they have foreign body sensation?
- Do they have ocular allergies?
- Do they have systemic diseases that may be associated with dry eye, such as rheumatoid arthritis, Sjögren's syndrome, or perimenopausal symptoms?
- Have they had a Bell's palsy, or prior eyelid surgery?

Prior LASIK patients may be at particularly higher risk as they have an anesthetic cornea. We generally recommend waiting at least 6 months after LASIK before proceeding with blepharoplasty.

During the exam, careful attention should be given to evaluating the tear film, tear evaporation, eyelid closure, and blink. Schirmer testing measures the basal tear secretion. While the reliability of Schirmer testing may be controversial, it can help identify those patients with severe dry eyes. A quicker and easier test is the Zone Quick Phenol Red (FCI Ophthalmics), where threads are placed in the inferior fornix (without anesthetic) for 15 seconds.

The most obvious cause of postblepharoplasty dry eye is frank lagophthalmos from too much tissue removal, lower lid retraction, or both. Corrective surgical procedures may include tarsorrhaphy, skin graft, spacer graft, and midface lift. Another more subtle and more common cause of dry eye is a decreased blink excursion where there will no be lagophtahlmos.

Fortunately, most cases of postblephaorplasty dry eye are transient and will resolve successfully on their own. Ongoing supportive measures should be tailored to the specific tear film problem.

Deficiency in the aqueous layer is easily treated with artificial tear supplements. There are many different brands on the market, and it may take a little trial and error to determine the best one for a particular patient. Punctal plugs (not intracanalicular!) can be helpful too.

Warm compresses with massage can help with meibomian gland dysfunction, which can worsen postoperatively, leading to increased tear evaporation. There are several products to improve meibomian gland dysfunction:

- Doxycycline
- Vitamin supplements such as Hydroeye® (sciencebasedhealth.com) containing omega-3 fatty acids
- Cod liver oil pills
- Flax seed oil pills
- Soy supplements

Rarely the conjunctival contribution (mucin from goblet cells) to the tear film can be the source of dry eye, and mucomyst drops can be helpful.

Suggested Reading

Korn BS,Kikkawa DO, Schanzlin DJ. Blepharoplasty in the post-laser in situ keratomileusis patient: preoperative considerations to avoid dry eye syndrome. Plast Reconstr Surg 2007;119:2232–2239.

Part IV

Lower Lid Blepharoplasty

Section One

Preoperative Considerations

39

Lower Eyelid Blepharoplasty: The Evaluation

John D. Siddens

Avoiding complications in performing a lower eyelid blepharoplasty may be based on the evaluation of the patient. By combining a thorough evaluation with proper history taking, many complications that result from this surgical procedure can be avoided.

1. Proper assessment of the patient is the first step in avoiding complications in lower eyelid blepharoplasty. Taking and recording the proper history can provide many clues important in the procedure. Of particular interest is the history of skin disease, sun exposure, anticoagulation therapy, vitamin and nutrition supplements, and previous surgery.
2. A psychiatric history is also important to ascertain the patient's expectations, both reasonable and unreasonable. Careful documentation of medicine used for psychiatric problems is necessary.
3. The procedure should be discussed with the patient at length and in detail. A description of the risks, complications, benefits, and goals is helpful to prepare the patient for what is to come. Informed consent should be presented to the patient and should be witnessed as it is signed. A copy may be given to the patient. If the surgery is not performed within 30 days, it is helpful to discuss the surgery again with the patient and have the document initialed and dated again.
4. Preoperative assessment should include a complete eye exam and visual acuity recording. Schirmer testing should be done when potential dry eye problems are considered. The use of mirrors for the patient to view him or herself and having the patient discuss their goals can help avoid postsurgical misunderstandings, especially when the surgeon provides realistic expectations with the patient. The use of brochures, websites, and other information can also increase the patient's understanding of expected surgical results.
5. It is helpful to have the chart and special notes handy when the procedure is to begin. Photographs may now be taken digitally and prints made which can be placed at bedside during the procedure. This provides a guide not only to what the patient looks like upright and not

sedated, but to the correct surgical site. Two specific photos are helpful in presurgical evaluation. An "eye box" photo (the edges beginning temporal to the lateral canthi and from just above the eyebrow to just above the tip of the nose) provides great detail of the eyelids (Figure 39.1). A full face or midface photo will help document eyelid and periocular features. The "tilt" photo helps to document the amount of orbital fat (Figure 39.2). Ask the patient to tilt the head forward, look upward, and take the photo from slightly above the nose. This demonstrates the amount and location of herniated orbital fat.

6. Skin evaluation begins with documentation of the amount and location of rhytids. Skin turgor and tone, as well as notation of abnormal pigmentation or lesions, are carefully documented. The presence of festoons or chronic eyelid edema may indicate chronic inflammation, which may reoccur postoperatively.

7. Several specific tests are documented to provide clues for successful surgery, including the gape test, snap back test, medial displacement test, and eyelid position measurements (MRD_1 and MRD_2).

8. Gape test: If the eyelid tone is normal, the lower eyelids will move upward when the patient is in upgaze. Even with the mouth open, the eyelid excursion should be close to normal. If lid laxity or retraction is present, the lids will not move upward, as demonstrated with increased scleral show (a positive gape test).

9. Lower eyelid laxity may be documented with a snap back test (Figure 39.3). This test involves grasping the lower eyelid, pulling it off the eye, and letting go. A quick "snap" of the lid back to the eye indicates a normal tendon tension. Lack of the lid returning to proper position, or return with a blink, may indicate a lax canthal tendon. The medial displacement test helps specify whether or not the medial canthal tendon is loose. Pulling the medial lower eyelid temporally will usually result in less than 2–4 mm of movement. Greater mobility indicates a lax medial canthal tendon.

10. To provide reproducible measurements, the margin-reflex distance in primary gaze (MRD_1) documents the distance from the upper eyelid margin to the corneal light reflex. The normal measurement is 3–4 mm or greater. Similarly, the margin-reflex distance in primary gaze II (MRD_2) documents the distance from the lower eyelid margin to the corneal light reflex, usually measured as 3–5 mm.

11. Location of herniated orbital fat and identification of orbicularis muscle hypertrophy can also be valuable clues to avoid complications in lower lid repair. Of particular note is the location and amount of the lateral fat pad. This pad often hides under the lateral rim, a much more difficult location to reach surgically.

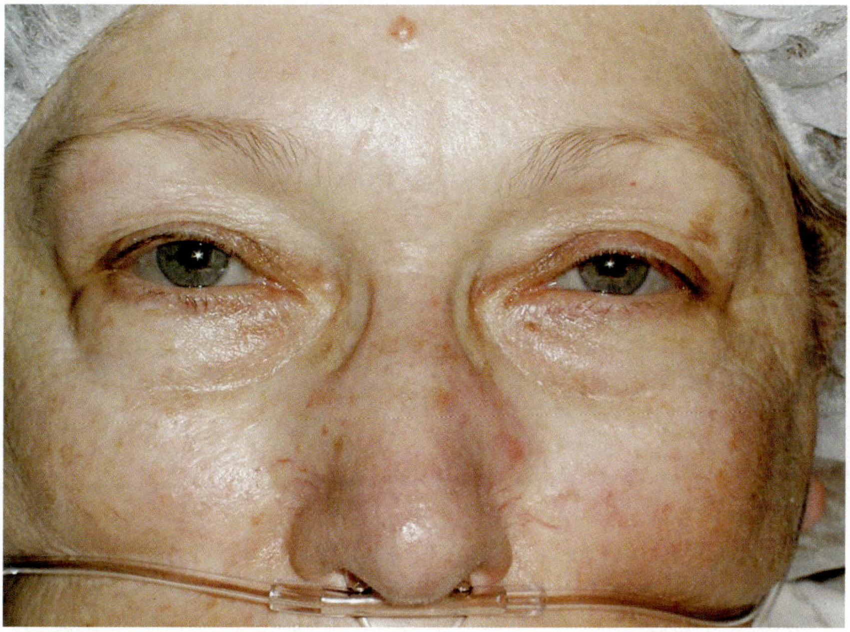

Figure 39.1. "Eyebox" photo showing eyes, eyelids, and periorbital area.

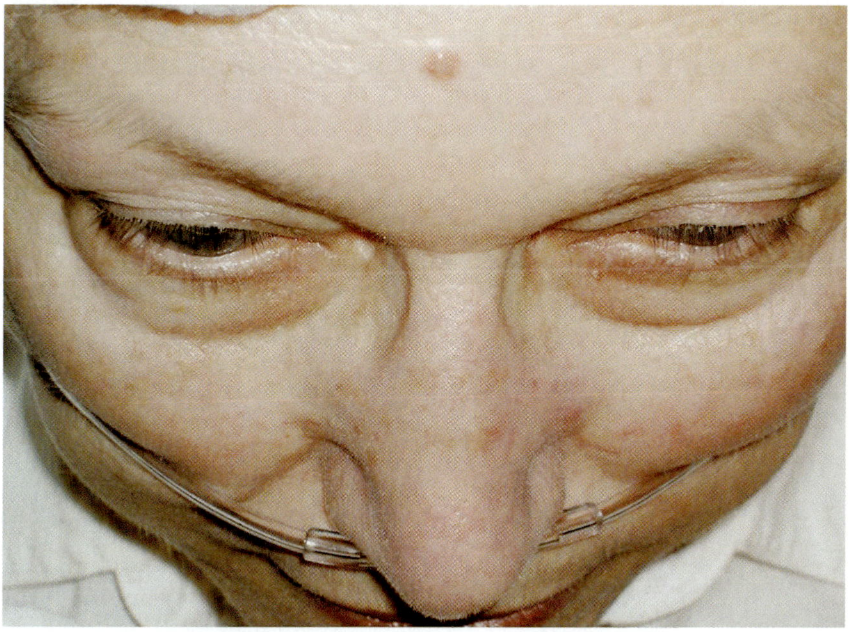

Figure 39.2. "Tilt" photo helps to show orbital fat.

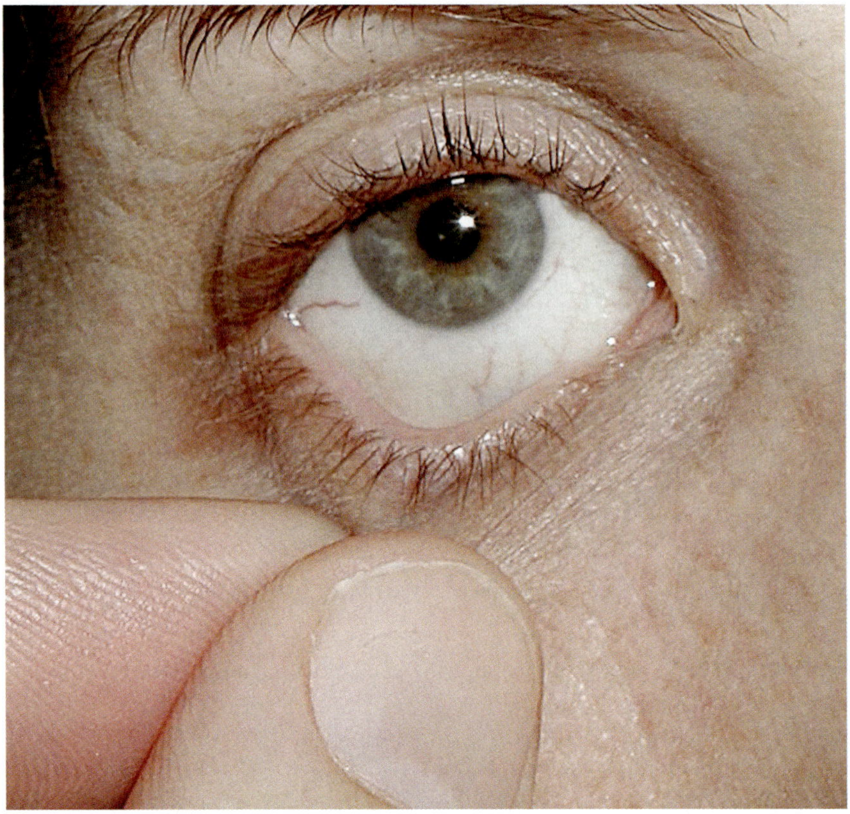

Figure 39.3. Eyelid pulled away from globe in snapback test.

40

Lower Eyelid Blepharoplasty Evaluation: Avoid the Cookie Cutter Approach

Sheri L. DeMartelaere, Todd R. Shepler, Sean M. Blaydon, Russell W. Neuhaus, and John W. Shore

The cookie cutter approach to lower eyelid blepharoplasty should be discouraged. Abnormal anatomic relationships should first be determined before an appropriate surgical plan can be established. Each individual patient will have characteristic anatomic problems that require different surgical techniques to correct.

- The amount of excess skin is evaluated. This should be done while the patient looks upward. This places the lower eyelid skin on stretch, and any excess skin with the lid in this position can be excised with less risk of producing cicatricial retraction or ectropion after lower eyelid blepharoplasty.
- Herniated orbital fat is noted by looking for areas of fullness in the lower eyelid as the patient looks straight ahead and then in upgaze. Gentle pressure can be applied to the globe through the upper eyelid to make these areas of fat prolapse more prominent. These areas of fullness may be absent when the patient is lying supine at the time of surgery.
- Look for lower eyelid laxity and ectropion that may need to be addressed at the time of surgery.
- Pull the lower eyelid away from the eye. The eyelid should not be able to be pulled more than 6 mm from the globe.
- The snap-back test can be performed by pulling the lower eyelid downward and observing how quickly it snaps back against the globe. In involutional ectropion the eyelid may not snap back until the patient blinks. Any ectropion secondary to laxity of the lower eyelid can sometimes best be seen at the slit lamp.
- Laxity of the lower eyelid at the lateral canthus can be evaluated by pulling the lateral lower eyelid towards the nose. The lateral canthus should move only minimally with this maneuver.

- Laxity of the medial canthal tendon can be similarly evaluated by pulling the medial lower eyelid laterally. If the lower punctum approaches the corneal limbus with this maneuver, then there is significant medial canthal laxity.
- Look for any punctal eversion and atresia that may need to be corrected at the time of ectropion repair.
  - Assess the relationship of the lower eyelid with the mid-face. One should pay particular attention to the presence of suborbicularis oculi fat (SOOF) and malar fat pad descent, prominent tear trough deformities, and adequate maxillary bony support of the lower eyelid and globe.
  - Lower eyelid retraction should be identified preoperatively. The etiology of the retraction should be established, such as cicatricial skin changes versus poor bony support and prominence of the globe.

Section Two

Lower Blepharoplasty Procedure Pearls

41

Three-Step Technique for Lower Lid Blepharoplasty

Joseph A. Mauriello, Jr.

The three-step technique for lower lid blepharoplasty has been utilized and modified since 1998.[1–4] It produces predictable results. Three and one-half mm of elevation of the eyelid/cheek skin interface is achieved.[1–4] The steps include:

- Transconjunctival removal of orbital fat
- "V" suture lateral lower eyelid horizontal tightening technique after creation of the eyelid (skin muscle)–cheek flap with the carbon dioxide laser
- Resuspension of the anterior lamella and adjacent malar fat pad to the lateral orbital periosteum

Step 1: Transconjunctival Fat Removal

Orbital fat is removed to the level of the inferior orbital rim. Overzealous fat removal is discouraged. The conjunctival incision is made across the entire lower lid in the conjunctival cul de sac. It extends medially below the caruncle in order to address the large medial fat pad. A residual central eyelid bulge is usually due to fat that surrounds the inferior oblique muscle. This fat has its own orbital septum that is incised, and the fat is removed without injuring the adjacent inferior oblique muscle. The conjunctival wound is closed with two or three interrupted 6-0 plain catgut sutures to theoretically restore eyelid anatomy and prevent pyogenic granuloma on the raw conjunctival surgically incised edge.

Step 2: "V" Suture Lateral Lower Eyelid Horizontal Tightening After Creation of the Eyelid (skin muscle)–Cheek Flap with the Carbon Dioxide Laser

Lower lids require horizontal lid tightening in order to achieve eyelid stability so that elevation of the eyelid/cheek skin interface is achieved without lid pulldown. The "v" suture technique vertically elevates the lateral aspect of the lower lid and prevents postoperative lower lid retraction. A subciliary incision is made with a #15 blade 5 mm medial to the lateral commissure and 5 mm lateral to it (Figure 41.1A). The initial dissection in the eyelid region involves skin only inferiorly, as much as technically feasible, to the level of the lower tarsal border in order to preserve pretarsal orbicularis muscle. The dissection is continued between the skin–muscle layer and the underlying orbital septum. The carbon dioxide laser is used as a cutting device to dissect inferiorly over the inferior orbital rim, laterally over the lateral orbital rim and under the malar fat pad (subcutaneous thickening of fat). Areas of redundant lower eyelid tissue including the malar folds may be treated focally with the defocused laser in order to effect immediate tightening of the overlying anterior lamella. In addition, gradual tightening continues for 6 months after surgery.[1–5] Subcutaneous fat should be treated judiciously in order to avoid fat necrosis. In patients with minimal redundant skin or negative vector orbits, the laser should only be used as a cutting device. Use of the defocused laser in such patients is avoided in order to prevent contracture and lower lid pulldown. The medial aspect of the lower eyelid skin muscle dissection is completed with a Stevens scissors since the laser cannot be visualized in this area. The entire skin–orbicularis oculi muscle flap is raised with a portion of the malar fat pad. Orbital fat excision can be reassessed once the skin–muscle flap is elevated. When the skin–muscle flap is pulled superiorly and pressure is placed on the globe, residual fat becomes evident.

The "v" suture technique involves two bites of a double-armed horizontal mattress 5-0 polydiaxanone (PDS) suture (Figure 41.1B). The two bites form a "v" so that the eyelid margin is tightened more than the lower tarsal border (Figure 41.1B). The first vertical bite creates the medial arm of the "v." A bite is taken approximately 4–5 mm medial to the lateral commissure and penetrates partial thickness tarsus by entering and exiting its anterior surface from inferior (at the tarsal base) to superior. This bite exits 2 mm below the eyelid margin and should not incorporate the superior skin edge of the subciliary wound. The bite of the second arm of the suture is taken from superior to inferior through the anterior tarsus and lateral to the first bite to form the "v." The distance between the open arms of the "v" is determined by the amount of horizontal laxity. Rarely, two such sutures are necessary to sufficiently tighten lax lower lids. In such cases, a tarsal strip for enhanced tightening should be considered. The "v" suture traverses partial thickness tarsus and exits adjacent to the initial bite of the first arm of the suture at the base of the tarsus to create the apex of the "v." Angling this second bite inferiorly towards the lower tarsal border creates the modified "v." When the arms of the suture are tied at the base of the tarsus, the arms of the "v," a "wave," or puckering of the lateral lower eyelid margin is evident (Figure 41.1C). The lateral eyelid hugs the globe, elevates the lateral lower lid margin to prevent lower lid retraction, and corrects mild to moderate horizontal eyelid laxity. The suture is tied at the bottom of the "v" to prevent prolapse or erosion of the knot through the subciliary wound.

Step 3: Resuspension of the Anterior Lamella and Adjacent Malar Fat Pad to the Lateral Orbital Periosteum

The previously undermined skin–orbicularis muscle and malar fat flap are now mobilized superiorly by grasping the superior edge of the orbicularis muscle (Figure 41.2A,B). A horizontal bite of the orbicularis muscle is taken with a 5-0 Vicryl (polygalactin) suture to resuspend the flap. The flap is suspended to the orbital periosteum laterally (Figure 41.2C). When this suture is properly placed, the skin appears flattened with minimal tension and the upper cheek is mobilized superiorly. Additional undermining may be necessary, and the suture may be replaced. Any excess skin is excised from the superior edge of the skin muscle flap. The amount of skin that is necessary to excise is usually only 1–2 mm of skin measured vertically. Any redundant orbicularis muscle at the superior edge of the skin–muscle flap that now overlies the tarsal plate just medial to the placement of the 5-0 Vicryl suture is then excised to avoid bunching. The skin edges are closed with an absorbable 6-0 plain catgut.

Steri-strips are placed while the recumbent patient looks up in order to support the lower lid, effectively "dam" the fat back into the orbit, and tamponade any postoperative edema. Steri-strips maintain the lower lid and cheek structures in a superior overcorrected position for 7–14 days after surgery. After the steri-strips are applied, there appears to be redundant lower lid skin, but the edema eyelid and laser tightening over time assures an improved result. Intravenous corticosteroids (8 mg of dexamethasone) the day of surgery and oral corticosteroids (prednisone, 60 mg/day) for the first 3 postoperative days reduce edema and facial distortion. Postoperative head elevation and liberal use of ice compresses allow the lateral canthus to heal in a relatively upward position.

Rationale for the Three-Step Procedure

Horizontal tightening by the "v" suture lateral lower eyelid technique elevates the lower eyelid margin by creating the "wave." This upward enhancement is complemented by the skin–orbicularis oculi and adjacent malar fat pad resuspension that reduces downward traction on the lateral canthus. Elevation and repositioning of this sphincter-like orbicularis muscle supports the lower lid, and malar fat and serves to reposit the orbital contents posteriorly. During the 6 months after surgery, a tug of war occurs between the lower eyelid margin and the undermined eyelid/cheek skin interface. The eyelid margin always wins if the above steps are performed appropriately and conservatively. The thermal damage induced by the laser affords gradual elevation of the eyelid/cheek skin interface (Figure 41.3).

Pearls

1. Avoid use of laser with thin skin because of possible thermal damage to overlying skin.
2. Avoid overzealous use of defocused laser in patients with mild to moderate skin redundancy to prevent postoperative anterior lamellar contracture and consequent lower eyelid retraction.
3. Chemosis is unusual with this technique and, if present, resolves with a short course of topical corticosteriods.
4. The technique may be learned and gradually improved with conservative performance of each step until experienced is gained by the surgeon.
5. Final results require 6 months. Patience is required.

A

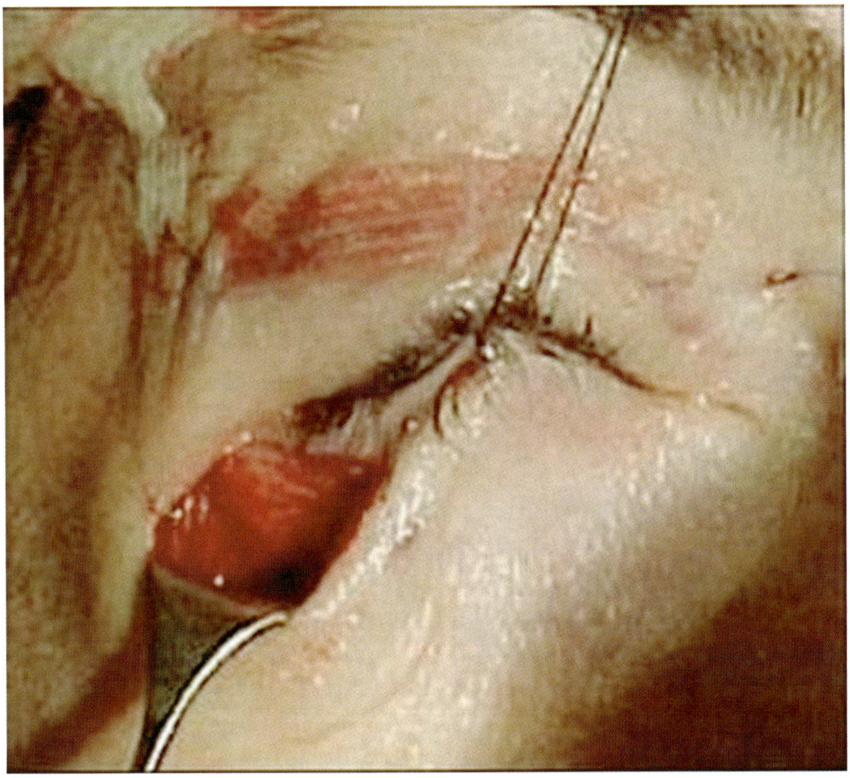

Figure 41.1. (A) Skin muscle flap is undermined through a small lateral subciliary incision that extends beyond lateral canthus. (B) The "v" horizontal mattress suture horizontally shortens the lower eyelid and also serves to elevate the lower eyelid margin. (C) Note the "wave" that gradually flattens, usually within 2 weeks after surgery.

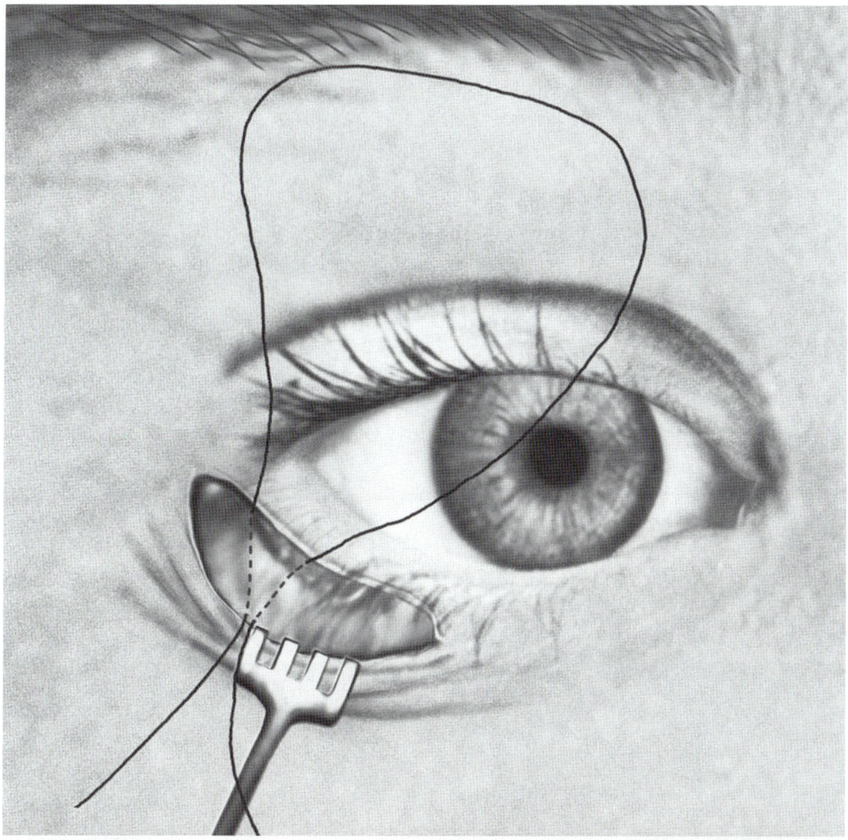

B

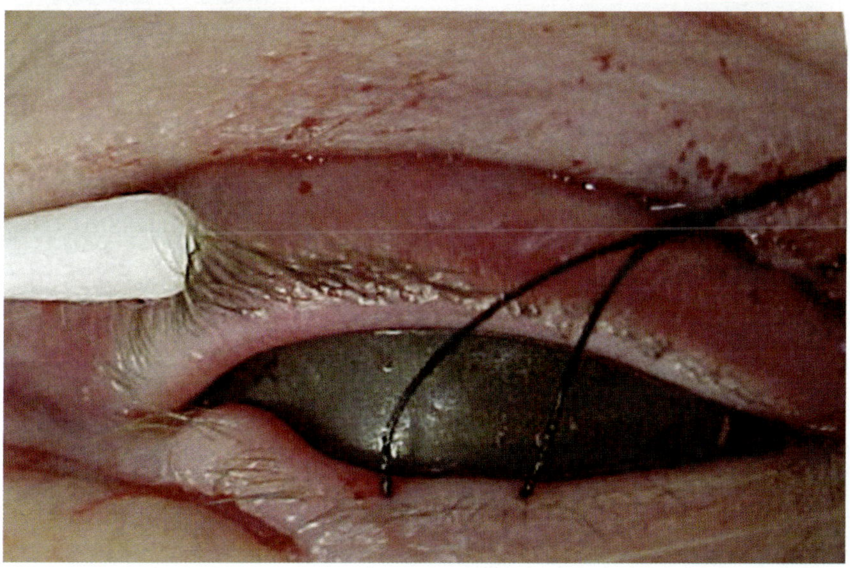

C

Figure 41.1. (*Continued*)

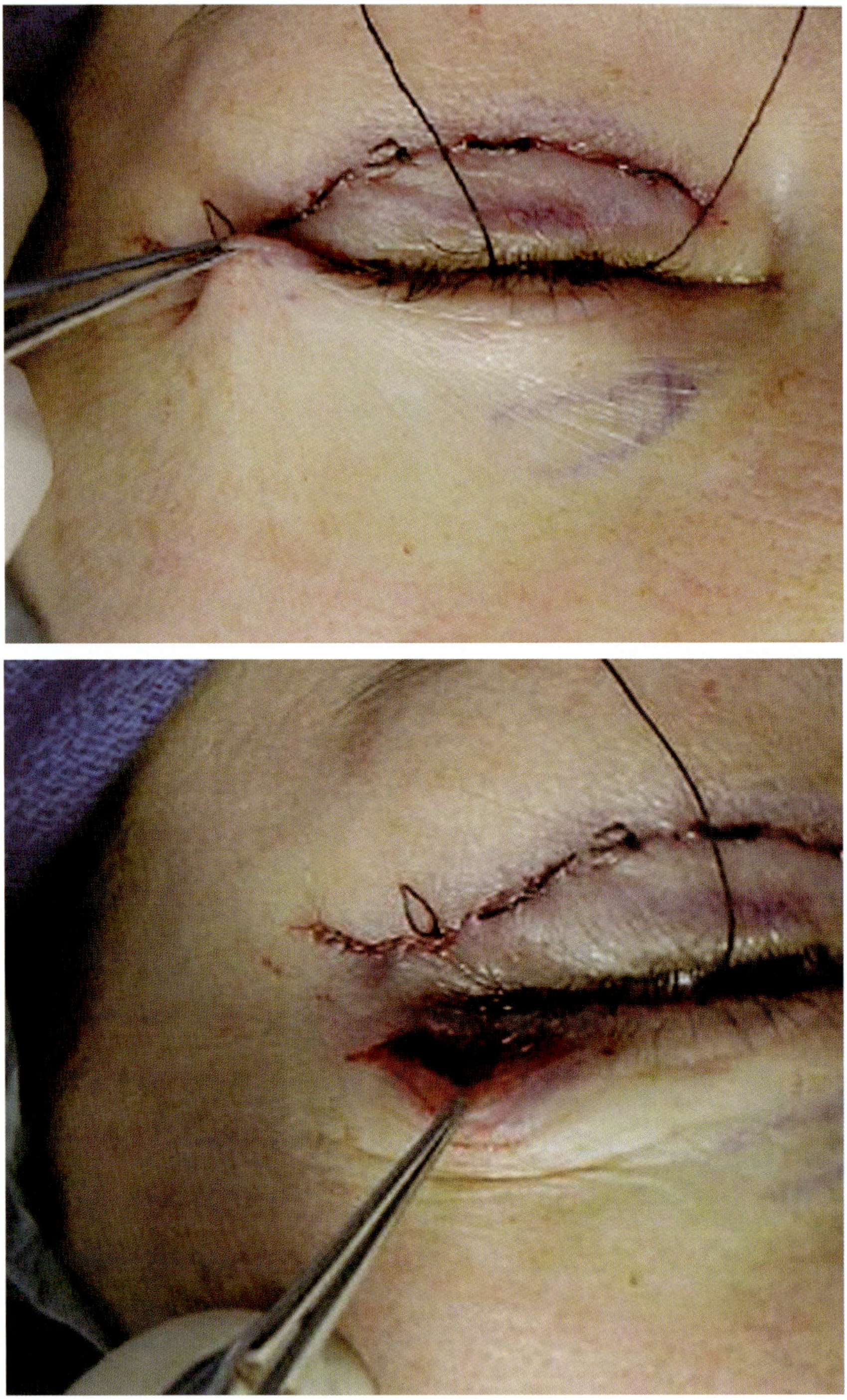

A

B

Figure 41.2. (A,B) The optimum point to fixate the skin–muscle flap is assessed. (C) Resuspension of skin–muscle layer to lateral orbital rim just beyond the lateral canthus is accomplished with a 5-0 Vicryl suture. Any residual redundant lower lid skin tightens over time due to thermal damage to the orbicularis muscle from the defocused CO_2 laser.

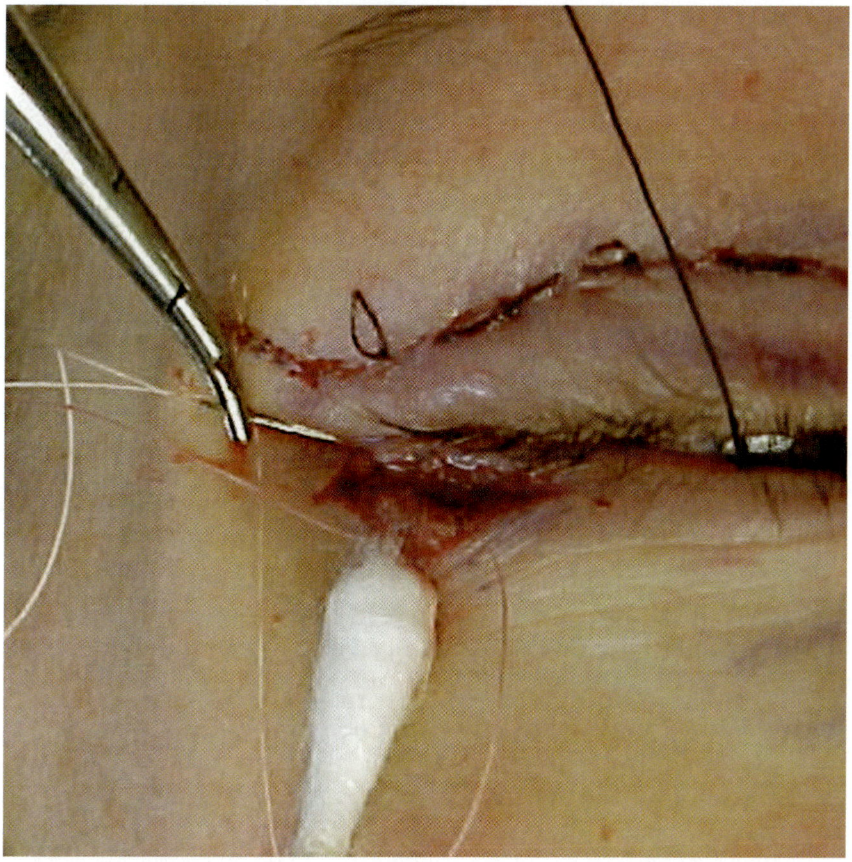

C

Figure 41.2. (*Continued*)

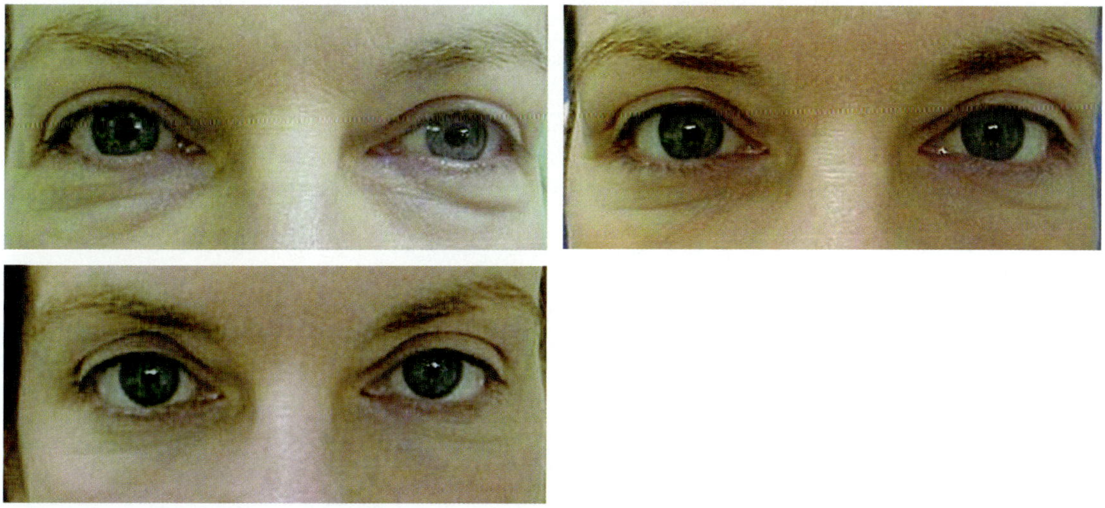

A B C

Figure 41.3. (A) Preoperative photograph of patient undergoing lower blepharoplasty using three-step technique as well as upper blepharoplasty. (B) Result 3 months after surgery. (C) Note increased elevation of the eyelid skin and cheek skin interface 6 months after surgery compared to result 3 months after surgery in (B).

References

1. Mauriello JA. Surgical technique: three-step technique for lower blepharoplasty. Ophthal Plast Reconstr Surg 2003;19:470–476.
2. Mauriello JA. Upper and lower blepharoplasty with combined blepharoptosis repair. In: Mauriello JA (ed.). Techniques of Cosmetic Eyelid Surgery. A Case Study Approach. Lippincott Philadelphia: Williams & Wilkins, 2004: 28–66.
3. Mauriello JA. Three-step technique for lower blepharoplasty. Annual Spring Meeting of the American Society of Ophthalmic Plastic and Reconstructive Surgery, Ponte Vedre, FL, June 17, 2004.
4. Mauriello JA. Check elevation and reduction of malar folds with minimal skin excision by treating the orbicularis oculi muscle with carbon dioxide laser during dosmetic lower blepharoplasty. Poster Presentation, American Society of Ophthalmic Plastic and Reconstructive Surgery, Chicago, IL, October 14–15, 2005.
5. Seckel BR, Kovanda CJ, Cetrulo CL, Passmore AK, Meneses PG, White T. Laser blepharoplasty with transconjunctival orbicularis muscle/septum tightening and periocular skin resurfacing: a safe and advantageous technique. Plast Reconstruc Surg 2000;106:1121–1141.

42

Lower Eyelid Blepharoplasty: Procedure Pearls and Pitfalls

John D. Siddens

1. If at all possible, a transconjunctival incision is preferable to a transcutaneous incision, especially if the mid-face is not being addressed.
2. A transconjunctival incision can be performed with a CO_2 laser, a radiofrequency unit, a monopolar tip, or even carefully with a high-temperature cautery.
3. Be conservative when removing herniated orbital fat. Draping or repositioning fat over the rim is often preferable to significant fat excision.
4. Meticulous hemostasis is critical in lower eyelid blepharoplasty. We recommend the clamp, cut, and cautery technique using a small hemostat, Westcott scissors, and the bipolar cautery, respectively.
5. If there is excessive skin laxity in an older patient, skin removal can be useful if done conservatively and in conjunction with a horizontal tightening of the lower eyelid. The fat should still be addressed through a transconjunctival incision. We never remove herniated fat through a transcutaneous incision.
6. Beware of creating a "lateral canthal syndrome" (Figure 42.1). This is caused by excessive skin removal and/or orienting the lateral skin too vertically.
7. If the patient is a CO_2 laser candidate, this is a preferred way to tighten the lower eyelid skin. Patient selection is critical as this should only be performed on the lighter skin types, and we need to warn the patients of possible persistant erythema or pigment changes.
8. Pretreat CO_2 laser patients with an anti-HSV medication, and avoid performing laser to tan patients.

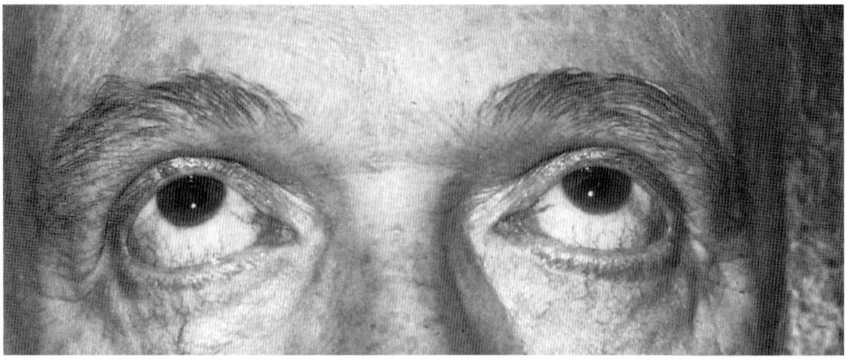

Figure 42.1. Lateral canthal syndrome.

43

Lower Blepharoplasty: The Bilamelar Approach

Guy G. Massry

In lower blepharoplasty surgery, the goal is to address skin, muscle, and fat. The order is important: fat-muscle-skin. I call my preferred method "bilamelar blepharoplasty."

The fat is addressed transconjunctivally through an incision 5 mm below the tarsus inferior to the point of fusion between the eyelid retractors and the orbital septum. The fat can be excised or repositioned or a combination of the two can be performed.

The orbicularis muscle can be tightened with an orbicularis strap technique. A subciliary incision is made across the lateral two-thirds of the lid. Laterally, a strap of orbicularis is created. It is then secured to the lateral orbital rim periosteum with 2–3 buried sutures. The skin, miscle, and septum are thus tightened. Skin excision and closure follows.

If a pinch skin excision is to be performed by itself, a transconjunctival retractor lysis allows the eyelid to elevate and counteracts any downward traction as the skin heals. A temporal intermarginal tarsorrhaphy of 5-0 chromic gut will further oppose downward traction in the first week.

44

The Skin in Lower Lid Blepharoplasty: General Principles

Guy Ben Simon and John D. McCann

In cases of fat removal or repositioning or pseudoherniation of orbital fat, enhancement of the deficient suborbital portion of the malar complex is the principal component of modern lower eyelid blepharoplasty. Skin removal is usually unnecessary since there is typically inelasticity rather than actual excess of skin. The widely preferred approach is transconjunctival incision, which results in less eyelid retraction, less scleral show, and less postoperative ectropion than other methods. Some surgeons prefer a transcutaneous approach in patients who have hypertrophy of the orbicularis oculi muscle and therefore require muscle excision.

Wrinkles and excess of vertical skin can be dealt with by skin-resurfacing techniques such as chemical peeling and CO_2 or erbium—YAG laser resurfacing. These techniques are applicable in patients with Fitzpatrick skin types I–III. Patients with darker skin are at risk of pigmentary changes; these can be managed by the pinch technique. Excess skin is crushed using a straight hemostat 1–2 mm subciliary and excised. Care must be taken to excise as little as possible of the orbicularis muscle. The skin is closed with a running suture. Regardless of the timing of laser treatment, transconjunctival blepharoplasty with adjunctive CO_2 laser resurfacing results in improvement of lower eyelid bulging and skin wrinkling.

45

Incising the Septum over the Nasal, Central, and Lateral Fat Pads in Lower Blepharoplasty

Jemshed A. Khan

The fat pads should be free from any encumbering structures. The overlying orbital septum specifically must be divided for each fat pad before the fat can freely prolapse. The lateral fat pad may be more difficult to mobilize because the overlying septum may be adherent to the inferior lateral orbital rim.

Nasal fat pad:

- Ballote the globe to bring the fat pad forward.
- Make an "X"-shaped incision over the nasal fat pad.
- Deepen the incision until fat prolapses.

Central fat pad:

- Ballotement of the globe to bring the fat pad forward.
- Make a horizontal 10- to 12-mm incision over the central fat pad.
- Place the incision 2–3 mm superior to the inferior orbital rim.
- Deepen the incision until fat prolapses.

Lateral fat pad:

- Expose the lateral fat pad.
- Divide the fat pad from the underlying lower eyelid retractors.
- Incise the overlying orbital septum.
- Divide the arcuate expansion if necessary (fibrous anterior band separating the central and lateral fat pads).

Reprinted with permission from: Chen WPD, Khan JA, McCord, Jr, CD. Color Atlas of Cosmetic Oculofacial Sugery. Philadelphia: Butterworth Heinemann/Elsevier, 2004.

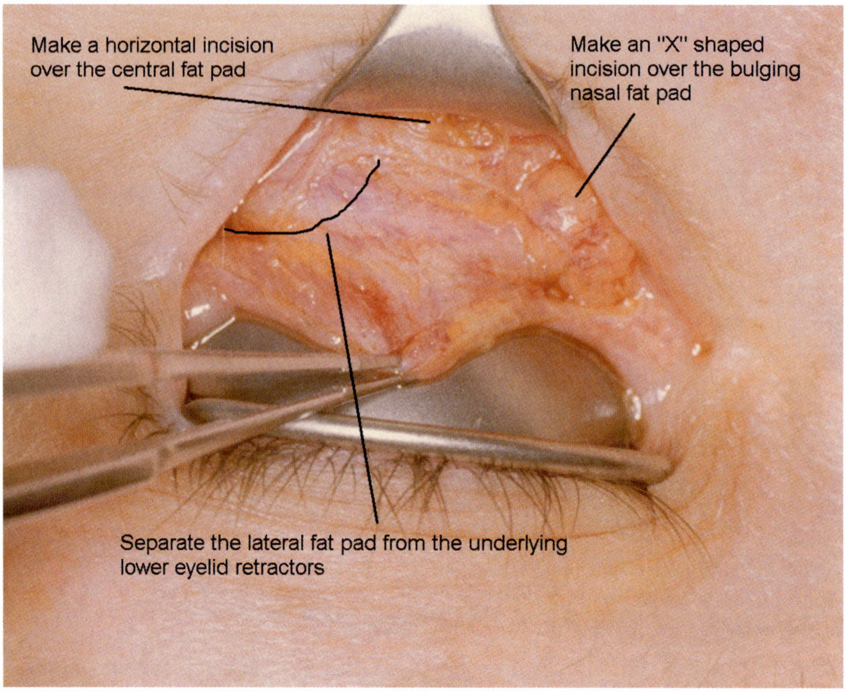

Figure 45.1. Separate incisions are placed over each fat pad.

46

Prolapsing the Inferior Fat Pads and Fornix in Lower Blepharoplasty

Jemshed A. Khan

The successful transconjunctival incision depends on adequate prolapse and exposure of the conjunctival fornix. The lower eyelid margin is retracted by the assistant with two fingers. Retraction of the lower eyelid margin requires that the pads of the assistant's fingers be placed directly upon the eyelid margin itself in order to exert sufficient inferior traction. At the same time, ballottement of the globe so as to prolapse the fat and conjunctiva anteriorly. When performed successfully, a liberal horizontal roll of prolapsing fat and overlying conjunctiva will present itself reliably and visibly. The use of the titanium Khan-Jaeger plate enables the surgeon to ballottement of the globe posteriorly in order to prolapse the fat anteriorly while also protecting the globe. Ballottement can also be achieved with a cotton-tipped applicator on the metal contact lens.

Key Points

- Begin at the inferior border of the lateral tip of the caruncle.
- Continue laterally.
- Stay 4 mm below the base of the tarsal plate.
- Continue to within 2 mm of the lateral canthal angle.
- Angle the beam towards the inferior the orbital rim.

Reprinted with permission from: Chen WPD, Khan JA, McCord, Jr, CD. Color Atlas of Cosmetic Oculofacial Sugery. Philadelphia: Butterworth Heinemann/ Elsevier, 2004.

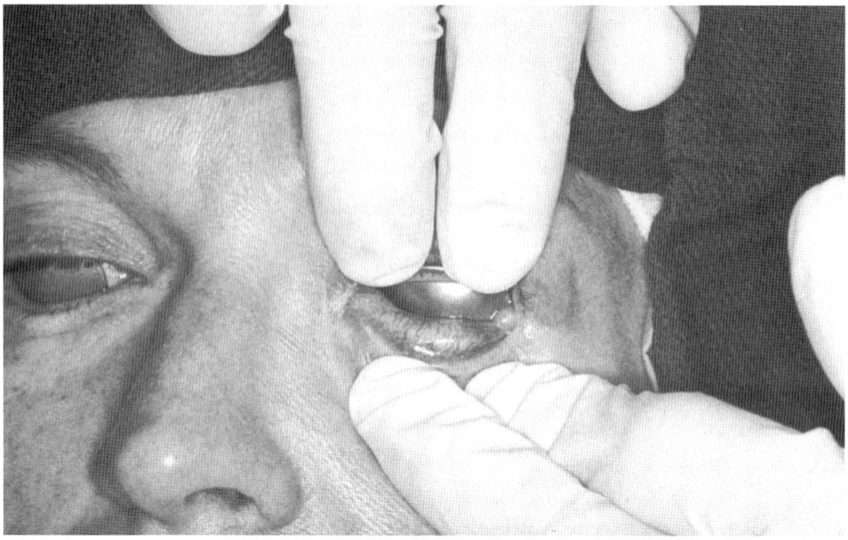

A

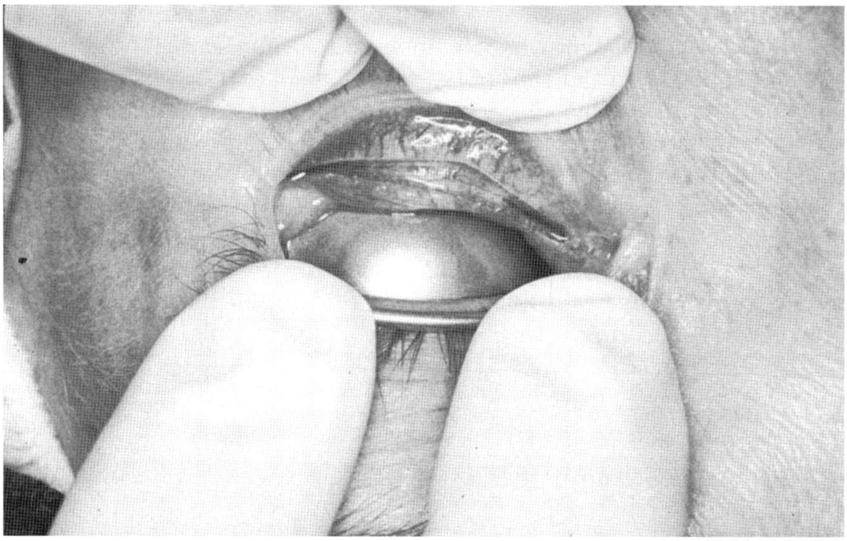

B

Figure 46.1. Demonstration of proper technique for fully prolapsing the inferior fornix. Note ballotte of globe and positioning of assistant's fingers on the eyelid margin. Globe may be balloted posteriorly with Jaeger plate or with cotton-tipped applicator on the metal scleral contact lens. Assistant retracts lower eyelid margin with two fingers.

47

Identifying the Inferior Oblique in Transconjunctival Blepharoplasty

Jemshed A. Khan

Prior to embarking upon transconjunctival blepharoplasty, the inferior oblique muscle should be clearly visualized. The inferior oblique is reliably located in the cleft between the nasal and central fat pads. Using cotton-tipped applicators, the nasal and central fat pads can be easily separated to allow the inferior oblique to come into view. Once identified, one can safely proceed with excision of the fat pads.

The inferior oblique muscle originates from the periosteum adjacent to the proximal bony nasolacrimal duct and passes inferior to the nasal fat pad and superior to the central fat pad. Arising from the inferior oblique is an expansion of connective tissue that sometimes restrains the contiguous fat of the central and lateral fat pads. This tissue, the arcuate expansion, may be divided if necessary.

Key Points

Recommended Instruments[1]:

- Khan-Jaeger Laser Eyelid Plate
- Castroviejo 0.5 mm toothed platform tying forceps
- Desmarres retractor (dull finish)
- Bipolar cautery, hemostat (fine curved)
- Protective metal scleral contact lens
- The inferior oblique can always be located between the nasal and central fat pads
- If the fat is restrained between the central and lateral fat pads, look for and divide the anteriorly located fibrous band of tissue (arcuate expansion)

The lateral fat pad is easier to remove once separated from the underlying lower eyelid retractor

Reprinted with permission from: Chen WPD, Khan JA, McCord, Jr, CD. Color Atlas of Cosmetic Oculofacial Sugery. Philadelphia; Butterworth Heinemann/ Elsevier, 2004.

[1] Storz Instrument Company, St Louis, MO

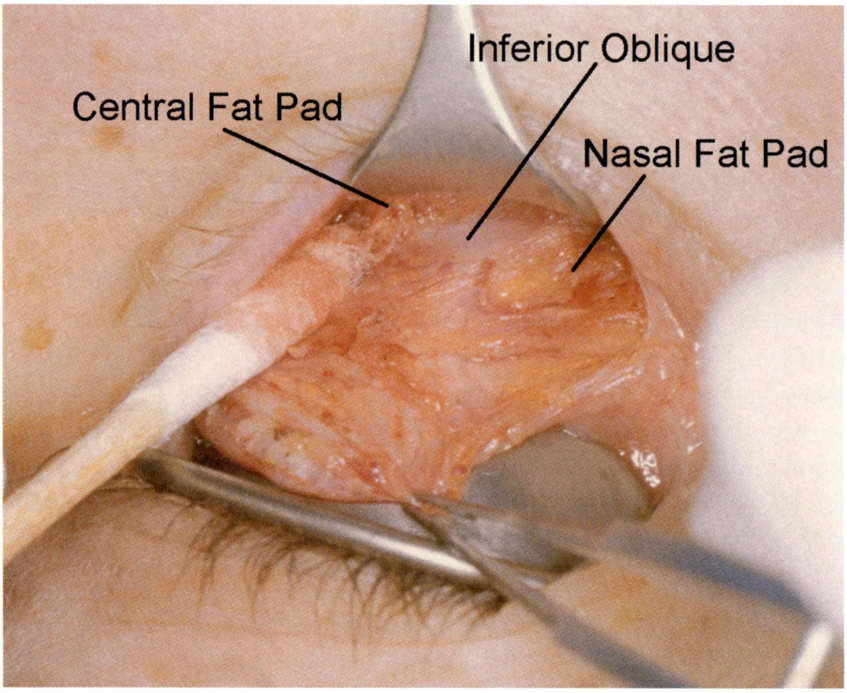

Figure 47.1. Inferior oblique muscle is reliably located in the cleft or separation between the nasal and central fat pads.

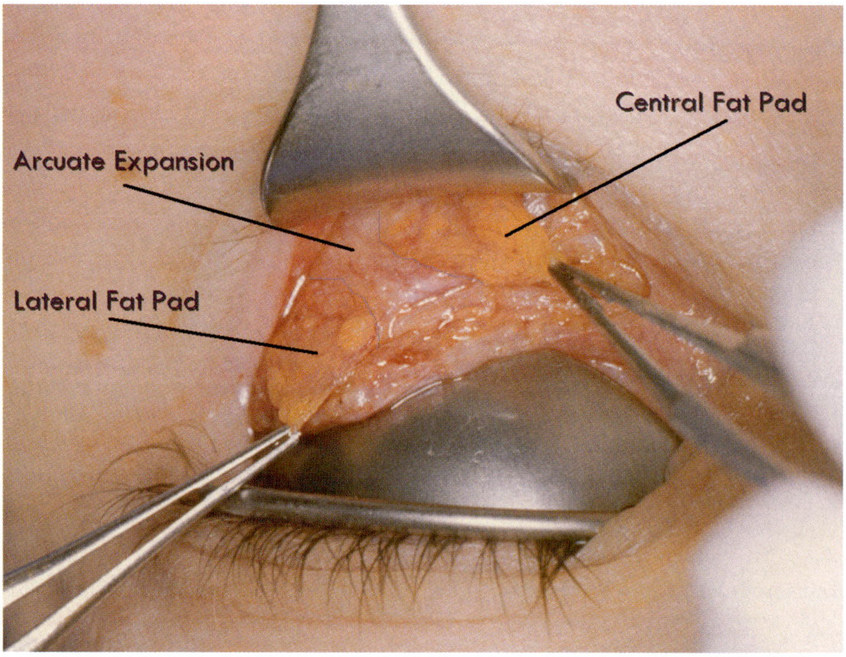

Figure 47.2. The arcuate expansion sometimes constrains the central and temporal fat pads.

48

Achieving Symmetry in Lower Blepharoplasty Fat Removal

Jemshed A. Khan

These tips will make fat removal in a purely subtractive transconjunctival lower blepharoplasty procedure more symmetric to avoid postoperative surprises.

Divide Each Fat Pad Flush with the Orbital Rim—Nasal and Central Fat Pads

Using the symmetric positions of the paired inferior orbital rims as a guide is a key to achieving postoperative symmetry in lower blepharoplasty. When deciding exactly where to transect the herniating lower eyelid fat, use the bony inferior orbital rim as the sole landmark. One can grasp the herniating fat with a hemostat which rests upon the orbital rim, and then one can comfortably proceed with excision of the fat. If piecemeal excision is used to remove the protruding fat, it is important to immediately perform ballottement and see if any more fat easily comes forward past the inferior orbital rim.

Divide Each Fat Pad Flush with the Orbital Rim—Lateral Fat Pad

Positioning a hemostat properly in addressing the fat pad in the tight lateral area requires diligence and experience, especially when it comes to positioning the hemostat. Not uncommonly, there is more fat prolapse immediately following the first excision. Also, there may still be a residual temporal bulge of fat that requires further division of the septum. Diligence and patience are necessary to achieve adequate temporal fat excision.

Reposition the Eyelid and Ballottement to Look for Any Residual Bulging Fat

The final and important step is balloting. Often one may find residual fat that was overlooked earlier in the procedure. Such fat may not come forward until later in the procedure because it had been constrained by cautery or clamping of the overlying fat.

- Ballottement by applying firm pressure against the globe.
- Examine the contours of both lower eyelids.
- Look for any bulging or asymmetry.
- Excise further fat as needed.
- Look for and cauterize any bleeding points.

Tug upward on the eyelid to prevent inversion or overriding of the wound.

No suture is used.

Remove eye shield.

Place ointment.

Reassure patient.

Reprinted with permission from: Chen WPD, Khan JA, McCord, Jr, CD. Color Atlas of Cosmetic Oculofacial Sugery. Philadelphia: Butterworth Heinemann/ Elsevier, 2004.

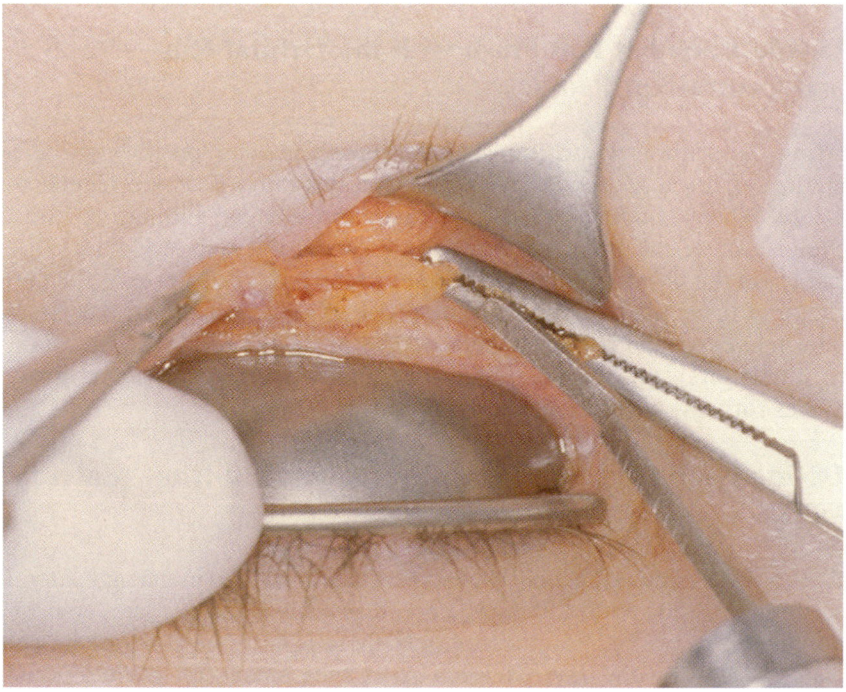

Figure 48.1. The lateral fat pad is transected flush with the inferior orbital rim and requires use of a metal desmarres, moist cotton tip, or hemostat as a backstop

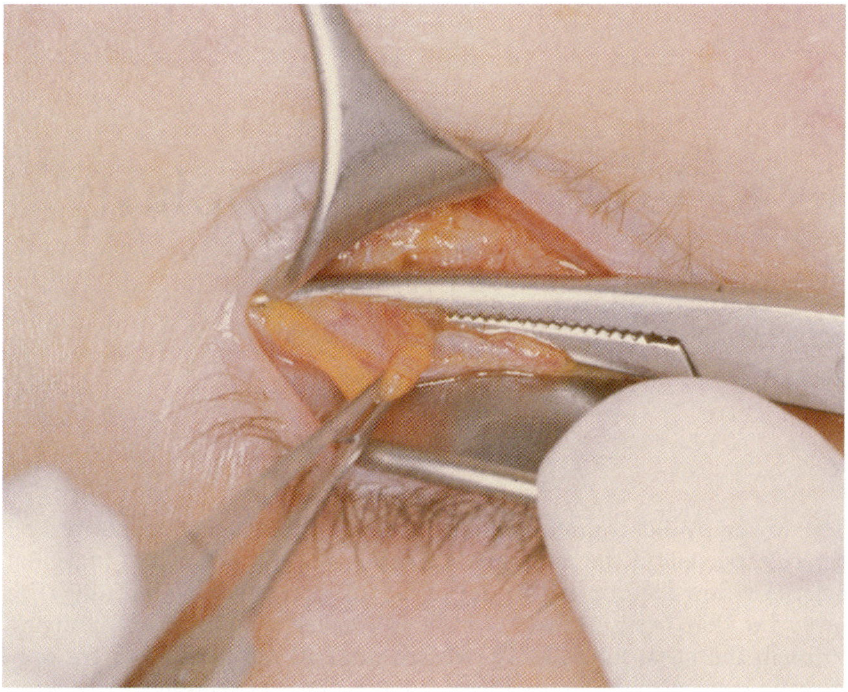

Figure 48.2. Finger pressure is applied to the protective shield in order to retropulse the globe and prolapse forward any residual excess fat.

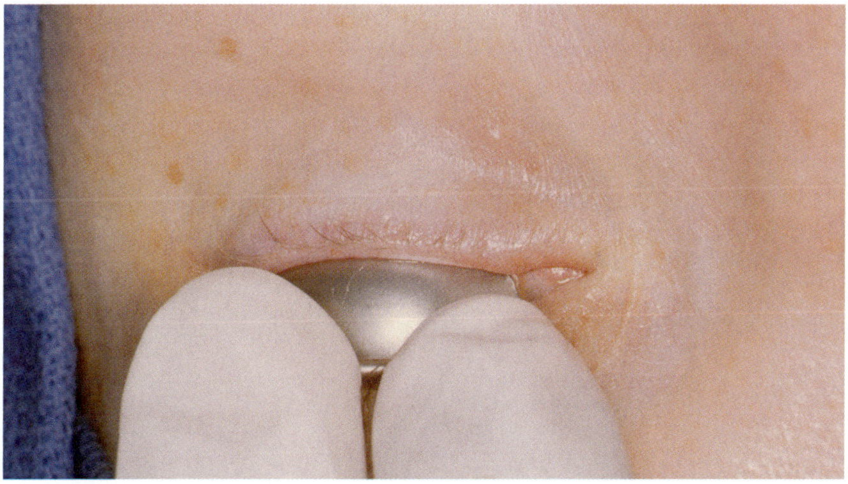

Figure 48.3. Appearance at end of procedure.

49

Hemostasis in Lower Blepharoplasty

Erin L. Holloman and Sterling S. Baker

The lower eyelid transconjunctival blepharoplasty can be performed safely, especially if the anatomy is clear. Avoid the prominent marginal arteries below the inferior border of the tarsus if possible. Carefully trim away fat that presents itself. There is usually a large vessel coursing through the nasal fat pads. The vessel, not cut, will not bleed. Try only sculpting away globules of lower lid fat, always avoiding the vessels, instead of clamping the fat paids and cauterizing excessively.

Absolute hemostasis in this area before closing is always in the surgeon's favor. The palpebral conjunctival incision does not have to be sutured closed as long as the eyelid is repositioned correctly.

50

The Treatment of Festoons in Lower Blepharoplasty

Sheri L. DeMartelaere, Todd R. Shepler, Sean M. Blaydon, Russell W. Neuhaus, and John W. Shore

Festoons or "malar bags" are thought to be involutional attenuation of the skin and underlying orbital orbicularis oculi muscle. Edema often accumulates in this area. Standard blepharoplasty techniques will not address festoons, if present, and may make them worse for a time due to persistent edema in this area.

In severe cases of festoons, one approach is direct excision (Figures 50.1 and 50.2). This approach needs to be entertained with caution as the result is a visible scar and frequently there is prolonged postoperative edema, often requiring 6 months or more to resolve. Any lower eyelid laxity, steatoblepharon, and dermatochalasis must be addressed first, otherwise one risks lower lid retraction and/or ectropion postoperatively. Thus, this is often a staged procedure, with the first step being lower eyelid blepharoplasty with correction of any lower eyelid laxity via standard horizontal lower lid tightening (HLLT) procedures. Lower eyelid retraction should also be addressed and may require a lower eyelid spacer graft, SOOF, or mid-face lifting. Three to 6 months later, the remaining festoons can be directly excised with local advancement flap repair. The incision is made at the crease at the inferior edge of the festoons (marked with patient upright). The skin is then undermined superiorly to the lash line of the lower eyelid, draped, and trimmed to fit the defect. Preoperative (Figure 50.3) and postoperative (Figure 50.4) results can be excellent.

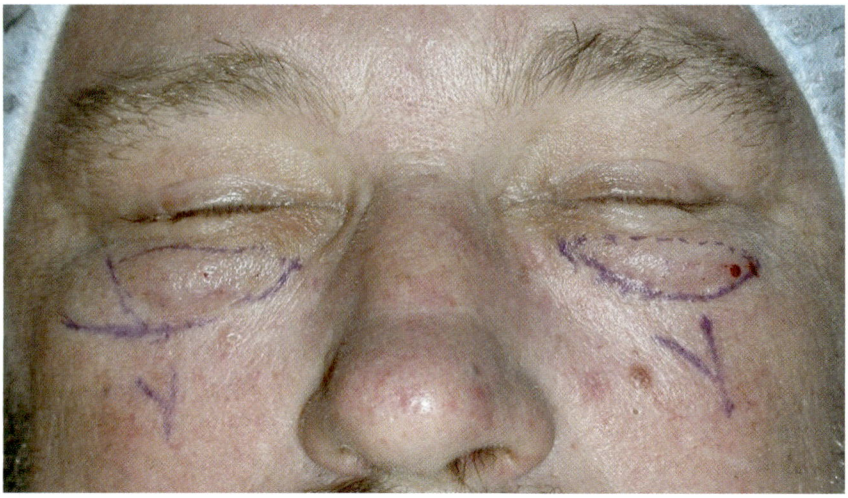

Figure 50.1. Planned incisions and undermining.

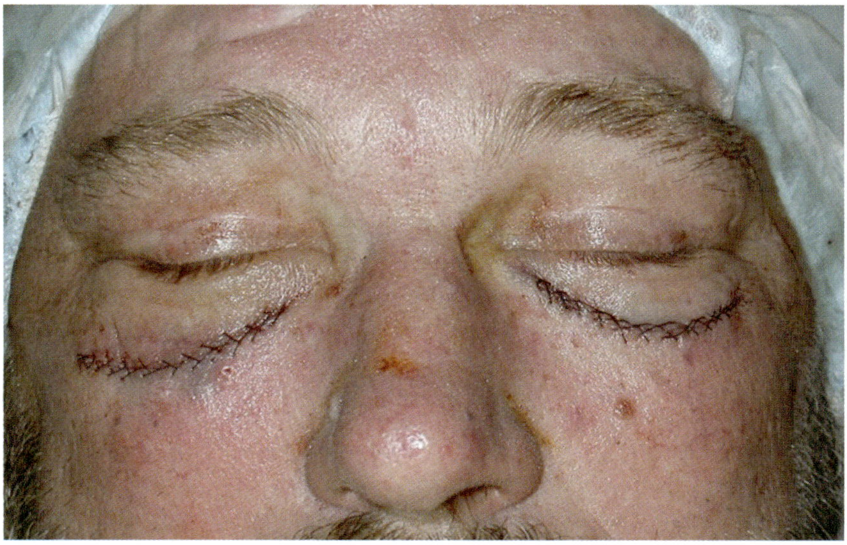

Figure 50.2. Closure.

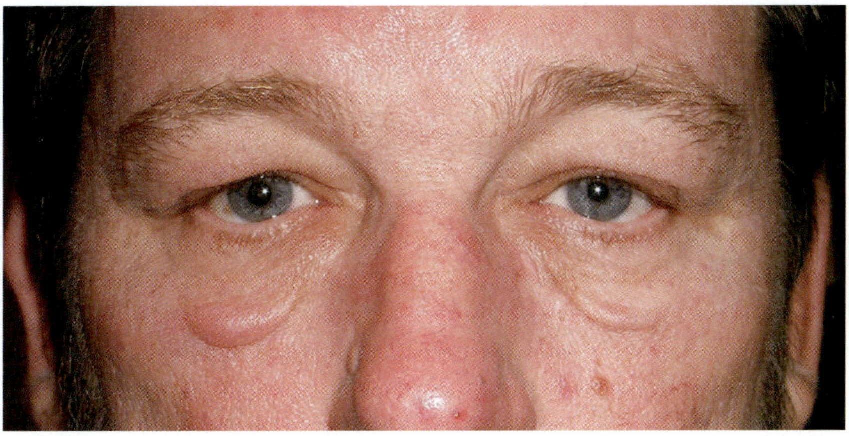

Figure 50.3. Preoperative appearance.

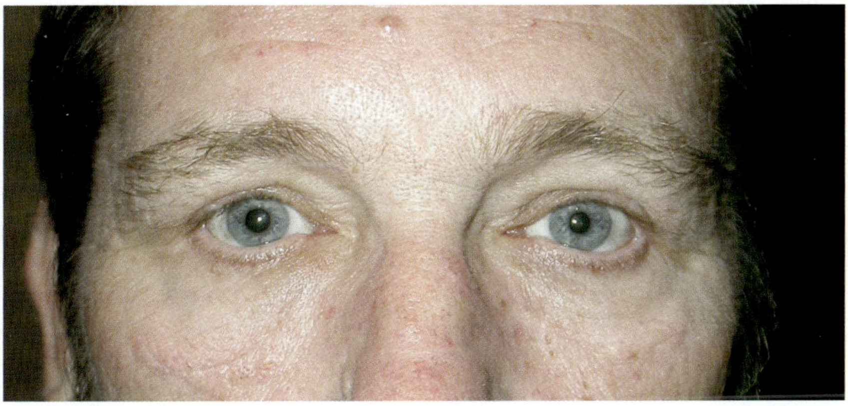

Figure 50.4. One-year postoperative appearance.

Section Three

Fat Repositioning in Lower Blepharoplasty

51

Fat Repositioning in Lower Blepharoplasty: Less Is More

Sheri L. DeMartelaere, Todd R. Shepler, Sean M. Blaydon, Russell W. Neuhaus, and John W. Shore

Techniques in lower eyelid blepharoplasty have moved to "less is more." We have moved away from fat excision and have a better appreciation for "fat enhancement" in our goal to soften any tear trough deformities and to minimize the hollow orbit appearance. More emphasis is now being placed on fat repositioning and elimination of the bony prominence of the inferior orbital rim. Fat repositioning is particularly useful in those patients with moderate medial and central fat prolapse, but with a hollow tear trough deformity. There has to be enough orbital fat in order to reposition it over the orbital rim. In patients where there is a prominent tear trough deformity but a paucity of anterior fat, a tear trough implant may be more appropriate to build up the bony support. Fat repositioning over the inferior orbital rim may be inadequate to fill in the hollowness if there is significant descent of the SOOF and/or malar fat pad. In these cases a lower eyelid blepharoplasty may need to be combined with a mid-face or SOOF lift to adequately deal with the contour defects.

52

Fat Repositioning in Lower Lid Blepharoplasty: General Principles

Guy Ben Simon and John D. McCann

In young people the eyelid–cheek complex is a single smooth convex profile. Aging causes descent of the globe and pseudoherniation of intraorbital fat, producing a double convex or tear trough deformity on the eyelid profile and a nasojugal groove at the medial aspect of the lower eyelid. With advancing age this depression appears more prominent because of attenuation and descent of the orbicularis oculi and cheek fat, resulting in skeletonization of the orbital area and revealing the topographical contour of the inferior orbital rim. Simple removal of orbital fat can result in a hollow appearance of the lower eyelid.

Preservation of the lower orbital fat is a new concept in facial rejuvenation, designed to prevent the hollow appearance that may follow the removal of excess fat in lower eyelid blepharoplasty. Such preservation creates a smooth transition to the malar eminence, blending nicely into the upper face. Aging causes progressive exposure of the underlying skeletal anatomy in the periorbital area, unlike in the lower facial area, where thicker soft tissue continues to cover bony landmarks.

The basic surgical technique includes release of the arcus marginalis and advancing of the subseptal fat beyond the infraorbital rim and underneath the orbicularis muscle. The fat pedicles are temporarily externalized to the midface by suturing. They can be placed in the sub- or supra-periosteal planes, with no apparent effect on aesthetic results. This technique camouflages the lower orbital rim anatomy and provides more youthful rejuvenation of the midface.

Other methods suggested to correct tear trough deformity include orbital fat removal, fat injections or grafts, and alloplastic cheek implants. In general, transconjunctival fat repositioning results in leveling of the tear trough deformity, a smooth contour of the lower eyelid, and high patient satisfaction.

53

Transconjunctival Lower Lid Blepharoplasty with and Without Fat Repositioning

Guy G. Massry and Paul S. Nassif

The title of this chapter is descriptive in that it reviews a posterior eyelid (conjunctival) approach to cosmetic rejuvenation of the lower eyelid. The designation of the procedure as transconjunctival is important in that it differentiates surgery from the more traditional transcutaneous (through the skin) approach. Transconjunctival blepharoplasty has become the most common approach to cosmetic lower lid surgery over the last decade.[1] Since I have been in practice, I have only rarely performed transcutaneous lower blepharoplasty, and not at all in the last 7 years. This is because, in my critical evaluation of this surgery and in my hands, the posterior eyelid approach yields excellent results, with high patient satisfaction and fewer complications.

It must be emphasized that the term transconjunctival refers to a surgical approach to handling lower eyelid fat. There are a variety of adjunctive techniques (canthoplasty, skin pinch, muscle strap) which I may include in surgery which warrant cutaneous incisions and muscle manipulation. In this chapter I will only describe fat excision and repositioning as these other techniques are described elsewhere.

My emphasis in the chapter will be on the specific technique of subperiosteal fat repositioning.[1–3] This is my preferred method of cosmetic lower lid rejuvenation as the incidence of lower lid hollowness (skeletonized look) is reduced.[1] With aging there is a change in the lower lid–cheek continuum. Lower lid fat becomes more prominent and the cheek descends.[4] This combination of changes leads to a groove overlying the inferior orbital rim, which we refer to as the tear trough. Often times, I add fat grafting to the lower lid hollows (to areas where I could not reposition fat) to augment the fat repositioning result.

Surgical Technique

In cases of fat repositioning, the tear trough is demarcated preoperatively. In addition, the amount of nasal and central fat to reposition is assessed. I rarely reposition lateral fat, as the amount of fat present is generally not adequate to fill the lateral orbital rim depression.

I have found that, as opposed to upper lid blepharoplasty, potential patient discomfort is much more prevalent with lower lid surgery. This is especially true if fat is repositioned during surgery. Consequently, I perform lower lid blepharoplasty, without intravenous (IV) sedation, when fat is cauterized or excised only, in patients who I feel have the disposition to tolerate the procedure.

For cases performed under injections of local anesthesia only, I pretreat patients with 5–10 mg of oral Valium depending on the patient's history of sedative use, patient weight, and patient anxiety. I then instill a drop of topical Tetracaine into the lower cul-de-sacs of each eye. I place a small cotton pledget soaked in the same Tetracaine drops into the lower cul-de-sacs and ask the patient to close his/her eyes. I call this step the "Tetracaine bath." After waiting 5 minutes, I remove the Tetracaine pledgets. This technique has allowed injection of local anesthetic in the majority of patients without discomfort. In patients receiving IV sedation, I skip this step as IV analgesia, sedation, and anxiolytics negate the need for significant preinjection conjunctival anesthesia.

I inject 2–3 cc of xylocaine 1% with 1:100,000 epinephrine transconjunctivally. I pull the lower lid inferiorly with my index finger while simultaneously compressing (balloting) the globe through the upper eyelid. This maneuver pushes the inferior cul-de-sac forward while increasing the surface area of injectable conjuntiva. I incise the conjunctiva and lower lid retractors 5 mm below the tarsus from the punctum nasally to the most temporal portion of the lower lid (Figure 53.1). It is important to incise tissue 5 mm below tarsus, as this level is inferior to tarsus enough to access the fat pads without violating the septum. Avoid incisions too low, as this may lead to persistent chemosis postoperatively. I continue incising tissue until fat is exposed (Figure 53.2). I engage the conjunctiva and retractors with a 4–0 silk suture and secure the suture under tension to the head drape with a hemostat. The traction suture is critical. It provides protection to the cornea by covering it with the conjunctiva and retractors. In addition, it allows greater surgical space exposure by putting tissues on stretch. I use a cotton-tipped applicator to bluntly dissect inferiorly to the orbital rim. This allows the fat pads and inferior oblique muscle to delineate themselves well. I incise the tip of the nasal and central fat and dissect them free of the inferior oblique muscle to assure that it will be undisturbed when manipulating the fat pads. I preserve this ligament (typically dense in persons under 50, and more attenuated thereafter) as it is a support for the globe. If I am excising fat, all three pads are reduced at this point. I cut the fat flush with the orbital rim with minimal pushing on the eye. If more fat is excised there is a strong tendency toward postoperative hollowness.

In cases of repositioning fat, I bluntly dissect the nasal and central fat pad from the inferior oblique muscle. All connective tissue attachments are severed. I hold the fat pads with toothed forceps at their tips. I pull on one fat pad while allowing the other to recess, and then reverse this process (Figure 53.3). This demonstrates that the fat pads can move freely beneath and around the inferior oblique muscle. I call this technique the "inverse shoeshine sign," because it mimics the inverse of shining a shoe. I also grasp the ends of each fat pedicle and splay the pedicle open to identify the width of area I can fill in with fat. I now retract the transconjunctival surface of the lower lid and all tissue over the orbital rim inferiorly, exposing the periosteum at the arcus marginalis (Figure 53.4). I cut the periosteum with the cutting mode of an electrocautery unit from just temporal to where the tear trough begins to the most nasal aspect of the orbital rim. I use a freer elevator to elevate the periosteum from the face of the maxilla for approximately 15 mm. Dissection is carried around the infraorbital neurovascular bundle. This dissection can lead to significant bleeding. In this instance, I pack the subperiosteal pockets with cotton pledgets soaked in 1:10,000 epinephrine. I now begin surgery on the other eye and allow the pledgets to take effect. After completing pledgeting on the second eye, I remove the pledgets from the first eye. I have found this pledgeting maneuver controls bleeding well. I bring a 4–0 Prolene suture on a FS-2 needle through the skin into the nasal pocket, feed it through the fat pedicle, and then bring the suture through the pocket and out the skin. I tie the suture over a cotton bolster (Figure 53.5), thus repositioning and fixating the fat pedicle over the tear trough. I repeat this step for the central fat pedicle. I then assure that forced ductions are free and allow the wound to heal by secondary intent.

Postoperative Care

Patients are instructed to apply ice compresses every hour (for 10 minutes) while awake for the first 48 hours after surgery. It is suggested to sleep as upright as possible for the first week after surgery. I typically recommend two to three pillows. A topical antibiotic steroid drop is applied three times a day for 1 week. In fat repositioning cases, an oral steroid preparation (Medrol dose pack) is prescribed and the Prolene sutures and cotton bolsters are removed 4–5 days after surgery

Complications

The most common complications of surgery are excessive bruising, swelling, chemosis, and subconjunctival hemorrhage. An over- or undercorrection of fat reduction can occur. This can lead to persistent fat prominence or hollowness. I have found this to be less common with fat-repositioning cases. When fat is repositioned, complications unique to this procedure can occur. These include diplopia (beyond the immediate postoperative period), fat granulomas, prolonged edema and chemosis, and tear trough irregularities. Diplopia is typically transient and related to edema or inferior oblique trauma. I usually treat this with higher dose oral steroids, which I taper over a 10-day period. This generally allows all cases to resolve over this time period. Fat granulomas are rare—less than 5% my of cases—and are treated with intralesional injections of low-dose and concentration steroids (Kenalogue 5 mg/ml, 0.1 cc). The granulomas usually resolve with one or two injections given 2–3 weeks apart. I have yet to have to excise a granuloma surgically. I treat prolonged edema and chemosis, as I do diplopia, with higher dose steroids.

Comments

My partner and I perform a significant volume of fat repositioning surgery in our practices. Our experience with the technique has been very rewarding (Figures 53.6 and 53.7). We have found this to be a highly reproducible and reliable surgery with high patient satisfaction. The following are the essential points to keep in mind when considering this surgery:

1. This is a fat preserving technique that reduces the incidence of post-operative lower lid hollowness.
2. This technique can be challenging and has a high learning curve.
3. The surgical space is small and tight, which may lead to difficulty in maneuvering instruments.
4. Experience with standard transconjunctival surgery is helpful.
5. Watching a number of procedures before attempting the technique is important.
6. There is a risk of diplopia, so be careful dissecting around the inferior oblique muscle and assure forced ductions are free.

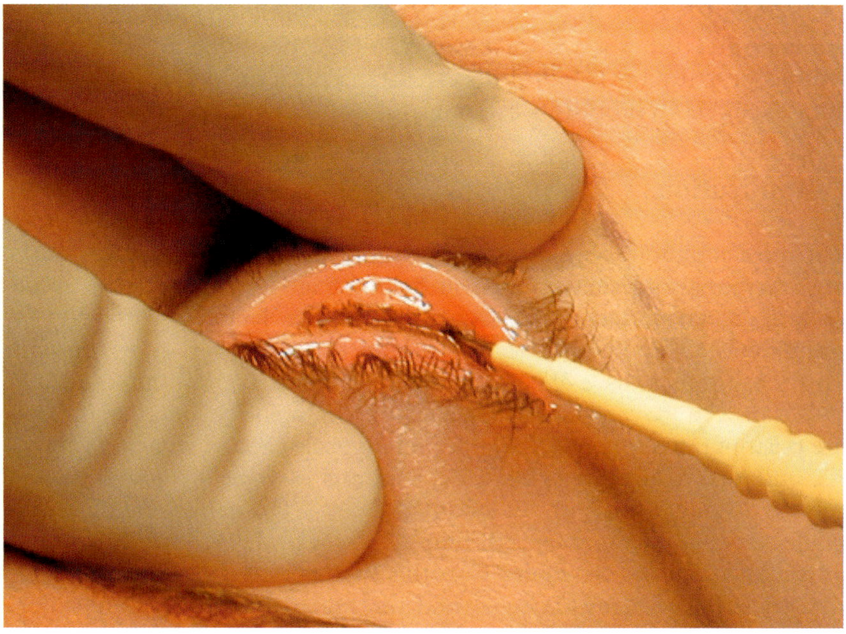

Figure 53.1. Transconjunctival incision.

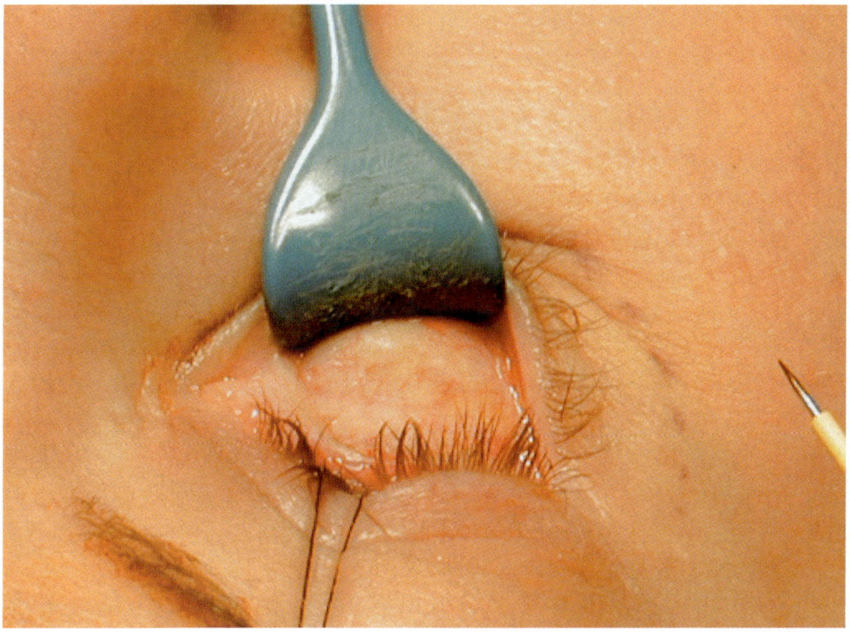

Figure 53.2. Fat exposed following completion of transconjunctival incision.

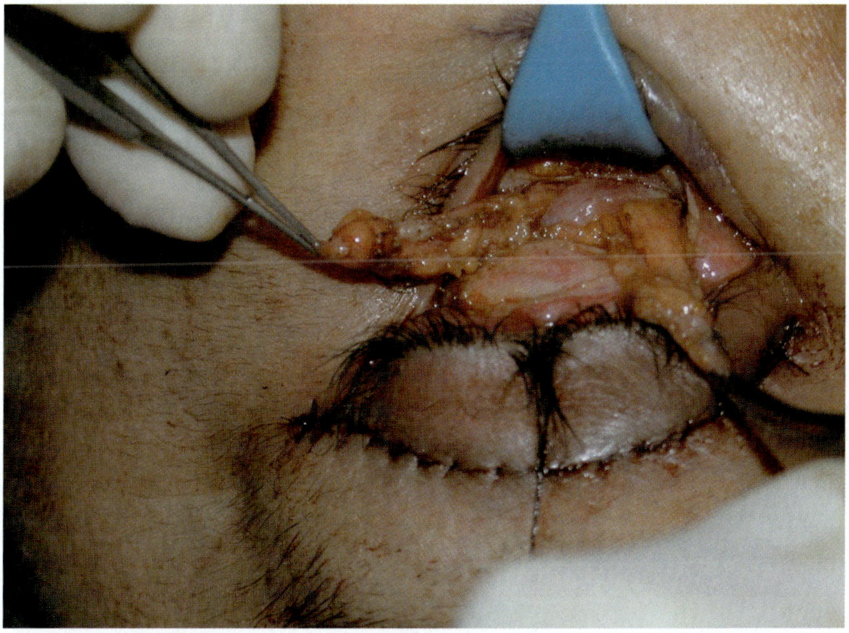

Figure 53.3. Fat pedicles freed of inferior oblique muscle.

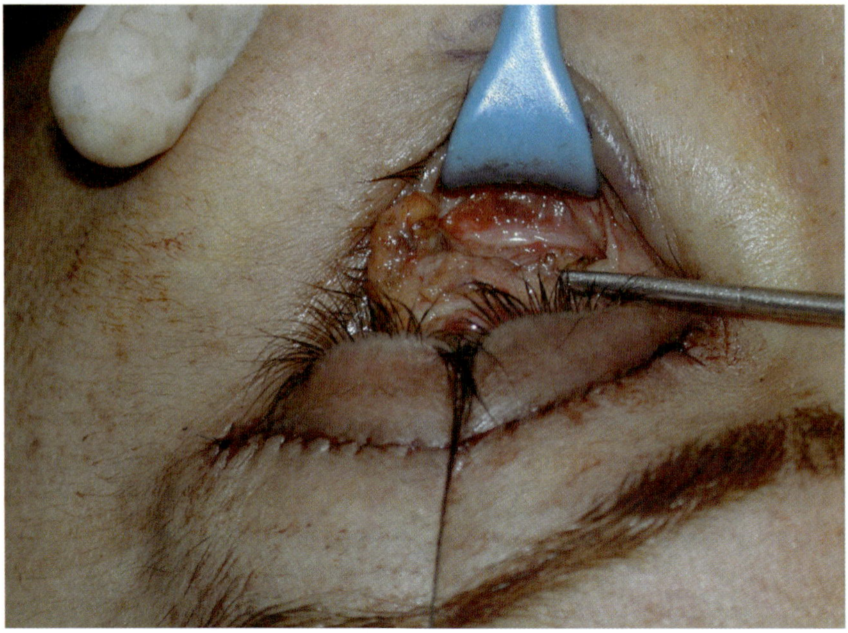

Figure 53.4. Orbital rim exposure.

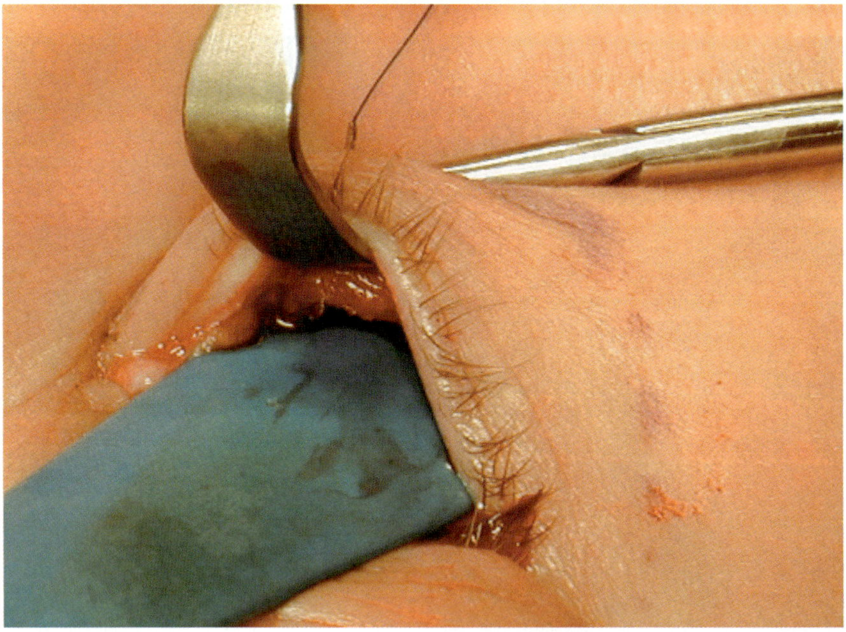

Figure 53.5. Passing suture from externally to secure fat with a bolster over the skin.

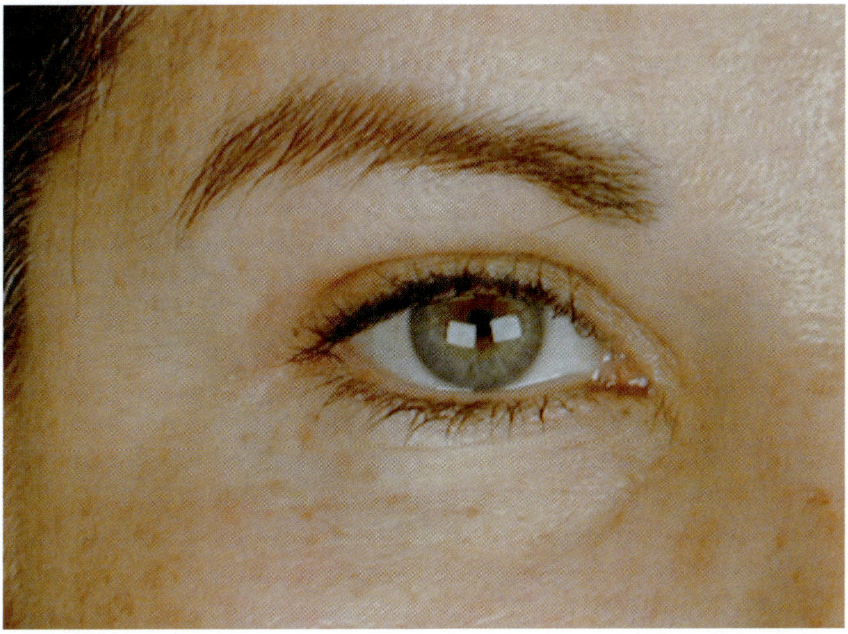

Figure 53.6. Lower lid blepharoplasty with fat repositioning. Note improved lower lid cheek contour and reduced tear trough.

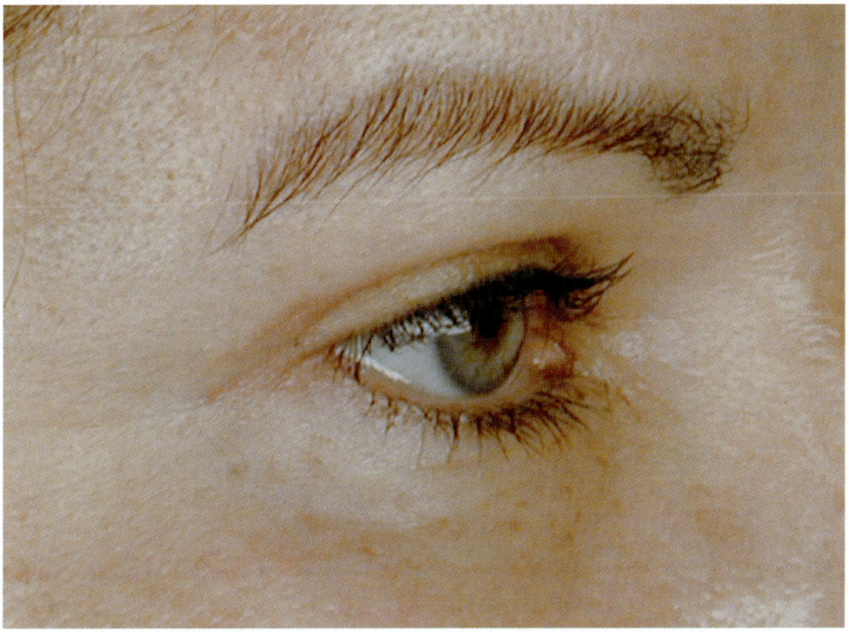

Figure 53.7. Oblique view of same patient in 53.6.

References

1. Nassif PSN. Lower blepharoplasty: transconjunctival blepharoplasty. Facial Plast Clin North Am 2005;13(4):553–559.
2. Hamra ST. Arcus marginalis release and orbital fat repositioning in midface rejuvination. Plastic Reconstr Surg 1995;92:354–362.
3. Hamra ST. The role of orbital fat preservation in facial aesthetic surgery. A new concept. Clin Plast Surg 1996;23:17–28.
4. Edelstein C, Goldberg RA, Shorr N, Balch KC. Transconjunctival approach to the arcus marginalis release. In: Mauriello JA (ed.). Unfavorable Results of Eyelid and Lacrimal Surgery. Boston: Butterworth Heinemann, 2000: 20–25.

54

Transconjunctival Lower Blepharoplasty with Intra-SOOF Fat Repositioning

Yasaman Mohadjer and John B. Holds

The increased recognition of anatomic factors associated with the tear trough deformity in the lower eyelids as well as an increased sensitivity of patients and surgeons to the secondary deformities associated with purely subtractive blepharoplasty surgery have led to a variety of conservative lower blepharoplasty techniques focused on the translocation or repositioning of fat to camouflage the anatomic tear trough.[1–3]

The authors have used two variations on an intra-SOOF fat repositioning over the past 6 years.[4] Generally excellent results have been obtained with correction of the tear trough deformity.

Patient Selection

The authors have found these fat-repositioning techniques to be applicable to the vast majority of their lower blepharoplasty patients. Preoperative examination should focus on the relevant anatomy, including the configuration of the tear trough as well as lid tone and laxity, midface configuration including globe prominence, and condition of the skin. Preoperative counseling should include discussion of surgical expectations. If laser skin resurfacing is to be performed as an adjunct procedure, a full discussion of the expectations and pre- and postoperative care must be undertaken.

Procedure

Except for special patient needs or requests, this technique of lower lid blepharoplasty may be carried out in the office-based procedure room with light oral sedation. The prominence of the fat pads and the edge of the tear trough, as well as the exit site of repositioning sutures and skin resurfacing zones, if indicated, are marked. Pledgets of topical tetracaine are placed in the inferior fornix. Local anesthetic consisting initially of 0.25% lidocaine with epinephrine buffered with sodium bicarbonate is injected through the inferior fornix. An infraorbital nerve block is important to achieve adequate anesthesia.

Metallic eye shields are placed. Lidocaine 2% with epinephrine is infiltrated to reinforce the anesthesia. A standard transconjunctival incision is made with a Luxar LX-20 CO_2 laser using a 0.4-mm tip. Dissection is carried anterior to the orbital septum down to the orbital rim exposing the periosteum at the arcus marginalis (Figure 54.1). Careful blunt dissection is completed in the plane of the SOOF from the orbital rim just anterior to the arcus marginalis to a level 8–12 mm below the orbital rim. Medially the SOOF thins with the muscle lying directly on the periosteum.

Each orbital fat pad is opened, and the fat is allowed to prolapse across the lid. A pedicle is developed in any pad to be repositioned, circumferentially releasing the fat to allow advancement. Gentle sculpting is done as necessary, most commonly only in the temporal fat pad (Figure 54.2). One to three mattress sutures (one for each fat pad) of 5–0 nylon are passed from the cheek into the dissected intra-SOOF pocket. A robust bite is taken weaving through the fat pedicle, and each fat pad is each repositioned into the intra-SOOF plane (Figure 54.3). In many patients it is possible to undermine a broad intra-SOOF pocket along the central inferior orbital rim and reposition the central and medial fat pads with a single mattress suture. The polyproplyene sutures are passed through a foam bolster and tied on the skin.

Appropriate patients undergo light- or medium-depth erbium-YAG laser skin resurfacing with a dual-mode erbium-YAG laser (Sciton®) at the end of the procedure. Lateral canthopexy and direct excision of excess skin via a subciliary incision are performed as indicated.

Patients are treated with antibiotic ointment and a skin dressing postoperatively. Mild analgesics are prescribed. We normally do not prescribe oral antibiotics or antivirals unless there is a specific indication. Sutures and bolsters are removed in 7 days.

A more recent variation of the procedure has focused on releasing the orbital septum at the arcus marginalis and advancing the septum and fat en bloc into the intra-SOOF dissection described above. It is generally possible with this technique to suture the orbital fat and septum with multiple 5–0 polyglactin 910 (Vicryl-Ethicon) sutures using a P-2 needle. This variation allows a more comprehensive treatment of the tear trough in most patients and avoids the externalized bolsters and sutures.

Postoperative

Ophthalmic ointment is instilled and cold compresses placed. Skin resurfacing may indicate follow-up sooner; otherwise any external sutures are removed at 6 days. The repositioned fat often hardens and is palpable 10–20 days postoperatively, later softening with a natural correction of the tear trough.

Conclusion

This technique of fat repositioning blepharoplasty has yielded a pleasing improvement in the tear trough deformity with a revision rate comparable to other blepharoplasty techniques. Short- and long-term results are generally excellent. We recommend this approach for the surgical treatment of the tear trough deformity.

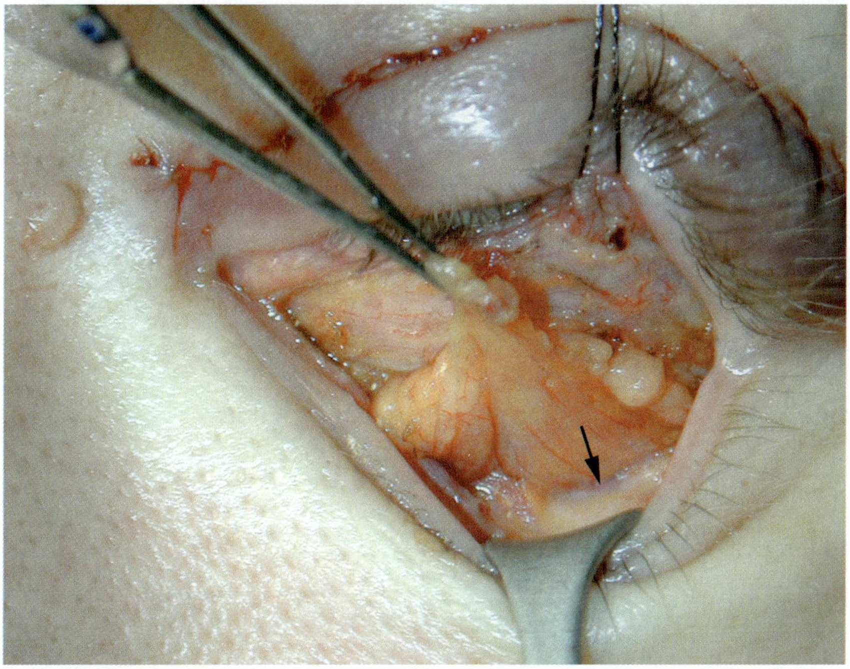

Figure 54.1. Transconjunctival exposure of orbital rim with central fat pad in forceps. Arcus maginalis shown with arrow.

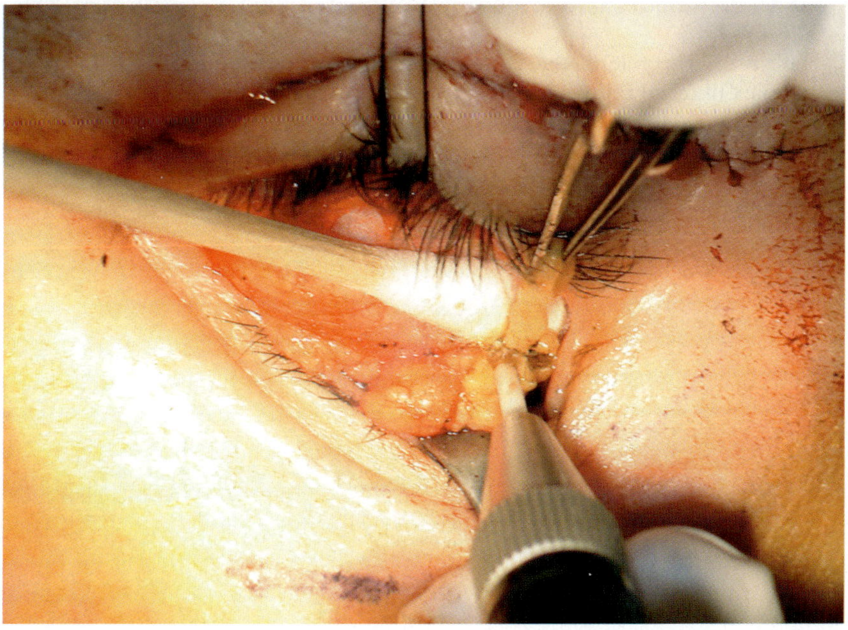

Figure 54.2. Some excision of temporal fat is generally needed.

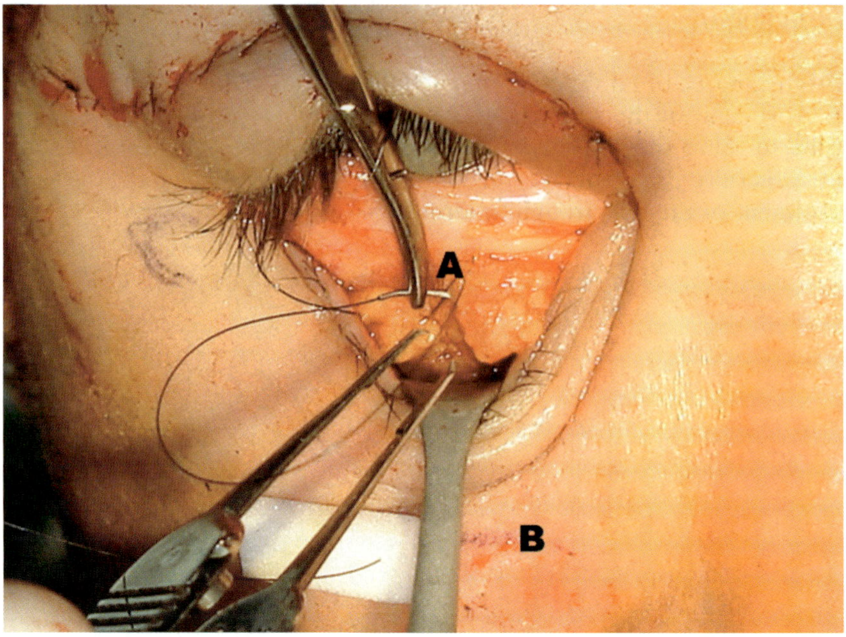

Figure 54.3. The polypropylene suture passes through the cheek into the intra-SOOF plane, across the fat pedicles (A), and exists the cheek (B).

References

1. Muzaffar AR, Mendelson BC, Adams WP. Surgical anatomy of the ligamentous attachments of the lower lid and lateral canthus. Plast Reconstr Surg 2002;110:873–884.
2. Goldberg RA. Transconjunctival orbital fat repositioning: transposition of orbital fat pedicles into a subperiosteal pocket. Plast Reconstr Surg 2000; 105:743–751.
3. Hamra ST. The role of the septal resent in creating a youthful eyelid-cheek complex in facial rejuvenation. Plast Reconstr Surg 2004;113:2124–2144.
4. Mohadjer Y, Holds JB. Cosmetic lower eyelid blepharoplasty with fat repositioning via intra-SOOF dissection: surgical technique and initial outcomes. Ophthal Plast Reconstr Surg 2006;22:409–413.

55

Lower Lid Blepharoplasty with Fat Repositioning Using a Foam Bolster

Eric A. Steele and Roger A. Dailey

The following is a modified transconjunctival blepharoplasty technique that has proved very effective in patients desiring rejuvenation of the lower eyelids that do not need skin or orbicularis resection.

A transconjunctival incision is made approximately 4 mm below the tarsus with a monopolar cutting cautery. This plane avoids the orbital septum, is inferior to the canaliculus medially, and allows a safe entry into the deeply situated fat compartments. The incision is made from the edge of the caruncle to the lateral canthus with the tip directed 1–2 mm posterior to the inferior orbital rim. A 4–0 silk suture (Alcon Surgical, Fort Worth, TX) is then placed through the edge of the lid retractors, and the tissue is retracted up over the globe and secured to the drape for the remainder of the procedure. The plane of dissection is toward the inferior orbital rim, with a desmarres retractor used to expose the fat pads and keep the septum away from the dissection. Care is used to avoid damaging the inferior oblique muscle. Cutting cautery is used create an intra-SOOF (Suborbicularis Oculi Fat) pocket, extending 10–15 mm below the orbital rim.

Attention is then directed to the fat pads, where the connective tissue septa are dissected with the cutting cautery to open the fat compartments and tease the fat forward as medial, central, and lateral pedicles. Rarely, a small amount of redundant fat is excised, but the goal of this procedure is to redrape the fat to create a pleasing contour. To this end, double-armed 4–0 PDS sutures (Ethicon, Somerville, NJ) are placed through the tip of each pedicle, and the needles are passed through the intra-SOOF pocket out through the skin below the tear trough and tied over a foam bolster. The straight PDS needles are bent to a 45° angle at the junction of their proximal and middle thirds to ease passage through the intra-SOOF pocket and skin. The foam bolster is created from the packaging of the 4–0 silk traction suture used during the procedure. These sutures are removed approximately 1 week postoperatively.

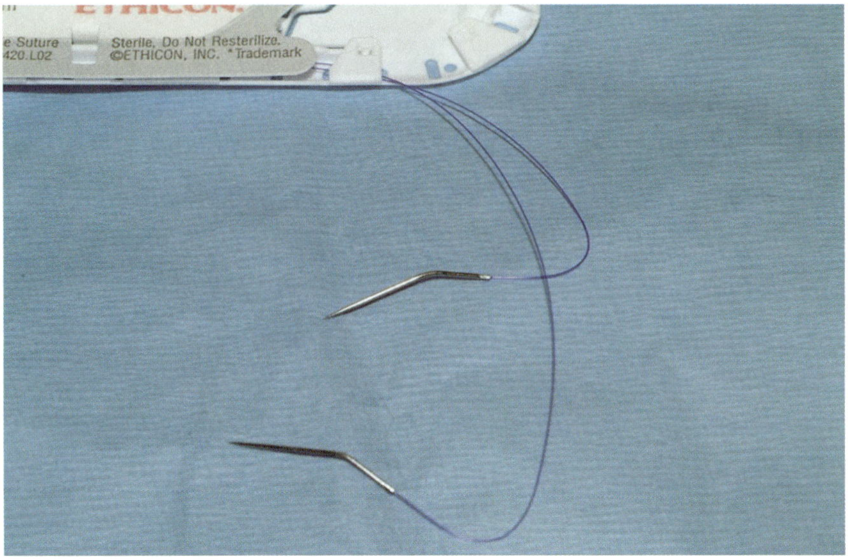

Figure 55.1. Straight PDS needles are bent to an advantageous angle using two needle drivers.

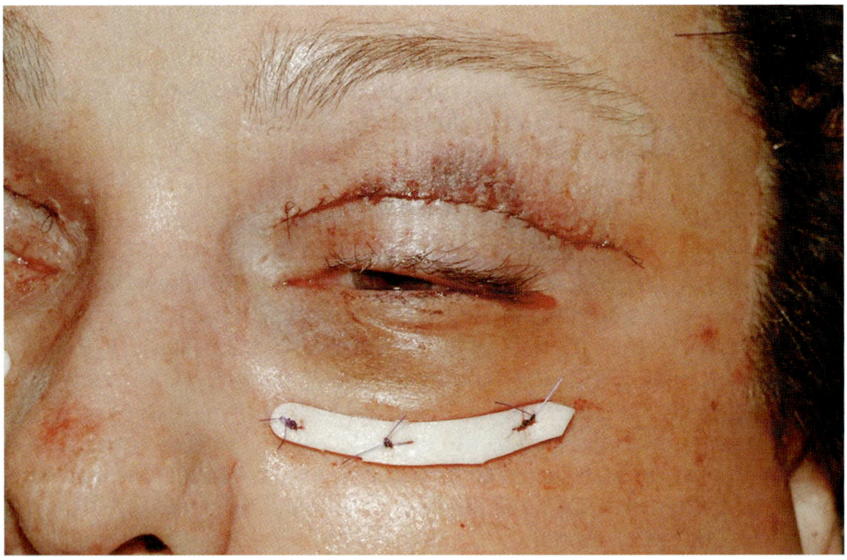

Figure 55.2. Foam bolster in place. The exposed sutures are connected to the orbital fat pedicles and are used to drape the orbital fat into the intra-SOOF pocket to create a pleasing contour.

Suggested Reading

Wobig JL, Dailey RA. Oculofacial Plastic Surgery. New York: Thieme, 2004.

56

Use of Tisseel in Lower Eyelid Blepharoplasty with Fat Repositioning

Asa D. Morton

Many techniques are employed in lower eyelid blepharoplasty. Eyelid surgeons are becoming more aware of the importance of blending the lid–cheek junction into a more uniform contour. Several options exsist for filling the tear trough and lid–cheek junction. Numerous hard and soft implants are commercially available, and these modalities are best suited to patients having poor projection of the inferior orbital rim and mid-face.

The use of orbital fat pedicles as a filler is gaining in popularity. The use of fat transposition can be incorporated with both transcutaneous and transconjunctival approaches to the lower eyelid. In either case a preseptal approach is utilized to expose the arcus marginalis along the entire inferior orbital rim. Periosteum is incised across the orbital rim, and a subperiosteal pocket is created approximately 1 cm deep across the external surface of the rim and onto the malar face (Figure 56.1). The arcus marginalis is opened to expose the medial, central, and lateral fat pads. The fat pad septae are lysed to allow the fat to flow over the orbital rim in a uniform fashion.

Tisseel (Fibrin Sealant) (Baxter Corporation, Ontario, Canada) is then prepared per manufacturer's instructions. Hemostasis is confirmed within the subperiosteal pocket. Cotton-tipped applicators may be left within the pocket to keep the area ready for application of Tisseel, which will begin to set rapidly following application (Figure 56.2). The 1-ml Tisseel package is adequate for both lower eyelids. When both lower eyelids are prepared, the Tisseel is applied deep into the subperiosteal pocket (Figure 56.3). The cotton-tipped applicators are used to push the prepared fat pedicals into the pocket. Care is taken to uniformly distribute the fat over the orbital rim and into area of greatest need of filling (Figure 56.4). The Tisseel will begin to gel within 30–45 seconds of application. Excess Tisseel is removed. The surgeon may proceed with orbicularis tightening and skin redraping as necessary. Conservative removal or sculpting of some fat may be necessary.

Other fat-capture techniques have been described to include the use of a percutaneous circular suture pass that pulls the leading edge of the fat into the subperiosteal pocket. Several of these sutures must be passed to allow for even distribution of the fat within the pocket. Certainly the cost of the Tisseel must be considered when compared to other techniques. This disadvantage may be negated by the decreased operative time associated with the use of Tisseel. Other possible benefits may include decreased postoperative edema and echymosis

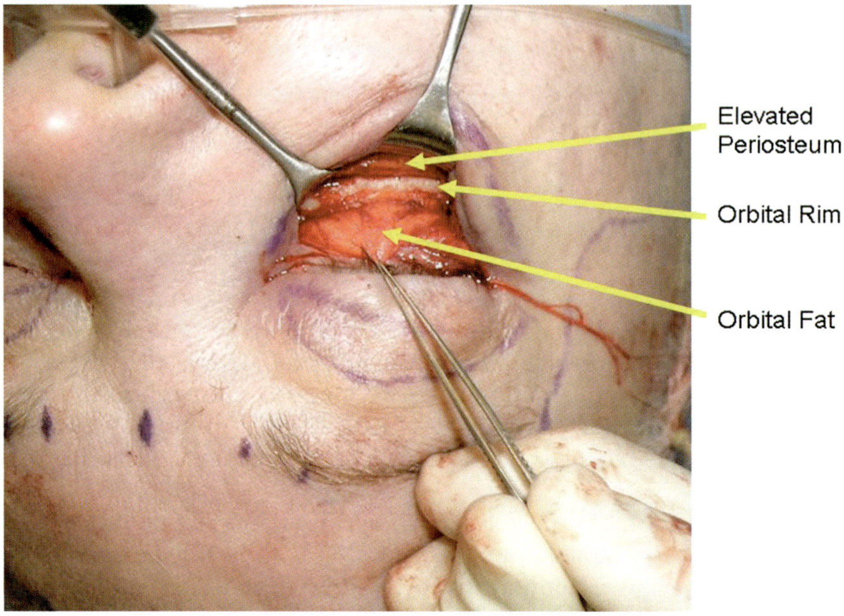

Figure 56.1. Creation of a subperiosteal pocket.

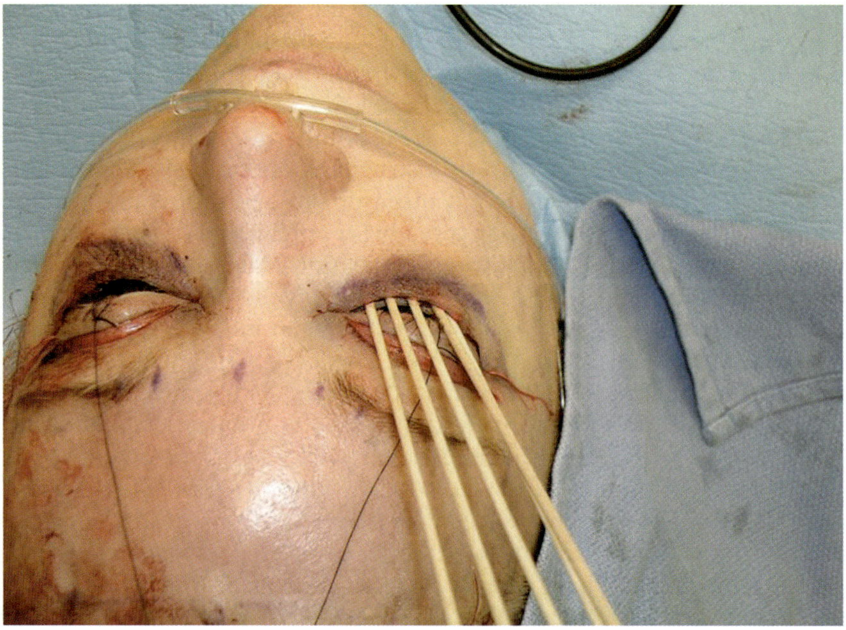

Figure 56.2. Orbital rim kept dry in preparation for Tisseel application using cotton-tipped applicators.

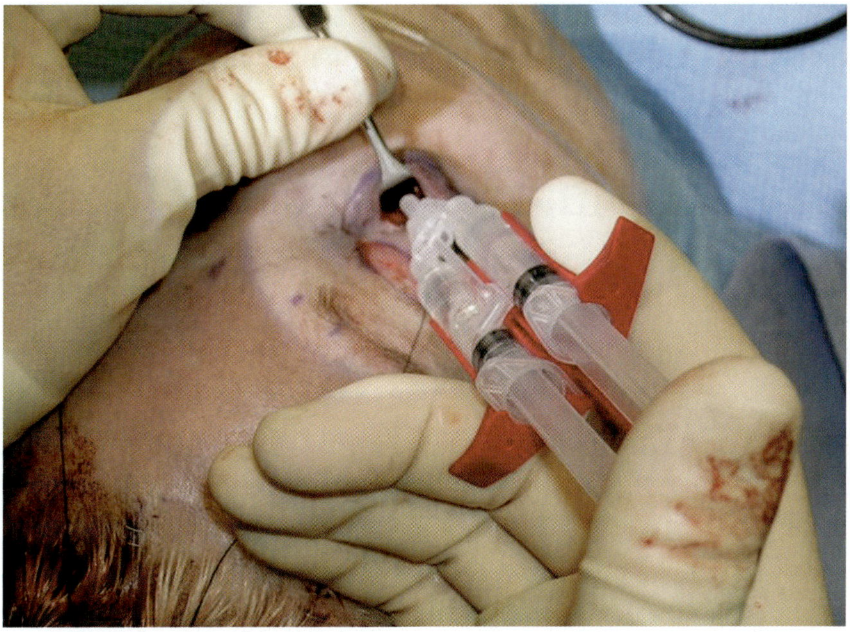

Figure 56.3. Tisseel (fibrin sealant) placed into subperiosteal pocket.

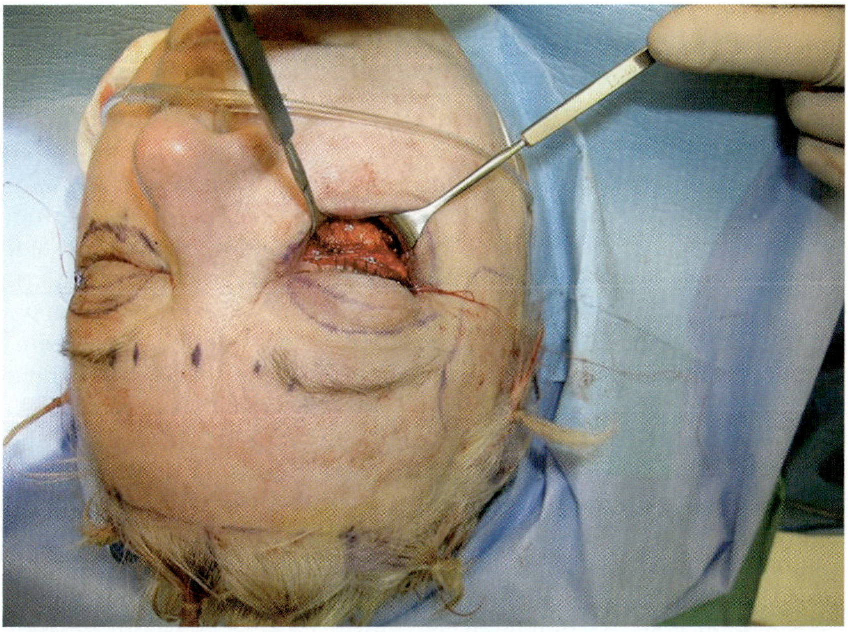

Figure 56.4. Fat pedicles are draped into subperiosteal pocket and held until fibrin sealant sets.

57

Lower Blepharoplasty with Fat Repositioning Without Sutures

John R. Burroughs and Richard L. Anderson

We seldom perform transcutaneous lower eyelid blepharoplasty due to the high incidence of lower eyelid retraction.

Most patients benefit from lower eyelid fat repositioning as compared to removal of excess skin of the lower eyelids.

To improve lower eyelid wrinkles and skin excess, we recommend a lower eyelid TCA peel (25–35%), which is safer and also helps pigmentation changes.

Fat-Repositioning Procedure

Through a transconjunctival incision, placed approximately at the midpoint between the inferior border of tarsus and the fornix, the septum can be accessed (Figure 57.1). Opening the septum and fat capsules should be done as inferiorly as possible so that the fat will drape inferiorly and fill the tear trough and the lower eyelid hollow areas. We have not found a need to suture the fat pads inferiorly, but an integral component is to release the preperiosteal attachments at the inferior orbital rim. This is best accomplished by blunt dissection and elevation of skin and the underlying tissues with the combination of Stevens scissors and a Sayer elevator (Figures 57.2–57.6). This release is carried below the rim (about 1 cm), which will help the fat fill the tear trough deformity. Undermining laterally and release of the orbital malar ligament in connection with the midface elevation, via upper blepharoplasty dissection provides opportunity for a more aggressive midface elevation. Fat sculpting should be kept to a minimum, and mostly involves the more superior fat that prolapses after the capsules are opened (Figure 57.7). Excessive lateral fat pads must be more aggressively sculpted as the lower eyelid trough deformity is usually less pronounced laterally, and lateral fat may protrude more after the septum is opened. After ensuring there are no sites of active bleeding, the conjunctiva is closed in the midline with a single 6–0 plain gut to avoid conjunctival adhesions. Excess lower eyelid skin removal, if needed, can be performed as a secondary procedure. The vast majority of patients do not require skin removal. The combination of TCA peel and lower eyelid fat repositioning with lateral canthopexy and/or lateral SOOF elevation provides an excellent aesthetic result and has high patient acceptance with fewer risks.

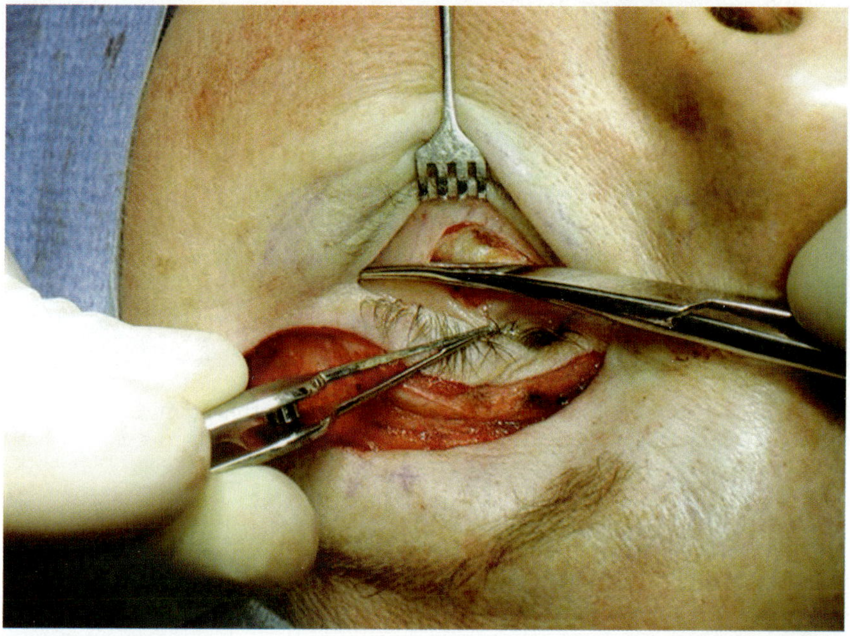

Figure 57.1. Making of transconjunctival incision with Stevens scissors at mid-fornix.

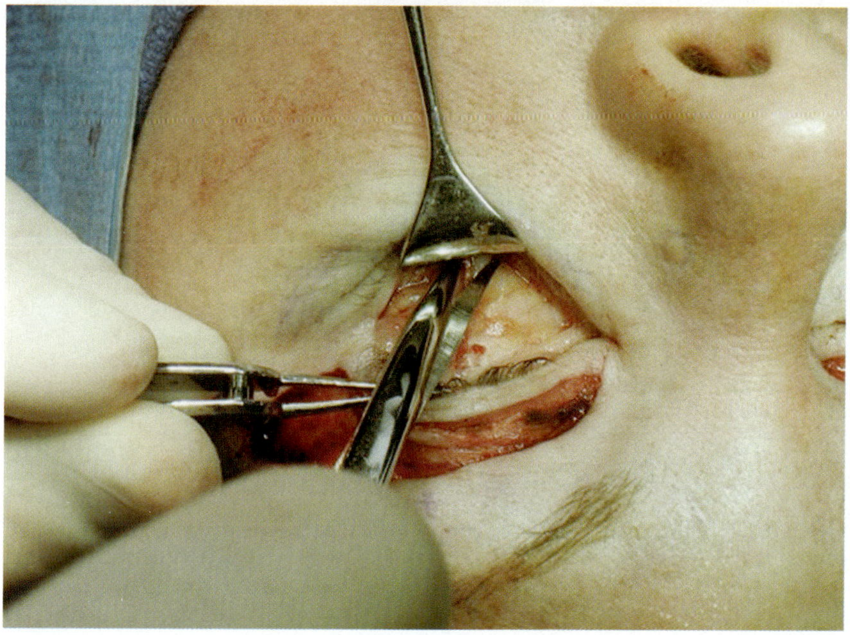

Figure 57.2. Opening of fat capsules inferiorly along the orbital rim, allowing fat to prolapse inferiorly.

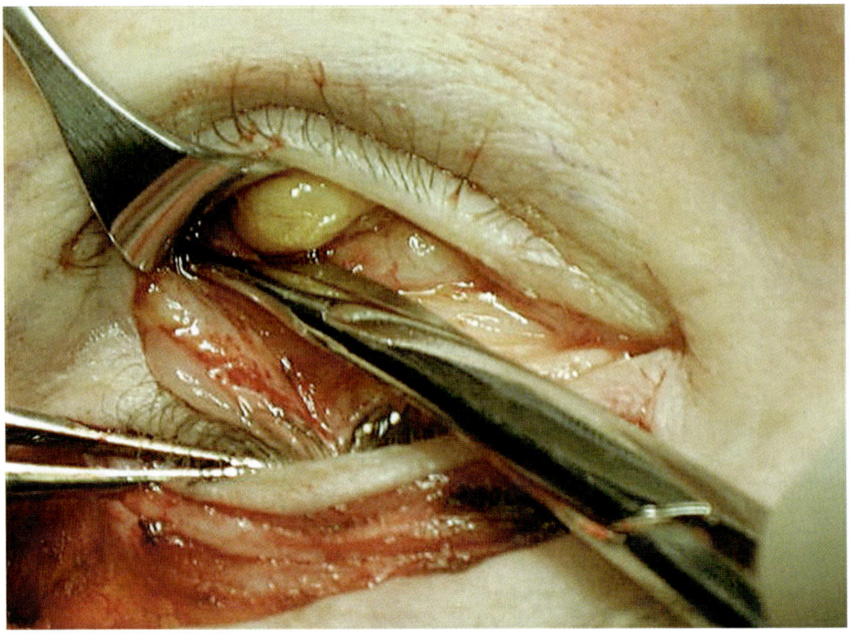

Figure 57.3. Opening of fat capsules inferiorly along orbital rim. Conservative sculpting of superiorly prolapsing fat may then be performed.

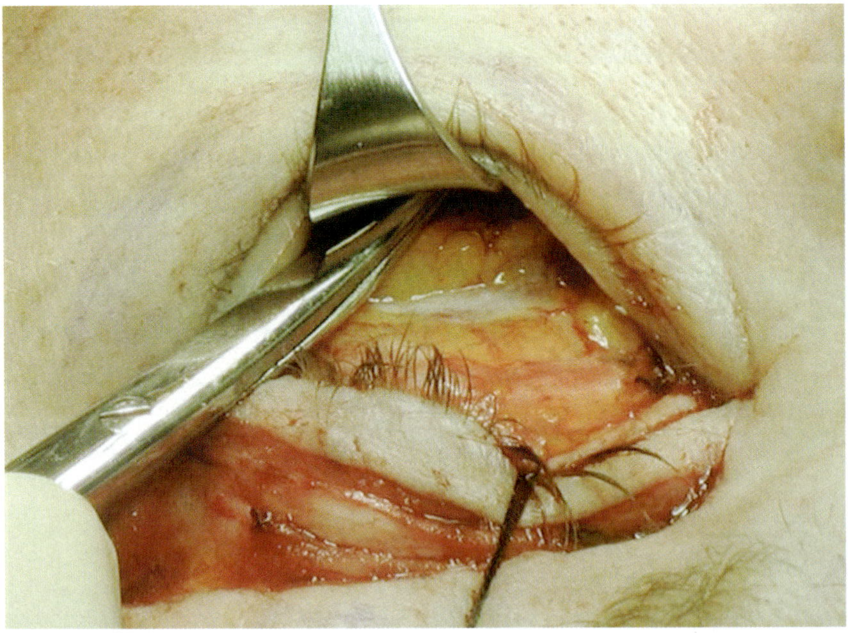

Figure 57.4. Beginning release of preperiosteal attachments along the inferior orbital rim.

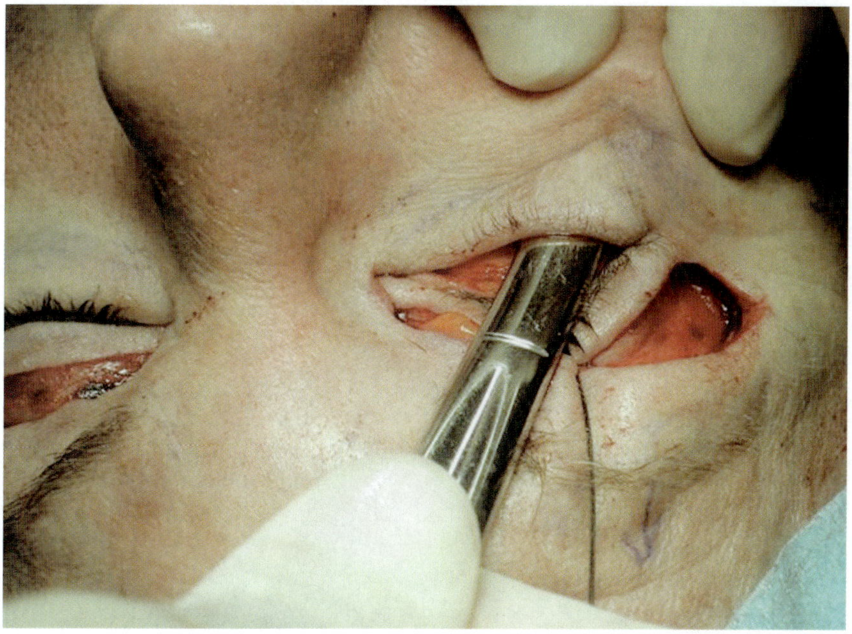

Figure 57.5. Utilization of Sayer elevator to release orbital rim preperiosteal orbicularis attachments, allowing inferiorly prolapsing orbital fat to fill the tear trough deformity.

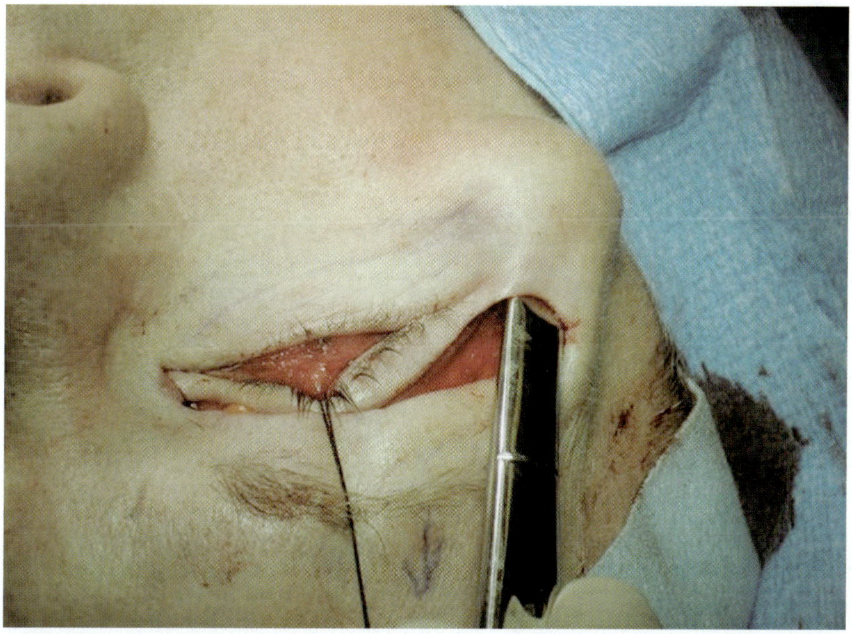

Figure 57.6. Complete release with Sayer elevator to approximately 1 cm below the orbital rim. The cheek fat pad and SOOF have been undermined supraperiosteally, thereby enabling midface elevation.

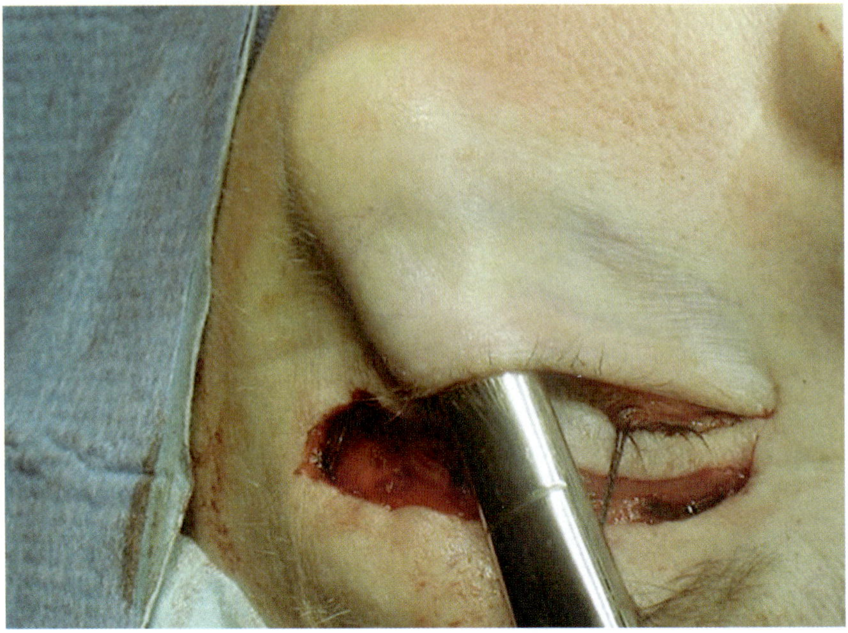

Figure 57.7. Utilization of Sayer elevator through transconjunctival incision to mobilize and elevate SOOF and lateral eyelid-check complex preperiosteally. This undermining joins that done through the lateral upper blepharoplasty incision (shown in Figure 57.6).

Section Four

Management of Postblepharoplasty Lid Retraction

58

Managing Postblepharoplasty Lower Eyelid Malposition

Michael T. Yen

Lower eyelid retraction and ectropion remains a challenging complication of cosmetic lower eyelid blepharoplasty. In addition to being cosmetically unacceptable, the eyelid malposition may be associated with ocular irritation, chronic tearing, and lagophthalmos with exposure keratitis.

Most cases of lower eyelid malposition after blepharoplasty are due to either cicatrix formation or an anterior lamellar shortage of the lower eyelid.[1] While some patients with mild ectropion and retraction may improve with time and eyelid massage, most patients require surgical correction to achieve acceptable functional and cosmetic improvements. Surgical repair of postblepharoplasty lower eyelid malposition should be graded depending on the severity of the malposition. For most cases that require surgical intervention, the lower eyelid malposition can be corrected by releasing the cicatrix (if present), providing additional support and recruiting anterior lamella to the eyelid with midface elevation, and horizontal tightening of the lower eyelid.

My preferred surgical approach to the midface is through a transconjunctival incision in the lower eyelid fornix.[2] A supraperiosteal midface lift is then performed by undermining suborbicularis oculi fat and malar fat pads and elevating the malar tissues with a broad flat elevator. Sharp dissection is avoided to reduce the risk of severing the zygomatico-facial and infraorbital neurovascular structures. The elevation may be extended down to the level of the nasolabial fold. Several 4–0 polyglactin 910 sutures are passed through the malar fat pad, engaging the superficial musculoaponeurotic system (SMAS), and elevated supero-temporally. If the sutures are placed too superficially, unacceptable dimpling of the cheeks will result. If the sutures do not engage the SMAS, adequate midface elevation is difficult to achieve. The sutures are secured to the periosteum along the orbital rim.

For moderate or severe lower eyelid retraction with middle lamellar scarring, a spacer graft is often required in addition to midface lifting and eyelid tightening.[1,3,4] This spacer graft provides additional support and vertical length to the middle lamella of the lower eyelid. My preferred spacer graft material is autogenous hard palate or acellular dermal grafts. Acellular dermis is easily obtained commercially and is less traumatic for patients as there is no separate donor site in the mouth to heal. However, there is less predictability of final eyelid height and position when compared to hard palate grafts. The hard palate graft is the gold standard for treatment of severe lower eyelid retraction or for cases inadequately corrected with acellular dermis. The dense collagen layers give the graft a firm consistency similar to tarsus, and the mucosal lining is less abrasive to the corneal epithelium than acellular dermis.[4] The grafts do not shrink, and the results are very predictable. The graft is harvested between the gingiva and the midline, where there is a well-defined submucosa allowing easy separation of the mucosa from the periosteum. The graft should be sized for the entire width of the lower eyelid and approximately 5 mm in height. The graft is dissected in the submucosal plane with a Freer elevator and should stop 3–4 mm short of the soft palate to avoid injury to the greater palatine vessels and to avoid fistula formation in the soft palate.

Lower eyelid malposition after cosmetic blepharoplasty can be very difficult to correct. As we have developed a better understanding of the anatomic relationship between the midface and lower eyelid, we are realizing that both need to be addressed to achieve optimal functional and cosmetic results. With successful midface lifting, eyelid spacer grafts are only required for severe lower eyelid retraction.

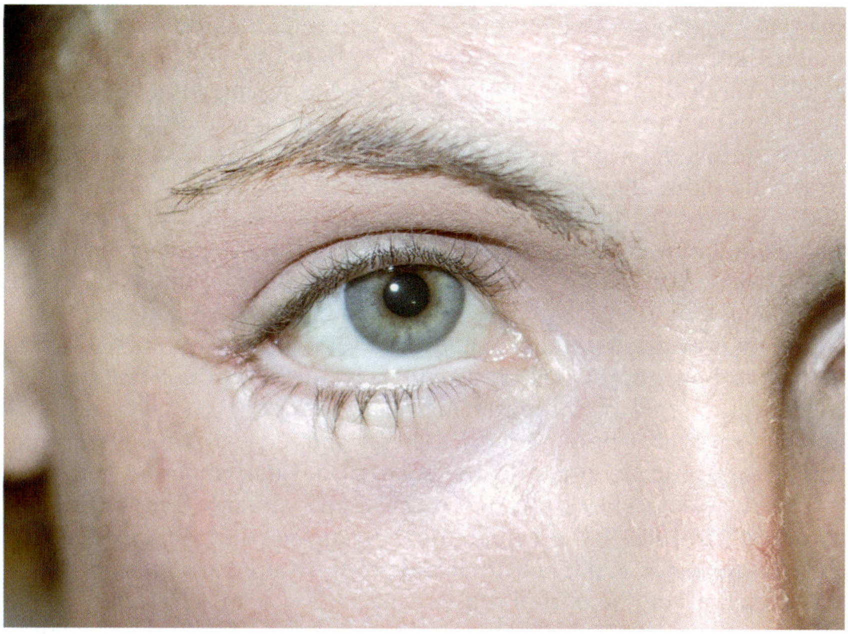

Figure 58.1. Retraction and lateral ectropion of the right lower eyelid after transcutaneous blepharoplasty.

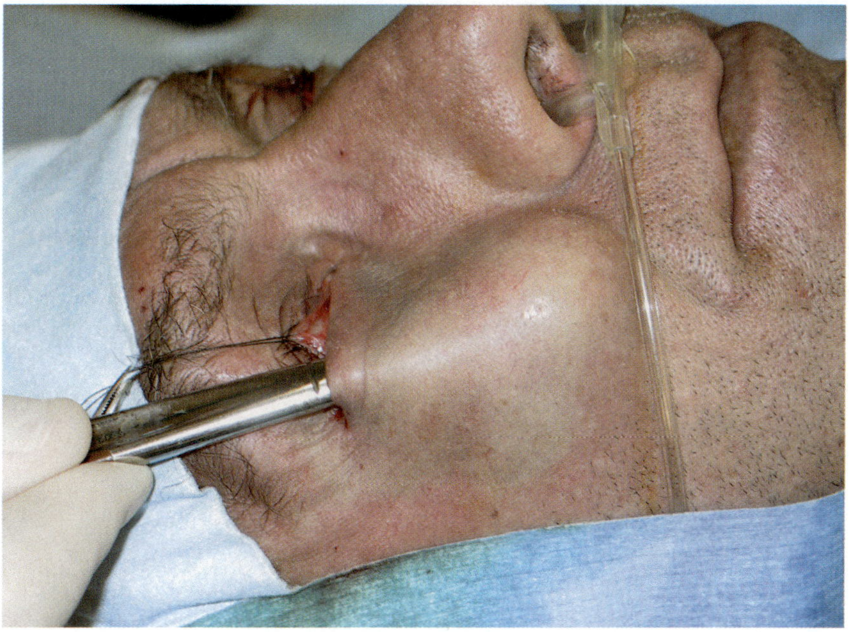

Figure 58.2. Using a broad flat (Sayre) elevator, the midface is elevated in the supra-periosteal plane down to the level of the nasolabial fold.

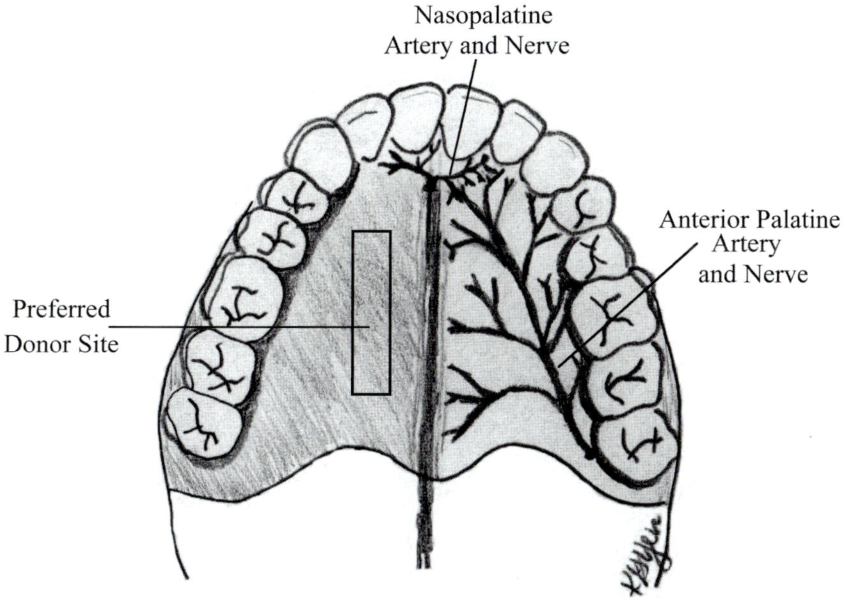

Figure 58.3. Harvesting of the hard palate graft should be between the gingiva and the midline and should stop 3–4 mm short of the soft palate to avoid injury to the greater palatine vessels and to avoid fistula formation in the soft palate.

References

1. Patel BCK, Patipa M, Anderson RL, McLeish W. Management of post-blepharoplasty lower eyelid retraction with hard palate grafts and lateral tarsal strip. Plast Reconstr Surg 1997;99:1251–11260.
2. Kim JK, Ellis DS, Stewart WB. Correction of lower eyelid retraction by transconjunctival retractor excision and lateral eyelid suspension. Ophthal Plast Reconstr Surg 1999;15:341–348.
3. Aldave AJ, Maus M, Rubin PA. Advances in the management of lower eyelid retraction. Facial Plast Surg 1999;15:213–224.
4. Kersten RC, Kulwin DR, Levartovsky S, et al. Management of lower-lid retraction with hard-palate mucosa grafting. Arch Ophthalmol 1990; 108:1339–1343.

59

Retroauricular Dermal Spacer Graft for Lower Lid Retraction Repair

Francesco P. Bernardini

In cases of ectropion/scleral show, another location to harvest valuable tissue that can be used as a posterior spacer to lift the lower eyelid is the retroauricolar area. Harvesting this spacer is quite simple, painless, without visible scar, and well accepted by the patients. It is like harvesting the skin from the retroauricolar region, only in this case we peel off the epidermis instead of the dermis. It is stiff enough to support the eyelid, works like Alloderm (but its cheaper), and avoids the pain and the prolonged healing time of the hard palate graft. I have used it satisfactorily in lower eyelid retraction, especially in patients with thyroid eye disease.

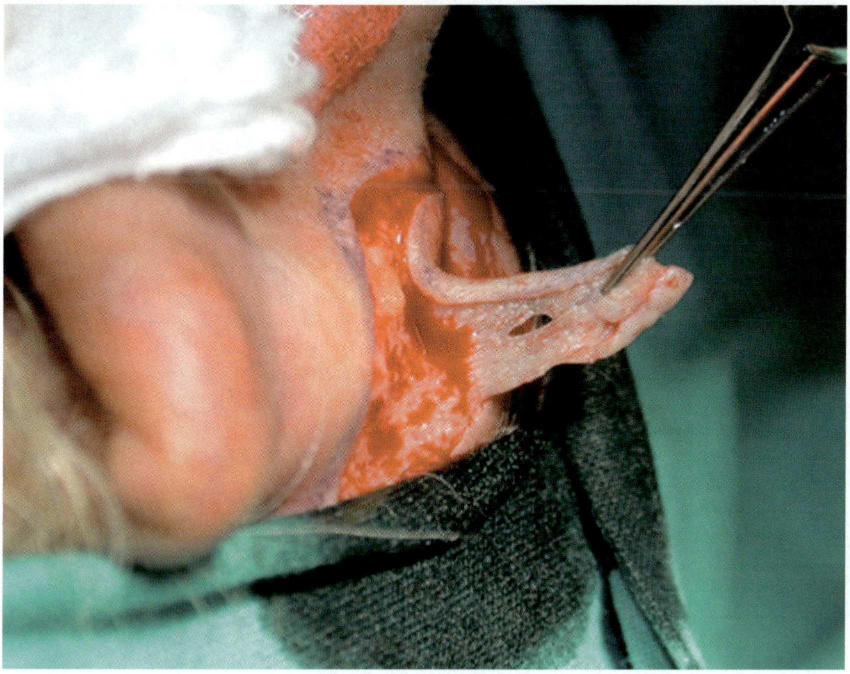

Figure 59.1. Excision of the superficial lay or the skin (epidermis).

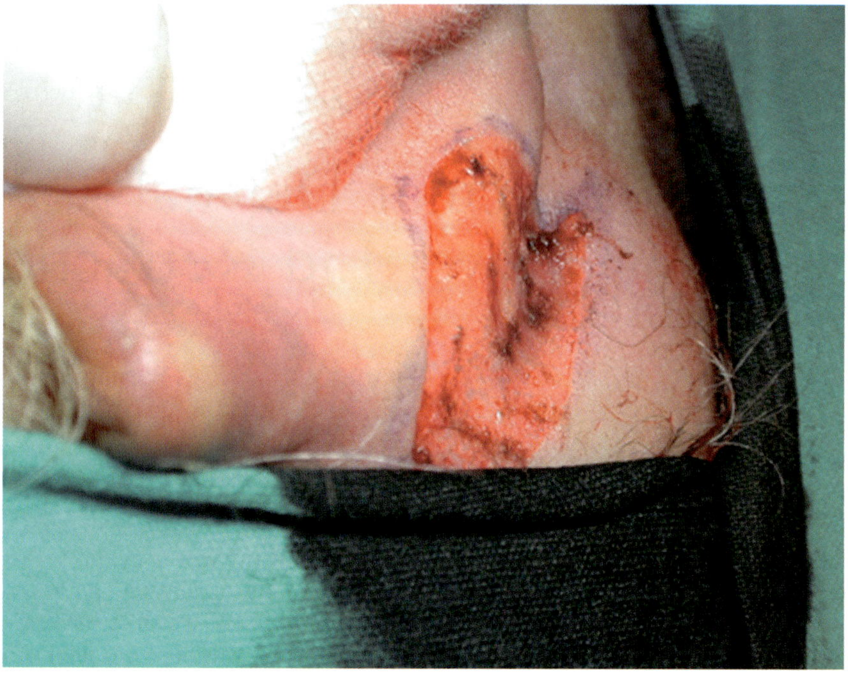

Figure 59.2. Deeper layer (dermis).

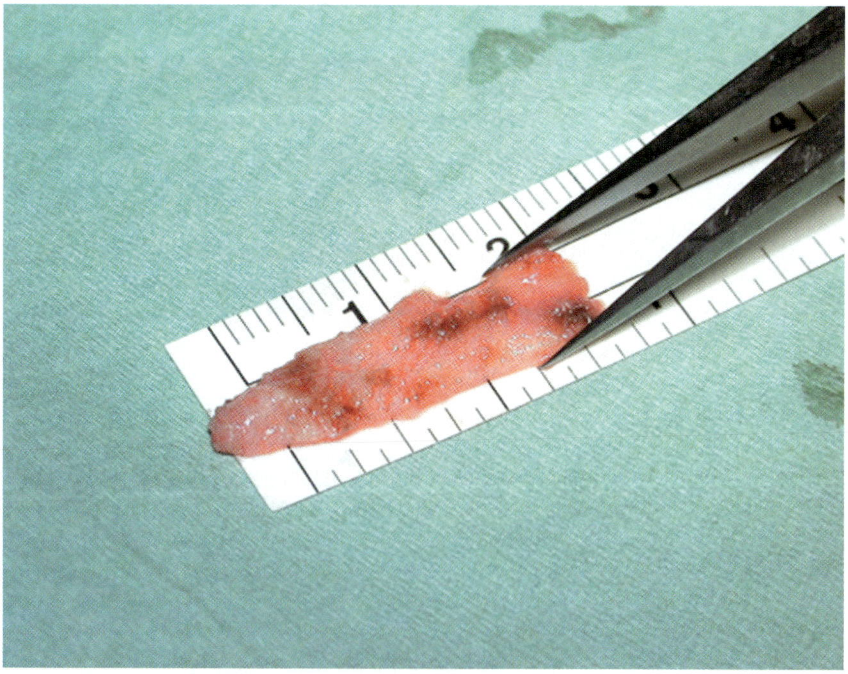

Figure 59.3. Dermal graft harvested.

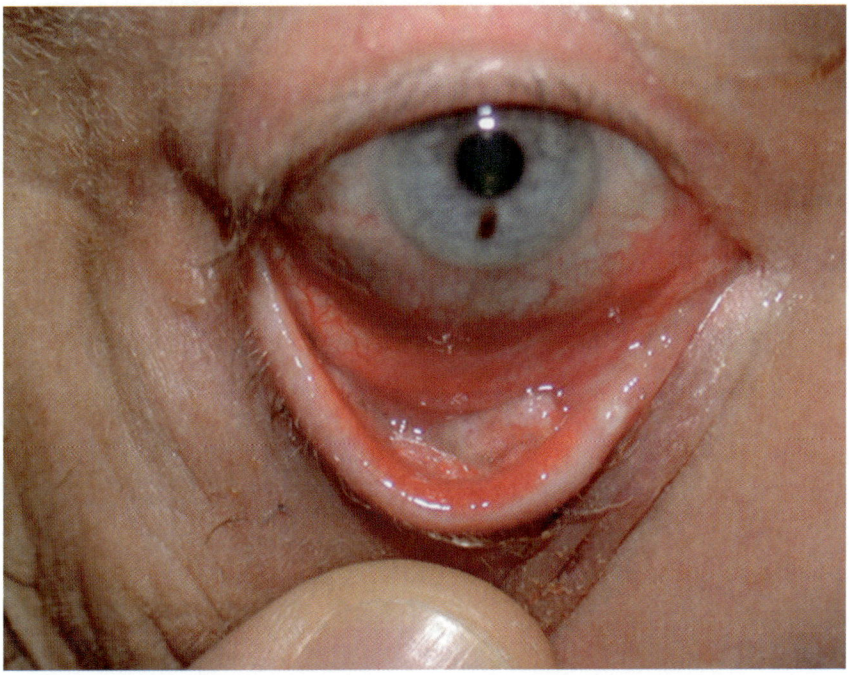

Figure 59.4. Dermal graft in position (long-term result).

60

Mid-Lower Eyelid Tarsoconjunctival Flap-Skin Graft: Treatment of Cicatricial Lower Lid Retraction

John Pak

One challenging and potentially disfiguring postoperative complication associated with lower eyelid blepharoplasty is lower eyelid retraction, defined as a downward malposition of the lower eyelid margin. Severe postblepharoplasty lower eyelid retraction has been reported in up to 20% of cases.[1–4] In severe lower eyelid retraction, cicatricial attachments develop between the anterior lamella of the lower eyelid to the inferior orbital rim (Figure 60.1).

Strategies in the surgical treatment of cicatricial lower lid retraction are challenging and commonly dissatisfying. Several surgical treatments, such as skin grafts, excision of cicatrix, midface lift, and tarsal strip, have been advocated to correct lower eyelid malposition in severe cicatricial lower lid retraction.[5–7] For the oculoplastic surgeon confronted with the arduous task of proficiently managing the severe lower eyelid retraction in order to improve the functional and aesthetic qualities of the post-blepharoplasty lower eyelid, the mid-lower eyelid tarsoconjunctival flap–skin graft is a powerful technique initially described by Putterman.[8]

Indications

Individuals presenting with the following signs of severe cicatricial lower lid retraction are appropriate candidates for this procedure: (1) retraction of lid associated with tethering of the lower lid to the orbital rim, (2) positive forced elevation test whereby the lower lid cannot be superiorly lifted, (3) binocularity, as the graft will obscure vision, (4) individuals who have not undergone previous tarsoconjunctival grafting of the ipsilateral upper lid, and (5) individuals who have undergone previous reconstructive surgeries (e.g., tarsal strip and mid-face lift).

Complications

Lower lid laxity, manifesting as mild to moderate ectropion developing after the flap is severed, can be appropriately managed by massaging the lower eyelid upward. In my experience, no corrective procedures have been required to treat lower lid ectropion as long as the skin graft is appropriately sized and no laxity is evident prior to surgery. Upper lid retraction may develop in the construction of the tarsoconjunctival graft.

Procedure

Stage 1

1. Inject the lower lid using lidocaine 2% with 1:100,000 units of epinephrine.
2. Create a subciliary mark 4 mm below the lower lid margin.
3. Place a 4–0 silk suture at the central aspect of the lid at the margin. This will serve as a useful traction suture.
4. Using a #15 Bard-parker blade, create an incision along the lower lid at the previously demarcated line. This incision must not be full thickness, but should incise to the suborbicularis space (Figure 60.2).
5. Evert the lower lid using a desmarres retractor and 4-0 silk suture.
6. Create an incision 4 mm below the lid margin at the conjunctival surface. The length of the incision must mirror the subciliary incision (Figure 60.3).
7. Using a sharp scissor, make a buttonhole along the conjunctival incision full thickness such that a union between the subciliary and conjunctival incisions is created.
8. Incise the remaining the tissue to completely unify the conjunctival and subciliary incisions (Figure 60.4).
9. Conservatively cauterize any bleeding vessels to reduce the chance of causing necrosis of the lid margin.
10. Create the tarsoconjuctival flap in the normal standard fashion.
11. Place the lower lid margin to a position slightly above the inferior limbus of the cornea.
12. Measure the size of the defect and obtain a full thickness skin graft (i.e., postauricular, eyelid skin, or supraclavicular).
13. Place the tarsoconjunctival graft below the lid margin and place the tarsal component next to the inferior edge of the conjunctival surface (Figure 60.5).
14. Suture the inferior edge of the tarsoconjunctival graft to the conjunctiva and inferior retractors using interrupted 6–0 vicryl sutures (Figure 60.6).
15. Place the full-thickness skin graft over the anterior lamellar defect and suture the edges together using 6–0 vicryl sutures (Figure 60.7).
16. Place a telfa bolster over the skin graft and lower lid, as previously described (Figure 60.8).[9]

Stage 2

1. Sever the conjunctival flap at 5–6 weeks after the first stage of the procedure (Figures 60.9 [preop] and 60.10 [postop]).
2. If any mild ectropion exists, instruct the patient to massage the lower lid upward multiple times.

Conclusions

The mid-lower eyelid tarsonconjunctival flap–skin graft is a powerful technique in the surgical armentarium for severe cicatricial lower eyelid retraction.[10] The procedure can result in excellent esthetic and functional outcomes, particularly in those situations where previous reconstructive efforts have failed.

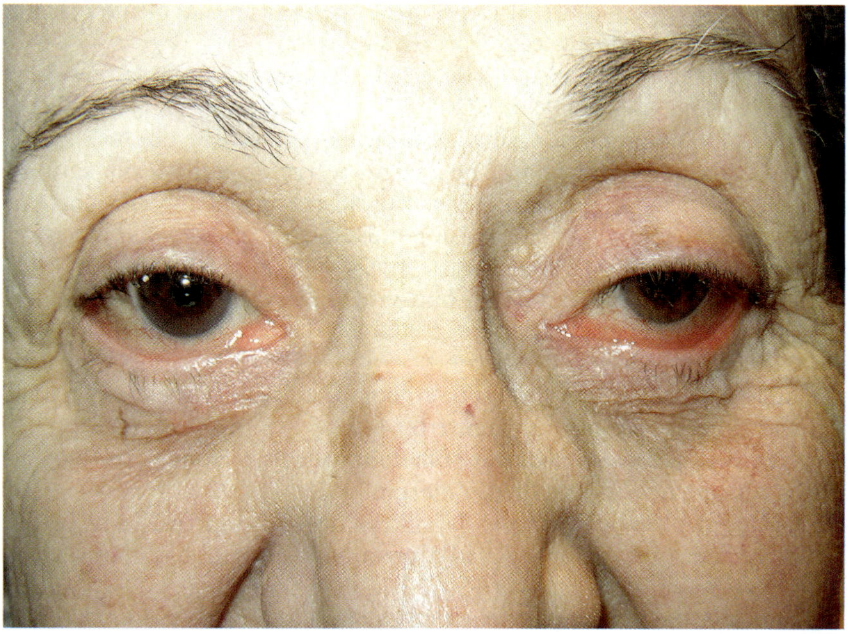

Figure 60.1. Bilateral lower eyelid cicatricial retraction.

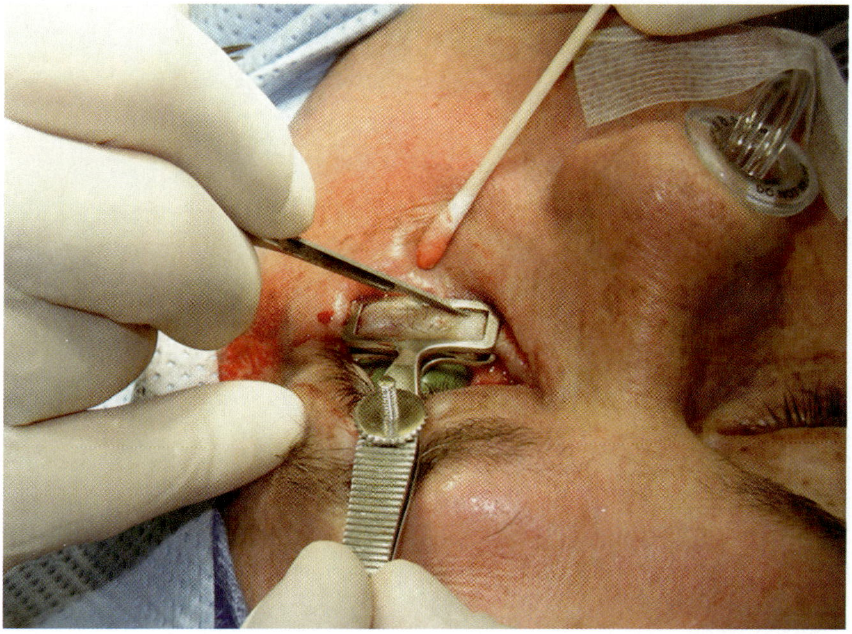

Figure 60.2. Incision of anterior lamellae.

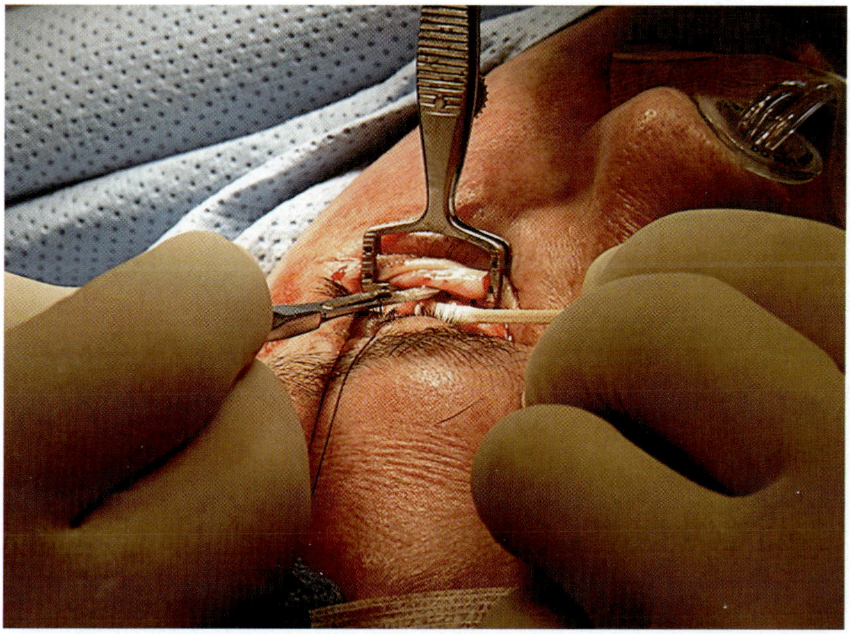

Figure 60.3. Incision of conjunctiva 4 mm below lid margin.

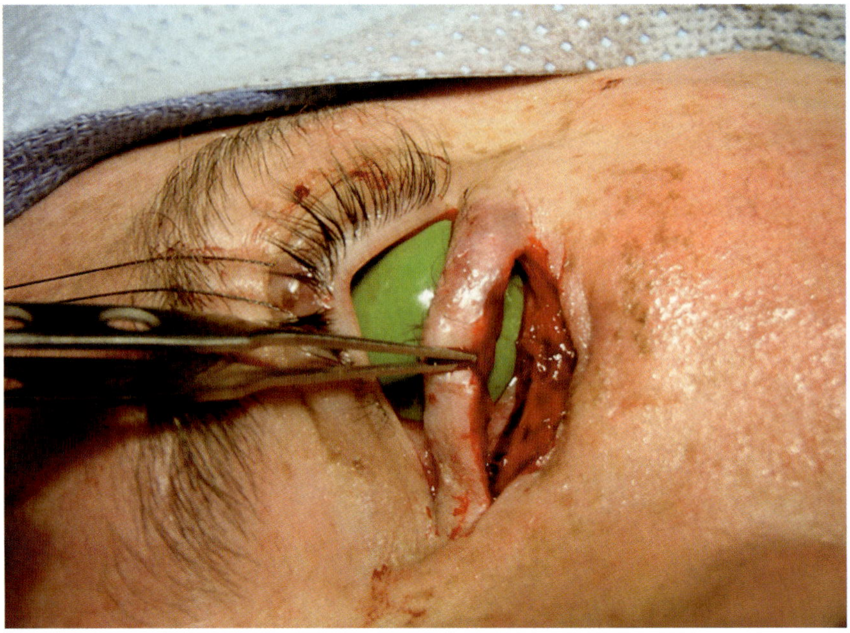

Figure 60.4. Unification of cutaneous and conjunctival incisions.

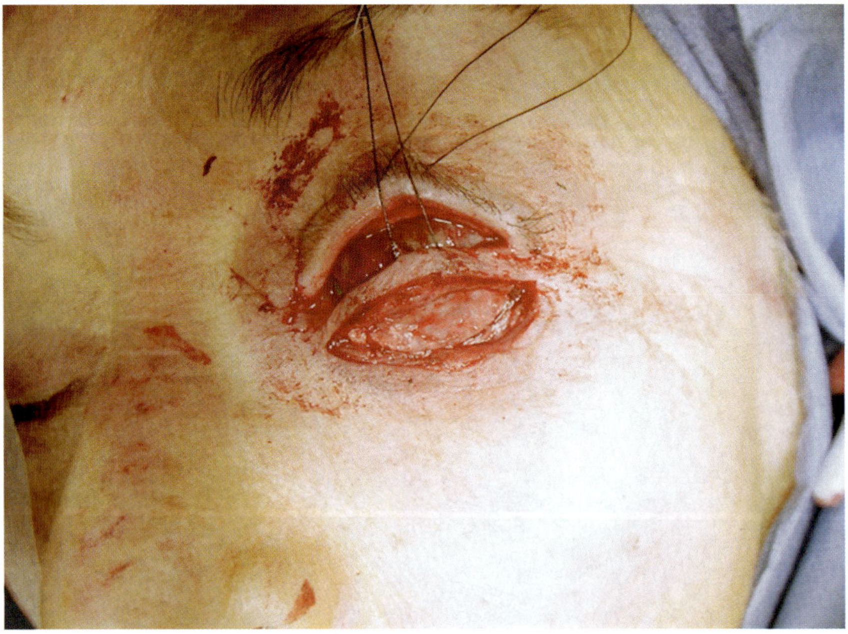

Figure 60.5. Position the transconjunctival graft.

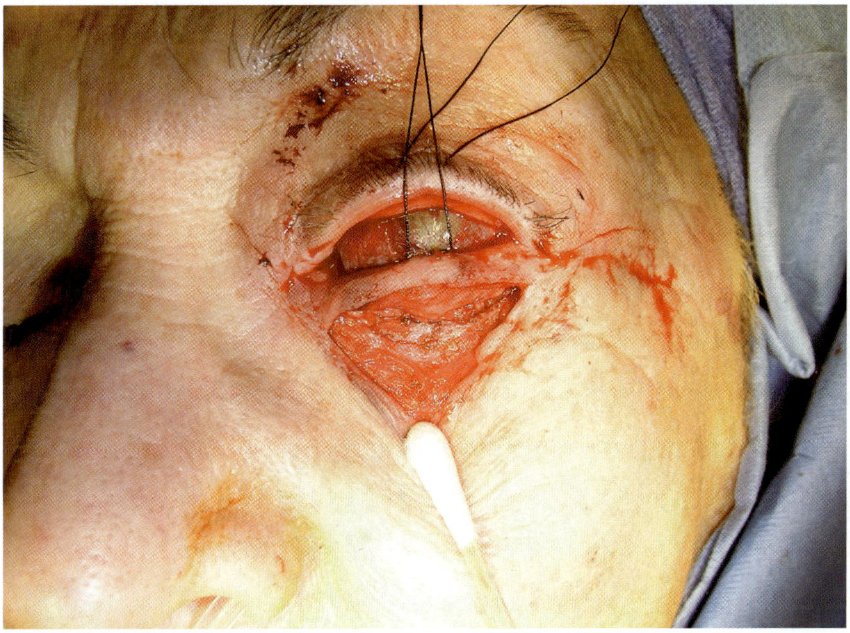

Figure 60.6. Suture for a conjunctival graft to conjunctiva and inferior retractors.

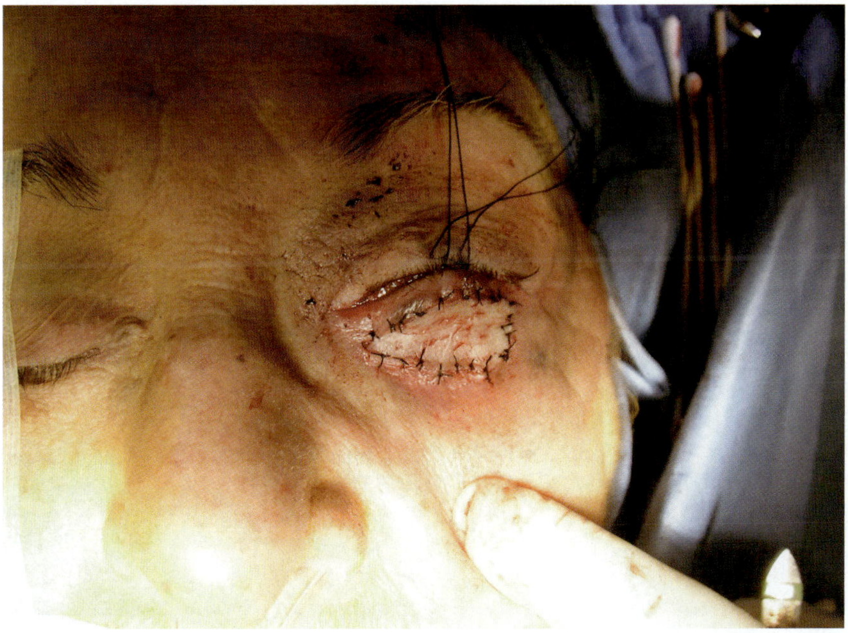

Figure 60.7. Placement of full-thickness skin graft to anterior defect.

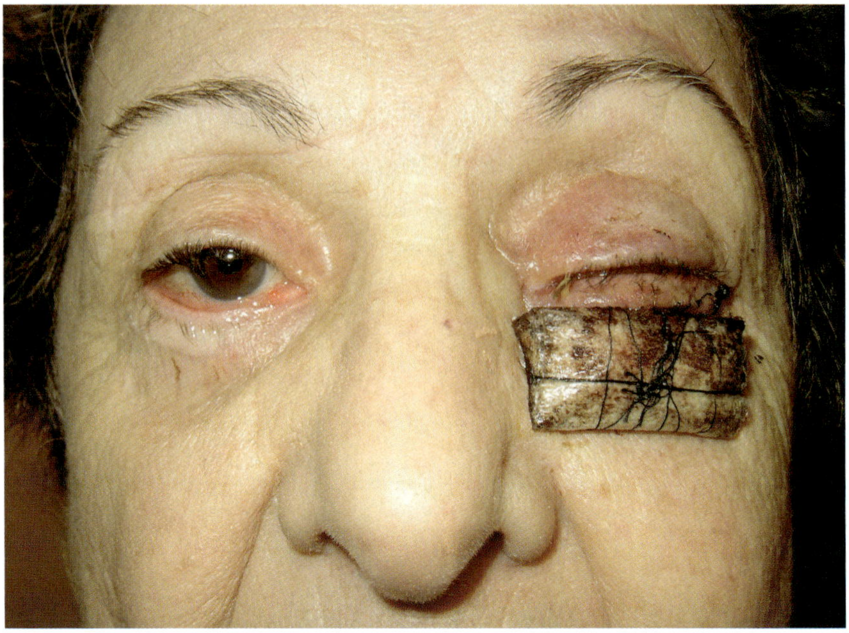

Figure 60.8. Secure skin graft adhesion with recipient bed using Telfa bolster.

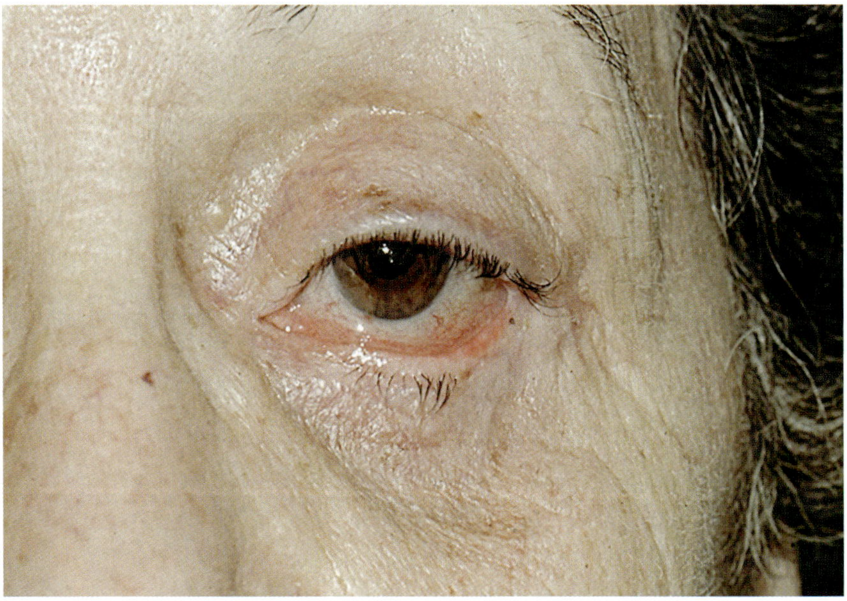

Figure 60.9. Preoperative photo of left lower eyelid.

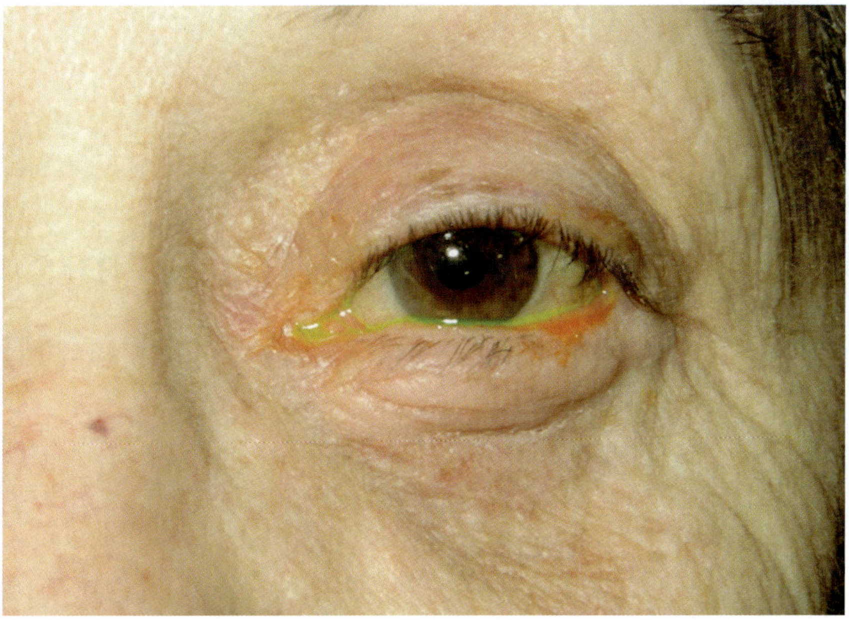

Figure 60.10. Postoperative photo of left lower eyelid.

References

1. McGraw BL, Adams PA. Postblepharoplasty ectropion. Arch Otol Head Surg 1991;117:852–856.
2. Lisman RD, Hyde K, Smith B. Complications of blepharoplasty. Clin Plast Surg. 1988;15(2):309–335.
3. Baylis HI, Goldberg RA, Groth MJ. Complications of lower eyelid blepharoplasty. In: Putterman AM, (ed.). Cosmetic Oculoplastic Surgery, 3rd ed. Philadelphia: WB Saunders, 1999:429–456.
4. Patipa M. The evaluation and management of lower eyelid retraction following cosmetic surgery. Plast Reconstr Surg. 2000;106(2):438–459.
5. Edelstein C, Balch K, Shorr N, Goldberg RA.The transeyelid subperiosteal midface- lift in the unhappy postblepharoplasty patient. Semin Ophthalmol 1998;13(3):107–114.
6. Shorr N, Fallor MK. "Madame Butterfly" procedure: combined cheek and lateral canthal suspension procedure for post-blepharoplasty, "round eye", and lower eyelid retraction. Ophthal Plast Reconstr Surg 1985;1(4): 229–235.
7. Jordan DR, Anderson RL. The lateral tarsal strip revisited: the enhanced tarsal strip. Arch Ophthalmol 1989;107:604.
8. Putterman AM. Lower eyelid full-thickness vertical lengthening. Am J Ophthalmol 1979;88(1):113–118.
9. Putterman AM. Bolster for the tarsoconjunctival flap-skin graft. Ophthalmol Plast Reconstr Surg 2002;18(6):466–467.
10. Pak J, Putterman AM. Treatment of cicatricial lower lid retraction using mid-lower eyelid tarsoconjunctival flap-skin graft. 2006 ASOPRS presentation.

61

Treatment of Postblepharoplasty Lower Eyelid Retraction with Dermis Fat Spacer Grafting

Bobby S. Korn and Don O. Kikkawa

Lower eyelid retraction is a potential complication following transcutaneous lower eyelid blepharoplasty. Several mechanisms contribute to postblepharoplasty eyelid retraction, including excess skin removal, exuberant scarring of the middle lamella, and unforeseen lower eyelid laxity. Several techniques have been described to treat postblepharoplasty eyelid retraction using a combination of mid-face lifting with or without posterior lamella spacer grafts. We described a new method of lower eyelid retraction using dermis fat as a posterior lamellar graft combined with mid-facial lifting.[1,2]

Surgical Technique

An elliptical mark is made over the donor site on the hip. A high-speed diamond burr is used to debride the epithelium until a fine, hyperemic surface is obtained. Sharp dissection is performed to remove the dermis and underlying adipose tissue. Attention is then turned to the lateral canthus, where a lateral canthotomy and inferior cantholysis is performed. The conjunctiva beneath the inferior tarsal border is incised with monopolar cautery. The dissection is then carried down to the inferior orbital rim, lysing all adhesions and liberating the orbitomalar ligament. Then the inferolateral suborbicularis oculi fat (SOOF) is imbricated with a 5-0 vicryl suture. Next, through an upper eyelid crease incision, blunt dissection is performed under the lateral canthal tissues with a mosquito clamp and this is used to pull the SOOF suture through the upper lid crease incision. Finally, the suture is fixated to the periosteum at the level of the frontozygomatic suture (Figure 61.1). The dermis fat spacer graft with the dermis side facing the ocular surface is then secured to the cut edges of the conjunctiva with 6-0 fast-absorbing gut suture (Figure 61.2). Any lower eyelid laxity is then addressed by a lateral tarsal strip procedure. A Frost suture is then placed over foam bolsters for 7–10 days. Figure 61.3 shows a patient after bilateral lower eyelid retraction repair with dermis fat spacer grafting and mid-face lifting.

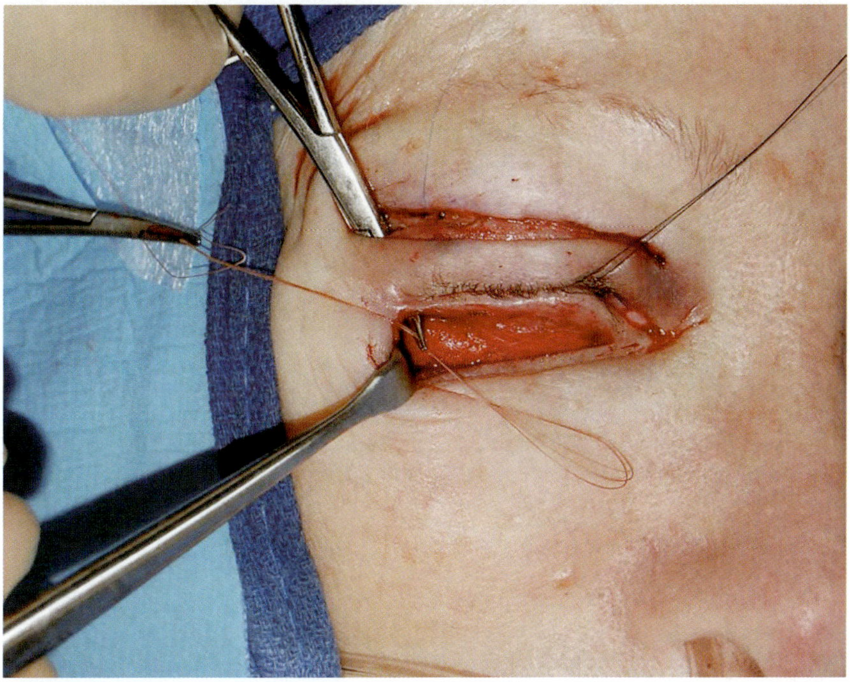

Figure 61.1. Fixation of SOOF suture through an upper eyelid crease incision. A 5-0 vicryl suture is used to secure the SOOF and this suture is then passed under the lateral canthal tissues with a curved hemostat. The suture is then fixated superolaterally to the periosteum at the level of the frontozygomatic suture.

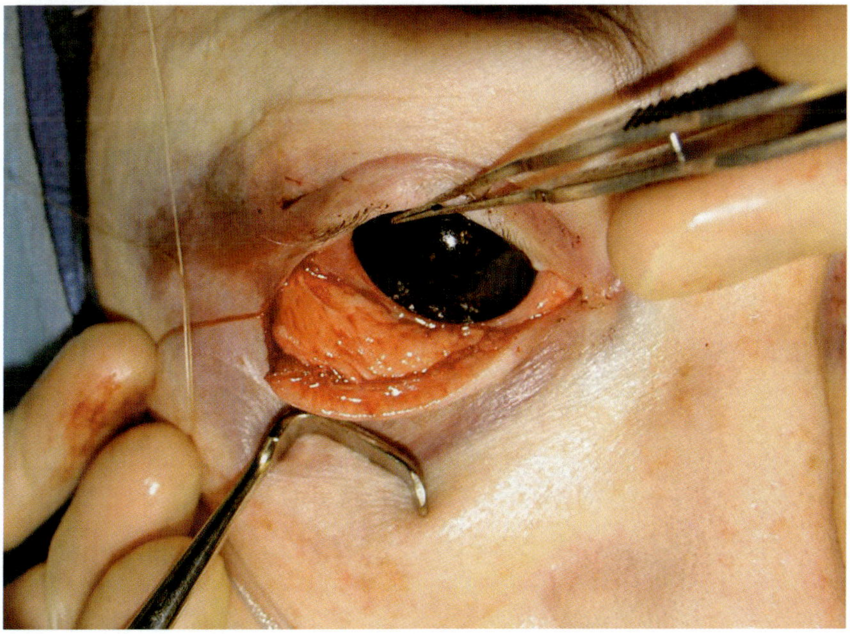

Figure 61.2. In situ placement of dermis fat graft. The dermis fat graft is oriented with the dermal side facing the ocular surface and the fat side directed towards the surgical bed. The graft is secured to the conjunctival edge with interrupted 6-0 fast abosorbing gut sutures.

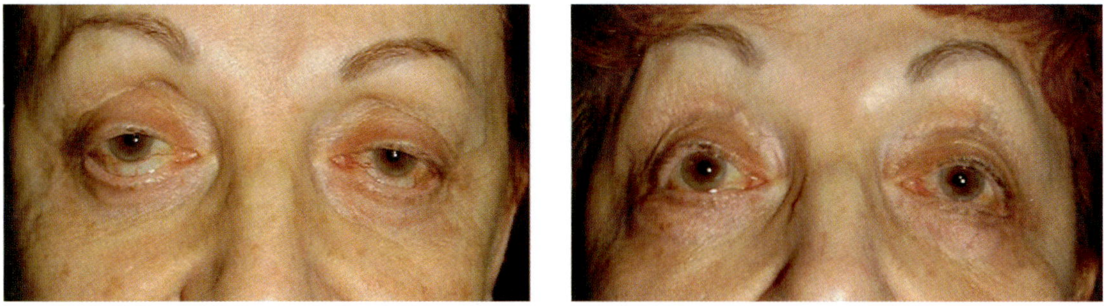

Figure 61.3. Preoperative and postoperative photographs of a patient before and after dermis fat grafting and midface lifting. On the left panel, the patient has postblepharoplasty lower eyelid retraction and exposure keratopathy. On the right panel, the patient has restoration of normal eyelid position after bilateral dermis fat grafting with midface lifting.

References

1. Kikkawa DO, Kim JW. Lower-eyelid blepharoplasty. Int Ophthalmol Clin 1997;37:163–178.
2. Korn BS, Kikkawa DO, Cohen SR, Hartstein MO, Annuziata, CC. Tratment of lower eyelid malposition with dermis fat grafting. Ophthalmology 2008; 115:744–751.

Part V

Forehead Rejuvenation

Section One

Preoperative Considerations

62

Which Browlift to Do?

Andrea N. Hass

In patient evaluation we must take note of the patient's hairline and hairstyle when evaluating him or her for a browlift.

Endoscopic technique works best in patients with a low to normal hairline. If the hair is thin but still along a normal hairline, endoscopic technique remains an option. The decision process is more difficult when a patient has a borderline high hairline. He or she may still be an endobrow candidate, but should not expect as tight a result as with a coronal-type browlift.

The patient with a high forehead presents the greatest challenge. An anterior-hairline coronal-type browlift is the best option for some of these patients. However, they need to be willing to wear bangs forever in case the scar is unsightly, and they need to be willing to accept potentially permanent numbness of the top of the head.

The patient with an extremely high or scarce hairline is not a candidate for either type of browlift. A direct browlift or trans-bleph browlift may be their only options, both of which have limitations. The direct browlift leaves the risk of an obvious scar on the brow, and the trans-bleph browlift provides only moderate improvement at best.

63

Browlifting: Patient Evaluation

Andrea N. Hass

No evaluation for upper lid blepharoplasty is complete without considering the role of the brow. In the past, a browlift was a daunting operation with a long ear-to-ear incision that was very bothersome to most patients, and thus avoided by many. With the availability of using endoscopic techniques and a few other options, browlifts are now much easier for patient and surgeon alike. This unit will discuss the evaluation process and current techniques for browlifting procedures.

Evaluation

As with any patient–doctor consultation, listening to the patient carefully to understand their concerns is paramount in making a patient happy postoperatively. Occasionally the patient will make this easy for us by demonstrating what bothers them. If they pull up on the brow to show the look they want, a browlift will be part of the equation; if they pull forward on excess skin, an upper lid blepharoplasty alone may suffice.

Often, however, the best plan is more elusive. While listening to patients, watch how they use their brows. Also watch carefully as they bring the mirror up to view themselves. Finally, look at their brow positions when their foreheads are completely relaxed.

At the same time, evaluate the upper lids. Do they have purely blepharochalasis, or are the brows contributing to the excess skin? Is there a significant lateral overhang of "skin" which is actually due to brow position? Do they have ptosis and are they raising their brows to compensate? Is there significant tissue fullness at the top of the nose when the brows are relaxed?

Once you have these answers in your mind, go over all of them with the patient, whether or not they have indicated an interest in a browlift. Working from top to bottom, review hairline position, brow rhytids, brow position (both where the patient holds it and when relaxed), and then upper lids. Try to demonstrate the desired position of the brow and how the upper lid would look both with and without a browlift.

The most complicated patient is the one with ptosis or severe blepharochalasis who raises his or her brow constantly in compensation. There is no way to determine whether or not this patient will relax the brow once the upper lids have been corrected. This is the time for careful discussion, so that should he or she decide not to do a browlift, it is understood that the postoperative brow position may be different from what he or she is used to. It is helpful to keep the possibility of a future browlift open to the patient and even more helpful if he or she understands this possibility prior to doing any surgery.

Many patients fear a "deer in the headlights" look postoperatively. These are typically those who use their frontalistone to compensate for heavy lids. These patients will find that after a browlift, the eyebrow tends to maintain its position, and the forehead above the brow is smoother and less wrinkled after the browlift. Patients who do not use the frontalis significantly tend to desire a higher brow position and are the easiest to please.

64

Preoperative Botox for Endoscopic Browlifting

Andrea N. Hass

Preoperatively for an endoscopic browlift is an excellent time to introduce a patient to the benefits of Botox. Over time, constant use of the brow depressor muscles (corrugator, procerus, and lateral orbicularis muscles) has worked with gravity to lower the brow to its current position. Temporary paralysis of these muscles allows the elevator muscles of the brow to work without counterbalance, thus making them relatively stronger.

In a borderline low brow, Botox may make enough of a difference to postpone a browlift for several years. In a truly low brow this will not make a big difference prior to a browlift. However, given 2–3 weeks prior to surgery, it will keep the patient from using those muscles to pull down against a freshly lifted brow. This allows the brow to heal with less stress during the first 2–3 months postoperatively. Once the Botox has worn off, it becomes up to the patient to decide whether to continue with the Botox. Encourage continued Botox at least every six months to maintain the results of the browlift as long as possible.

Section Two

Endoscopic Forehead Rejuvenation

65

Five Tips for Endoscopic Browlift

Sheri L. DeMartelaere, Todd R. Shepler, Sean M. Blaydon, Russell W. Neuhaus, and John W. Shore

1. Botulinum toxin type A injected in the glabellar area 1 week preoperatively can be a useful adjunct to promote wound healing in patients with hypertrophic corrugator and procerus muscles.
2. The endoscopic dissection is eased by use of a tumescent injection. We prefer to use a dilute local mixture (0.3 ml of 2% lidocaine with epinephrine 1:100,000 with 2.7 ml of normal saline) to slightly elevate the periosteum across the glabellar region. The 2% lidocaine with epinephrine 1:100,000 is drawn from a 50-ml vial in which 150 units of hyaluronidase and 5 ml of sodium bicarbonate 8.4% have been added.
3. An alternate "tumescent" technique is used to elevate the scalp across the forehead down to the glabellar area. A 50-ml vial of 2% lidocaine with 1:100,000 epinephrine is drawn up and injected into a liter bag of IV normal saline or lactated ringers (creates a mixture with 0.1% lidocaine and 1:2,000,000 or 0.5 µg/ml epinephrine). For an additional anti-inflammatory effect 4 ml of Kenalog 40 mg/ml can be added to the bag. IV tubing is placed through a tumescent pump or the IV bag placed in a pump-up IV infuser. A 25 g spinal needle is attached to the tubing then placed through skin and into the subperiosteal plane. Under pressure the dilute local mixture is injected and spread subperiosteally down to the level of the glabella.
4. Because of the increased risk of postoperative hematoma formation, contour deformities, or unsightly splaying of the brow heads, we no longer transect the procerus and corrugator muscles unless there is significant hypertrophy of muscles in this area.
5. Some patients experience prolonged postoperative nausea and vomiting. One liter of intravenous fluid given towards the end of the surgical case lessens the risk of dehydration postoperatively.

66

Anesthesia Options in Endoscopic Forehead Lifting

Andrew S. Eiseman

The decision to use general anesthesia or local anesthesia with monitored anesthesia care is usually left up to the patient. The procedure can be completed quite comfortably with intraveous sedation. However, if the endoscopic forehead elevation surgery is to be combined with other procedures, general anesthesia may be a better choice simply because of the length of time the patient will have to remain still if awake. Even if general anesthesia is chosen, local anesthesia is infiltrated under the forehead region to aid in hemostasis and to provide postoperative analgesia. There are two main options when administering the local anesthetic. The first option is local infiltration of the entire forehead region. The second option is a tumescent technique that places dilute anesthetic in the subperiosteal plane centrally and under the superficial temporal fascia laterally.

Local Infiltration

If local infiltration is to be used, the entire forehead flap should be anesthetized. A 25-gauge needle is used to block the supraorbital and surpratrochlear nerves, the superior orbital rims, and the lateral orbital rims with either 1% lidocaine or 0.5% lidocaine with 1:200,000 epinephrine. Some surgeons use 0.5% bupivacaine with 1:200,000 epinephrine to provide some postoperative analgesia as well. A slightly higher concentration of local anesthetic is used in these areas because they are typically the areas that cause the most discomfort for the patient during enoscopic dissection. The rest of the forehead flap and the scalp incisions are then anesthetized with 0.25% lidocaine with 1:400,000 epinephrine. One slight alteration to the above technique is to create a "vasoconstrictive" tourniquet by infiltrating 1% lidocaine with 1:200,000 epinephrine along the zygomatic arches and along the coronal line. Then 0.25% lidocaine with 1:200,000 epinephrine is infiltrated beneath the forehead and temporal scalp. Finally, some bupivacaine 0.5% with 1:200,000 epinephrine can be infiltrated along the superior orbital rims.

Fifteen to 20 minutes is then allowed to pass before dissection ensues to allow time for the epinephrine to take effect.

Tumescent Technique

The tumescent technique of infiltrating anesthetic for endoscopic forehead surgery has the benefit of not needing to repeatedly penetrate the scalp with a 25-gauge needle. Additionally, it can facilitate dissection by establishing the correct plane. To perform the tumescent technique, a dilute solution of local anesthetic is mixed by adding 50 ml of 2% lidocaine with 1:100,000 epinephrine to a liter of normal saline. This creates a mixture of local anesthetic with 0.1% lidocaine (1 mg/cc) and 1:2,000,000 epinephrine (0.5 μg/cc). Before this mixture is utilized, the superior orbital rims, the lateral orbital rims, and the supraorbital and supratrochlear nerves are anesthetized with either 1% lidocaine with 1:200,000 epinephrine or 0.5% bupivacaine with 1:200,000 epinephrine. A small amount of this solution is also infiltrated around the central scalp incision and the two temporal incisions. A liposuction straight (Pocar, Tulip Medical) is used to create an opening in the central scalp incision through periosteum. A 3.0-mm spatulated liposuction cannula is then placed on a Toomey syringe filled with 40 cc of the dilute mixture. The cannula is placed in the subperiosteal plane and approximately 120 cc of dilute local anesthestic is delivered to the central forehead region. Confirmation that the cannula is delivering the solution in the correct plane is achieved when a globular elevation of the area is noted. If the elevation appears to have multiple lobules the plane is probably too shallow. A similar technique is then utilized in both temporal regions. The straight punch is used to create openings along the temporal incision lines down to the level of the deep temporal fascia. A 2.5-mm standard liposuction cannula is then used to infiltrate approximately 20 cc in each temporal region. Attention is then addressed back to the central region where the local anesthetic solution that is in the subperiosteal plane is milked inferiorly by applying pressure with both thumbs and pushing inferiorly. When this is complete, 15–20 minutes is allowed to pass to allow time for the epinephrine to take effect.

An alternate tumescent technique can be utilized if liposuction cannulae are not available. A 22- or 23-gauge 3-inch spinal needle can be used to deliver the dilute anesthetic solution. Instead of using a syringe to inject the solution, the solution can be delivered by placing the bag of dilute anesthetic in the pressurized bag used by anesthesia to push fluids. The entire forehead, temporal area, and scalp can be tumesced with a continuous delivery device through several injection sites. Additional more concentrated anesthetic like 1% lidocaine with 1:100,000 epinephrine is still given along the superior orbital rims. When using this alternative technique, remember that the spinal needle has a sharp end and care must be taken to prevent inadvertent damage or bleeding during the administration of the anesthetic.

Avoiding Anesthetic Toxicity

To avoid toxicity from either the local anesthetic or from the epinephrine in the solution, the surgeon must keep track of the total dose administered. The maximum dose of lidocaine that can safely be administered is 4.5 mg/kgm which is approximately 300 mg for a 70-kg subject. If epinephrine is added to the lidocaine, 7 mg/kg can be safely usedm which is approximately 500 mg for a 70-kg subject.[1] A safe dose of epinephrine in the absence of an inhalational anesthetic is 3–5 μg/kg/hr.[2] For a 70-kg subject this would equate to 210–350 ml/hr of a 1:1000,000 solution of epinephrine that contains 1 μg/ml of epinephrine.

The following table gives the maximum safe doses for different concentrations of lidocaine with 1:200,000 epinephrine:

Anesthetic solution	Maximum safe dose
2.0% lidocaine with 1:200,000 epinephrine	25 cc[a]
1.0% lidocaine with 1:200,000 epinephrine	50 cc[a]
0.5% lidocaine with 1:200,000 epinephrine	70 cc[b]
0.25% lidocaine with 1:200,000 epinephrine	70 cc[b]

[a]Dose limited by lidocaine toxicity.
[b]Dose limited by epinephrine toxicity.

Tumescent Technique

If the tumescent technique is used, the epinephrine becomes toxic before the lidocaine does if 1:1000,000 epinephrine is used. Up to 350 cc/hr of 0.1% lidocaine with 1:1,000,000 epinephrine can be safely utilized. If 1:2,000,000 epinephrine is used, the lidocaine will become toxic before the epinephrine. Up to 500 cc/hr of 0.1% lidocaine with 1:2,000,000 epinephrine can be safely utilized. When the tumescent technique is used, the adjunctive local anesthetic that was injected into the superior orbital rims and along the supraorbital and supratrochlear nerves must also be added to the amount of tumescent solution used to prevent toxicity. Usually, 140–180 cc of tumescent solution is all that is needed to anesthetize the forehead region. This added to the more concentrated local anesthetic given falls well short of the maximum safe dose.

References

1. Xylocaine and xylocaine with epinephrine. In: Physicians'Desk Reference, 54th ed. Montvale, NJ: Medical Economics Company, 2000:638.
2. Steinsapir KD, Shorr N, Hoenig J, Goldberg RA, Baylis HI, Morrow D. The endoscopic forehead lift. Ophthal Plast Reconstr Surg 1998;14(2):107–118.

67

Endoscopic Forehead Rejuvenation: How to Set Up the Operating Room and Trouble Shooting

Asa D. Morton

1) Room assessment
   a) Determine most efficient setup for given room
   b) Viewing of monitor and positioning of light and camera cables important
   c) Ensure assistant or scrub will not interfere with view of monitor
2) Placement of the monitor and endotower
   a) One monitor
      i) At foot of bed or alongside at level of patients knees
      ii) Length of camera or light cable often insufficient for foot of bed placement
      iii) Prefer a cart with swing out table on top
         (1) Can position monitor over the patient while cart is off to the side of bed
         (1) Provides best viewing from either side of patient
   b) Two monitors
      i) A luxury; nice, but not necessary
      ii) One on either side of the bed at level of patient's knees
      iii) Ideal viewing for primary surgeon and assistant
3) Anesthesia
   a) Situated at foot of bed
4) Scrub and or assistant
   a) Situated on side of patient opposite monitor
   b) Back table
      i) Majority of equipment
      ii) Within easy reach
      iii) Placement doesn't interfere with surgeon's view of monitor
   c) Mayo stand
      i) Over the patient's chest
      ii) Holds endoscope and supports camera and light cable

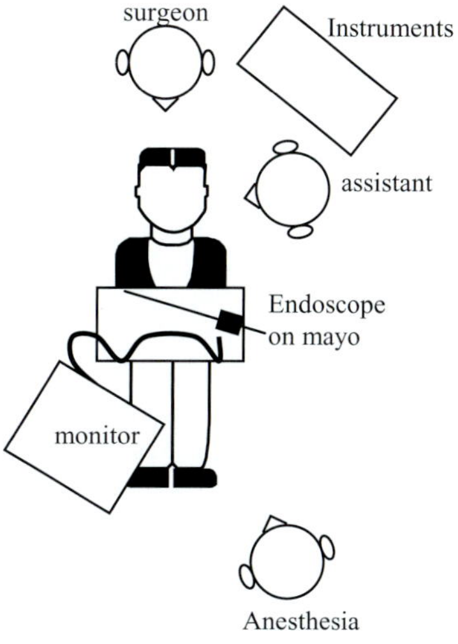

- iii) May keep a warm water thermos to holster the endoscope
  - (1) Decrease fogging by keeping scope closer to patient's body temp

5) Setup essentials
   - a) Know your electronics and specifics of camera connections
   - b) Sterilization
     - i) Cold (e.g., Steris) easiest on camera and light cable
     - ii) Can use sterile wrap (e.g., condom over cable) but makes it harder to manipulate
   - c) Drying and defogging
     - i) Ensure that all interfaces are dry—moisture in any of these areas will degrade image
       - (1) Camera coupler to scope eyepiece
       - (1) Camera cable to coupler
   - d) Confirm signal
     - i) Ideally before injecting or sedating patient
     - ii) The time to realize that the camera is not working is BEFORE you begin the procedure
6) Trouble-shooting tips
   - a) Picture not centered
     - i) Ensure that endoscope is seated and centered in the camera coupling ring
     - ii) Some monitors have an image magnification switch that may limit your peripheral viewing
   - b) No picture on monitor
     - i) Check for monitor power
     - ii) Check for cable from camera video out to monitor video in
   - c) Picture too dark
     - i) Auto iris on camera may be tricked by heme in the optical cavity
     - ii) Turn off and adjust light source power to appropriate level
   - d) Tissue color balance incorrect
     - i) Repeat white balance
   - e) Picture blurry or foggy
     - i) Check focus on camera coupler hand piece
     - ii) Blood on tip of endoscope
       - (1) Flush through irrigating port on the cannula
       - (1) Remove scope, wipe tip, and apply antifog
     - iii) Fluid has leaked into one of the other optical interfaces—check and clean:
       - (1) Camera coupler to scope eyepiece
       - (1) Camera cable to coupler

68

Endoscopic Forehead Rejuvenation: Equipment and Setup

Asa D. Morton

1) Endoscopic Video Setup
   a) Endoscope
      i) Types
         (1) 30° angle tip most useful
         (2) 4- and 5-mm-diameter shafts available
         (3) 17–20 cm in length
         (4) Has side connector for the light source
      ii) Cannulas
         (1) Match up with specific scope
         (2) Protects fragile scope from bending
         (3) Length and coupling mechanism must be compatible
         (4) Bill extends beyond tip of endoscope
            (a) Serves as retractor/elevator to create the optical cavity
            (b) Varied designs
               (i) Straight
                  1. Extension projects out beyond and parallel to the superior aspect of the endoscope
               (ii) Angled
                  1. Extension out beyond and angled up relative to the superior aspect of the endoscope
                  2. May give greater retraction but could limit placement into tighter spots
               (iii) Wide bill
                  1. Extension flares out laterally to support more tissue during retraction
         (5) Irrigating side port
            (a) Allows for attachment of syringe and pulsed irrigation to clear endoscope tip of heme
            (b) Sometimes useful for application of suction during cautery to clear smoke

- iii) Defog
    - (1) Helpful to keep the scope warm in a waterbath
    - (2) Antifogging solutions (FRED) available in the OR
        - (a) Can be applied to the tip of the scope
        - (b) Work well without the extra hassle of the water bath
- b) Camera
    - i) Coupler
        - (1) Attaches to the viewing end of scope
        - (2) Converts image to a signal that is processed by the camera box
    - ii) One vs. three chip systems
        - (1) Cost vs. clarity
        - (2) Most one-chip cameras provide more than adequate clarity and definition
    - iii) Focusing
        - (1) With system connected, place tip 1 cm from suture packet or other object with small lettering
        - (2) Adjust knob on coupler device
    - iv) White balance
        - (1) Flat white object is placed in front of endoscope, and when activated camera will auto adjust to provide most realistic color balance
    - v) Auto iris
        - (1) Most cameras have selection to allow camera to determine appropriate amount of illumination
        - (2) In some settings manual adjustment is helpful
            - (a) In a bloody field auto iris will underestimate the illumination needs
- c) Light source
    - i) Xenon is the preferred option
    - ii) Spend the money, skimp elsewhere if necessary
- d) Monitor
    - i) High-resolution 13- to 20-inch model preferable
    - ii) Although not essential, two monitors allow for ease of viewing from different surgical positions
- e) Recording source
    - i) Optional
    - ii) Vhs or still recorder

2) Hand instruments
- a) Essential
    - i) Periosteal elevator/dissector (central pocket)
        - (1) Straight
        - (2) Curved
    - ii) Temporal dissector
        - (1) Oval, dissects sideways as well as forward
        - (2) Separates superficial temporal fascia from superficial layer of the deep temporal fascia
    - iii) Periosteal spreader
        - (1) Upturned tip useful to spread periosteum after opening of arcus marginalis along superior and lateral orbital rim

- iv) Endoscopic scissors
  - (1) Right-handed surgeon can get by with only the left going
  - (2) Nice to have both right and left though
  - (3) Cutting periosteum
  - (4) Transecting corrugators and procerus
- v) Endoscopic grasping forceps
  - (1) Right-handed surgeon can get by with only the left going
  - (2) Nice to have both right and left though
  - (3) Dissecting out the corrugators from the supratrochlear nerve and vessel
  - (4) Stripping the corrugator and procerus
  - (5) Grabbing bleeding vessels to transmit externally applied cautery (instrument is insulated)
- vi) Nerve hook
  - (1) Come as right and left going
  - (2) Useful to dissect out the supraorbital and supratrochlear neurovascular bundles
  - (3) Also can be used to strip out the procerus

b) Nice to have instruments

3) Cautery
- a) External monopolar
  - i) Applied to insulated endo instruments
  - ii) Shielded frasier suction
    - (1) Red rubber covering
- b) Endoscopic suction coagulators
- c) Ellman RF suction coagulators

4) Boney fixation
- a) Drill motor or hand drill
- b) Anchors
  - i) Flush mount
- c) Screws
  - i) Permanent
  - ii) Bioabsorbable
- d) Posts
- e) Bone tunnel
  - i) Metal template
- f) K wire
- g) Tissue glue

5) Miscellaneous
- a) Skin hooks
  - i) Assist in introducing the endoscope
    - (1) Avoids blood on tip
  - ii) Temporal incision
    - (1) Elevates the superficial layers away from the deep
    - (2) Minimizes risk of dissection in the wrong plane
- b) Free needles
  - i) Straight or curved

69

Incision Technique for Endoscopic Forehead Elevation

Andrew S. Eiseman

Care must be taken when creating the incisions during endoscopic forehead elevation. Although the incisions are usually hidden within the hair line, meticulous surgical technique can limit both alopecia and scarring. Usually five incisions are made: one central, two paracentral, and two in the temporal region (Figure 69.1). All five incisions are made 1–2 cm within the hair line and are usually 1–2 cm in length.

Central Incision

The central incision is usually placed directly above the center of the glabella. It is 1–2 cm within the hair line and is usually made in a radial fashion 1–2 cm in length. The hair is either parted with the surgeon's fingers or can be confined with sterile clips or rubber bands. The incision is made with a number 15 blade scalpel parallel to the direction of the follicles to prevent damage and alopecia. It is carried down to the level of the bone through periosteum. Spot hemostasis can be accomplished with a bipolar cautery on as low a setting as required to stop bleeding. Minimizing cautery around the incision and the hair follicles can minimize thermal damage and postoperative alopecia. If preoperative alopecia in the area of the central incision exists, the incision can be placed within a forehead furrow in a horizontal direction.

Paracentral Incisions

The paracentral incisions are usually placed 2.5–3.5 cm lateral to the central incision. These incisions are used at the end of the surgery for fixation and therefore correspond to the area where maximal elevation of the brow is desired. For women, maximal elevation is usually desired between the lateral limbus and the lateral canthal area. These incisions are made the same way the central incision is made. A radial incision is made with a blade down to the level of the bone. The incisions are placed 1–2 cm within the hairline and are 1–2 cm in length. If a patient has preoperative alopecia in the area of the paracentral incisions, these incisions can be made along the temporal fringe of hair or along a horizontal forehead furrow.

Temporal Incisions

The temporal incisions are also placed 1–2 cm within the hair line and are made perpendicular to a line drawn from the nasal ala to the lateral canthus of the eye. These incisions are usually made a little longer than the other incisions and are 2.0–2.5 cm in length. They are created with a scalpel parallel to the hair follicles. The initial incision is made through skin and dermis only. Two skin hooks are then used to elevate the skin away from the deeper structures, and a blade is used to carefully cut through the wispy tissues down to the level of the shiny deep temporal fascia. The temporal incisions must be made carefully and cleanly to prevent disruption of the superficial temporal fascia that will be anchored to the deep temporal fascia to provide lateral brow lift. Also, a clean incision allows easier identification of the different tissue planes that is very important to prevent superficial dissection and damage to the facial nerve. To ensure that the deep temporal fascia has been found, a small nick can be placed in it to allow identification of the red temporalis muscle beneath. Once the temporalis muscle has been identified, gauze, cotton-tipped applicators, or the blunt back of the blade holder can be used to dissect a small pocket directly above the deep temporal fascia. Further dissection to create the temporal pocket is carried out directly above the deep temporal fascia to minimize risk to the overlying facial nerve.

Prevention of Alopecia

Alopecia around the incision sites is a concern and can be minimized by adhering to several techniques:

1. Instrument compression at the incision sites can cause alopecia. To minimize this, the incisions can be made slightly larger, especially when new to the endoscopic technique. Additionally, care should be taken when the instruments are torqued forward since this is also placing pressure on the incisions. To minimize this, ensure that the patient's head is placed at the end of the table.[1]
2. Compression at the site of fixation and anchoring to the scalp can occur, especially if 14-mm fixation screws are used. To minimize this, a two-layered closure of the galea and scalp is recommended as well as using additional fixation points to distribute the tension.
3. Excessive cautery can cause alopecia by thermally damaging the follicles. This can be minimized in several ways. First, the patient should discontinue use of all anticoagulants to include aspirin and nonsteroidal anti-inflammatory agents for at least 2 weeks before surgery to limit the amount of bleeding. Second, adequate use of local anesthetic containing epinephrine can reduce operative bleeding and require less cautery.

Finally, if cautery is required during the case, minimizing its use around the follicles and using the lowest power necessary can limit its damage.

4. Cutting across follicles with the blade can cause alopecia. Care should be taken when performing the incisions to stay parallel to the follicles to minimize damage.

5. Follicular shock (telogen effluvium) is a more diffuse temporary loss of normal club hairs possibly related to undermining of the scalp with disruption of the hair follicle blood supply and traction on the scalp. Keeping the dissection subperiosteal minimizes but does not completely remove this as a risk for alopecia. The hair usually grows back, but careful preoperative counseling about the risk of alopecia is important.

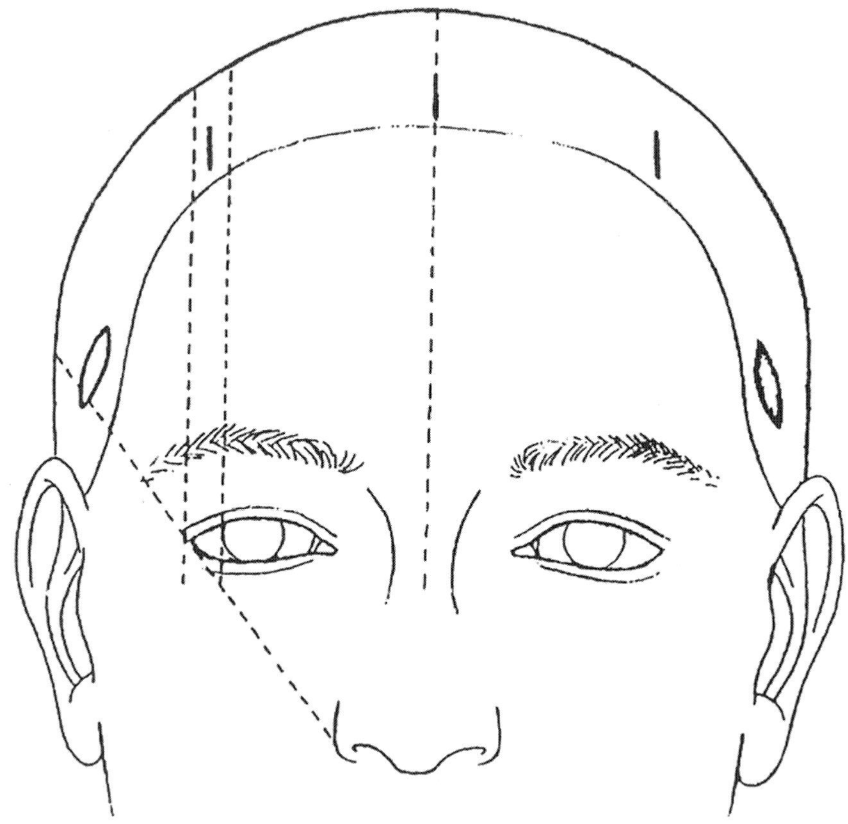

Figure 69.1. Usual five incision configuration for endoscopic browlift.

70

Endoscopic Forehead Elevation: Patient Marking and Preparation

Geva Mannor

Patient Marking:
- Number of incisions 3–6 depending on hair type and lift desired
- Balding patients—central incision may still be hidden
- Bald patients—central incision optional, other incision at hair fringe
- Incision length—1.5–3.5 cm
- Meticulous closure of long incision is preferred to traumatizing short incision
- Parasagital incision vector can define brow peak

Anatomic Landmarks:
- Supraorbital and supratrochlear bundles, VII branch, conjoined tendon

Individualized Landmarks:
- Corrugator and procerus muscles, rhytids

Hair Confinement:
- Wet or dry hair
- Rubber bands, hair clips
- Similar to "braids" little girls wear
- Port protectors

Prepping and Draping:
- Occiput should hang over head of bed
- Entire face, head, and hair should be prepped
- Entire face, head, and hair should be exposed
- Drape below chin and occiput

71

Endoscopic Midforehead Techniques: Improved Outcomes with Decreased Operative Time and Cost

Asa D. Morton

The design and implementation of any surgical procedure should first optimize outcome. Secondarily, procedural steps can be refined to maximize efficiency and minimize cost. Novel techniques for hair confinement and flap fixation adhering to these constructs are presented.

Optimum hair confinement provides for improved wound visualization and shorter operative times. A 4-cm open-ended cylinder is fashioned from the barrel of a 3 cc plastic syringe. A series of small dental rubber bands are double wrapped onto the barrel and rest parallel to each other. The hair is wet, combed, and parted to expose the incision sites. Alongside of each incision the hair is twisted into a tightly wrapped tuft. A small straight hemostat is then placed through the modified syringe barrel lumen and used to grasp the hair tuft 4 cm from the scalp. The hemostat is withdrawn pulling the hair tuft through the barrel. The hair tuft is pulled taut and the syringe barrel is held firmly against the scalp. The most proximal band is advanced off the barrel, capturing the hair tuft near the scalp. The procedure is repeated until all the incision sites are exposed. A small scissor can be used to snip the band free at case conclusion.

Numerous central flap fixation techniques have been described. Periosteal suture fixation bites placed anterior to the hairline may provide for better brow elevation while minimizing posterior shift of the hairline. The semicircular needle of the selected fixation suture is modified into the shape of a lazy "S" (author's preference 3-0 Mersilene with FS-1 needle) (Figure 71.1). The needle is loaded into a Webster needle driver with the tip directed back toward the surgeons hand and parallel to the instrument. The suture end of the needle is directed 180° from this position, running away from the surgeon's hand and parallel to the instrument tip. The loaded needle driver is inserted into the parasagital incision and directed down toward the brow (Figure 71.2A). The needle tip is palpated and directed to enter the periosteum approximately 2 cm inferior to the hairline. As the needle driver is withdrawn, a large slip of periosteum is captured and the needle directed to exit near the anterior apex of the incision and deep to the periosteum (Figure 71.2B).

For bone fixation a simple 1 × 4 mm titanium screw is used. It is placed near the posterior extent of the parasagital incision with the screw head left slightly elevated (Figure 71.3A). A #12 Frazier suction tip, just large enough to fit over the screw head, is essential to completing the fixation through a small 10mm incision. The Frazier suction tip is placed over the screw head and angled approximately 30° anterior to a vector perpendicular to the cranium. While the assistant holds the suction tip in this position, the surgeon ties the previously placed fixation suture around it (Figure 71.3B). The knot is rotated into the wound. The suction tip is angled posteriorly and gently twisted on the screw head. This encourages the suture loop to slip off and anchor on the exposed screw head. The rotational arc of the suction tip acts as a lever arm, adding a small amount of additional suture tension to suspend the flap (Figure 71.4).

Hair confinement improves wound exposure while minimizing the amount of hair that is dragged in to the wound. This confinement technique is quick and does not require special instrumentation. Rubber band removal at case completion is easily completed with scissors.

The central flap fixation technique allows for anterior and inferior placement of the periosteal fixation sutures. This translates to a more direct pull on the brow and better lift. Additionally, it may minimize posterior shift of the hairline.

Using simple titanium screws and the lever arm suture capture technique decreases cost, operative time, and wound size. Titanium screws are readily available and easy to place. Securing a suture over the small screw head can be difficult. The addition of a Frazier suction tip to guide the suture loop on to the screw head allows for a small incision and decreased operative time.

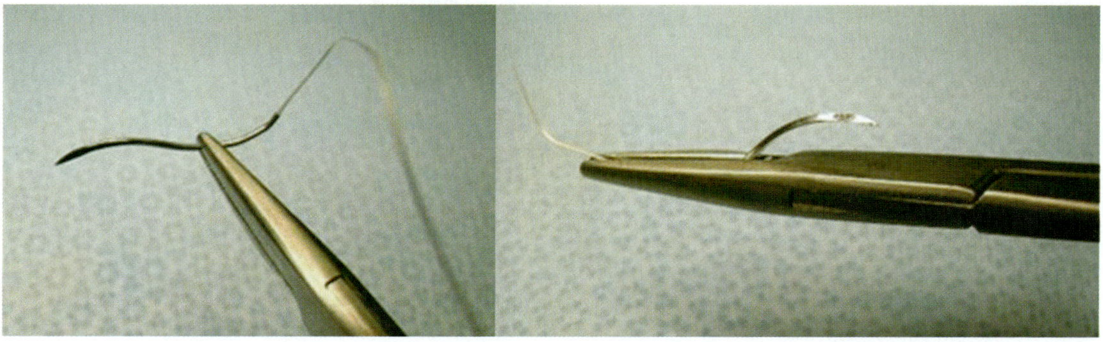

Figure 71.1. S-shaped bend in needle(left), then loaded into needle holder (right).

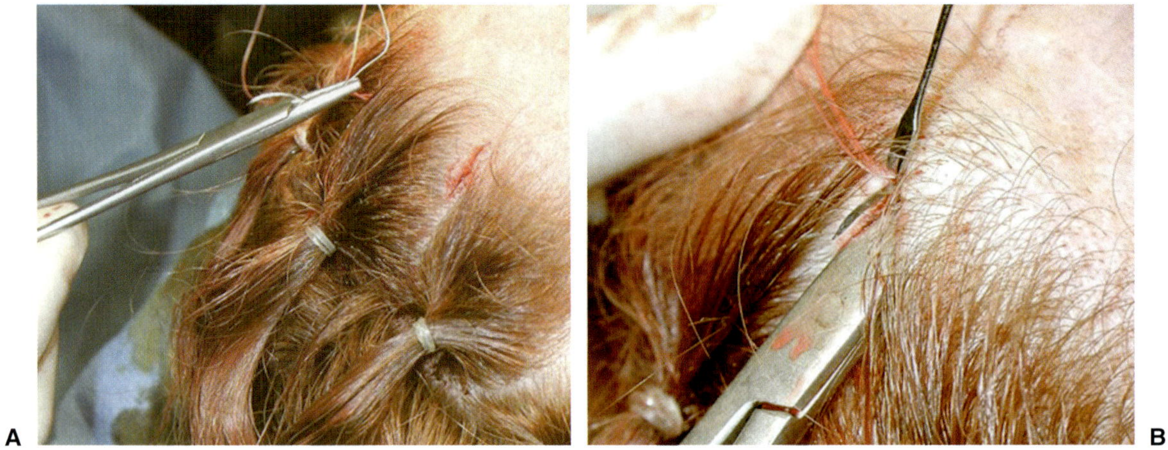

Figure 71.2. (A) Needle loaded to tag periosteium anterior to incision. (B) Needle on withdrawl ready to be retrieved.

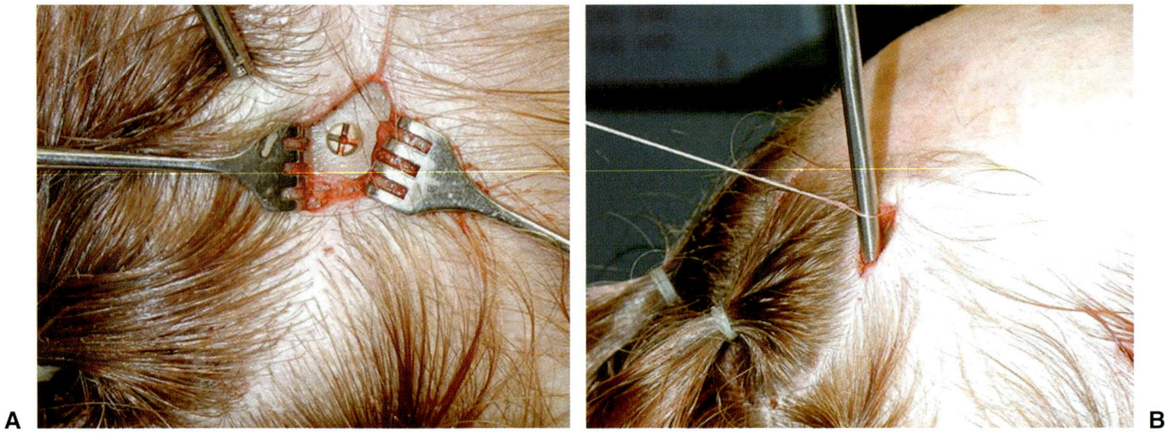

Figure 71.3. (A) Titanium screw placed through parasagittal incision. (B) Fixating suture tied over Frazier suction used to seal suture over screw.

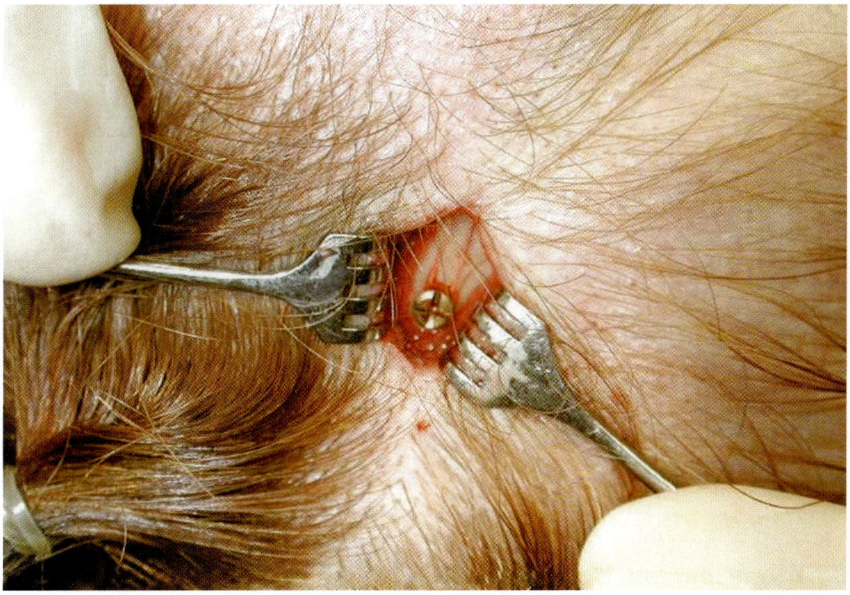

Figure 71.4. Mesilene suture shown seated over titanium screw.

72

Fifteen Principles of Enhanced Success in Endoscopic Browlift

Guy G. Massry

The endoscopic browlift can be a powerful surgical procedure. As surgery is performed within a closed space and with specialized instrumentation, attention to detail, knowledge of anatomy, and surgical experience is critical to attain successful results. Educate yourself with knowledge and practice.

With these basic principles in mind, I have found that that there are a number of caveats which both simplify the surgery and enhance surgical outcome:

1. In the majority of patients it is the tail of the brow that has become lax and ptotic. Elevating the body and head of the brow out of proportion to the tail yields unnatural results and unhappy patients. To accomplish this elevation, mark the temporal posthairline incision parallel to the tail of the brow. The marking should be an inch and one-half long and the same distance behind the temporal hairline.

2. I rarely perform paracentral boney fixation with screws or other means, as it has risks and is unnecessary with appropriate release.

If you choose paracentral boney fixation, the fixation point (and incision) should be somewhere between the lateral limbus and lateral canthus. The exact point will vary with individual anatomy.

3. Precise incisional markings are not necessary in our experience. We routinely use three incisions (one midline, two temporal). The anteroposterior midline incision is approximately 2 cm posterior to the hairline and 1 cm in length. Temporal incisions are 3 cm long 2 cm posterior to the hairline. The temporal incision is parallel to the tail of the brow, with its medial extent at the temporal conjoint fascia. It is not necessary to mark the incision before surgery.

4. Use high-volume, low-concentration local anesthetics. To avoid excess bleeding that will obscure the surgical view, inject 15–20 cc of 1% xylocaine with 1:100,000 epinephrine where bleeding will occur, to the incision sites, supraorbital rims, lateral canthus, and medial zygomatic arch. Inject 30–40 cc of 0.25% xylocaine with 1:800,000 epinephrine diffusely to the same areas and sites in between. This high-volume injection aids greatly in attaining appropriate hemostasis.

5. Avoid cautery subcutaneously at the incision sites to avoid hair loss. If bleeding occurs, reinject with the dilute solution mentioned above or with saline. If bleeding is brisk and cautery is necessary, do so conservatively.

6. When performing the temporal dissection, cut down to the white glistening surface of the deep temporal fascia. Entrance into and maintaining surgery within this plane will avoid inadvertent injury to the frontal branch of the facial nerve.

Be sure to connect the the temporal subaponeurotic plane with the central subperiosteal plane by dissecting in a temporal to central direction through the conjoint. This helps fascia to avoid inadvertent injury to the frontal branch of the facial nerve.

7. Be careful when performing glabellar muscle manipulation. Weakening the corrugators and procerus muscles will yield and elevated medial brow and will increase the interbrow distance. This may not be a desired effect. Discuss this with patients preoperatively, and proceed with caution. We tell the patient that the procedure elevates the ptotic brow, but does not eliminate frown lines (see caveat 15 regarding Botox).

8. In all cases, release the periosteum at the arcus marginalis along the entire supraorbital rim. This alone will yield a suboptimal brow release. It is also critical to spread and release the orbital portion of the orbicularis oculi muscle (the temporal brow depressor). We spread and release the muscle until the yellow brow fat pad is exposed. This allows unopposed elevation of the brow during the postoperative period and is the critical element in attaining appropriate temporal brow elevation. This step stabilizes long-term brow position and has obviated the need for paracentral boney fixation.

9. Postoperative dressings can increase periorbital swelling and eccymoses. It may be helpful to place a #10 French drain from one temporal incision to the opposite one, making sure the drain is situated inferiorly in the temporal incisions and along the orbital rim. The drain can be removed in 2 days and greatly reduces postoperative bruising and swelling.

10. Deep temporal fixation only (DTFO): I believe if appropriate release is achieved, only temporal fixation is needed in most cases. This is accomplished be securing the superficial to deep temporal fascia with two to three interrupted 2-0 PDS sutures.

11. Overcorrect brow height. This is necessary to compensate for the inevitable drop in postoperative height.

12. Close incisions at the skin only. Subcutaneous closure leads to hair loss.

13. Inject dilute Marcaine (bupivacaine) solution to the supraorbital nerve bundles postoperatively. This saves calls for pain control in the immediate postoperative period.

14. Botox is used pre- or postoperatively in the temporal brow area to weaken remaining orbicularis fibers and maintain brow height during healing.

15. Be careful when adding blepharoplasty to avoid creating an unnatural appearance and lagophthalmos. When we combine these

procedures, we do not excise orbicularis muscle. The browlift plus blepharoplasty adequately debulks the eyelid so orbicularis excision is superfluous and can only lead to difficulties.

Suggested Reading

Ramirez OM. Endoscopic subperiosteal browlift and facelift. Clin Plast Surg 1995;22:639–660.

Zimbler MS, Nassif PS. Adjunctive applications for botulinum toxin in facial aesthetic surgery. Facial Plast Surg Clin North Am 2003;11:477–482.

73

Dissection of Central Forehead and Temporal Pocket with Periosteal Release

Don O. Kikkawa

Dissection of Central Forehead Space and Scalp

A 15 blade is used to make incisions down to periosteum. Through the paracentral incisions, blunt elevator dissection in the subperiosteal plane is performed. The dissection extends laterally to the temporalis line and posterior to the vertex of the skull, permitting shifting of tissues posteriorly.

Much of the subperiosteal dissection can be performed safely and quickly in a blind fashion, taking care to stay directly on the bone. Blind dissection is stopped 2 cm above the superior orbital rim to avoid the supraorbital and supratrochlear nerves. It is best to palpate the supraorbital notch and mark a 2-cm area around nerve near the orbital rim. The supratrochlear nerves typically consist of multiple branches and are located medially to the supraorbital nerve. Temporally, dissection should stop before the temporalis line of fusion. The corrugator and procerus muscles can be identified under direct visualization in the glabellar region. The procerus fibers run vertically and the corrugator fibers run obliquely.

Initial dissection is best performed with the slightly curved endoforehead dissector. After initial dissection, a dissector with a greater curve is useful for lower on the forehead and nasal root. The parietal dissector can be used for posterior dissection. The endoscope can also be used to progress and dissect.

Dissection of Temporal Space

The temporal regions are then dissected. The flat pancake-shaped temporal dissector is best for this dissection. The frontal branch of the facial nerve lies in the superficial temporalis fascia (STF). Dissection should be done deep to this plane. Dissection in the wrong plane may result in paralysis of the frontalis muscle and superior orbicularis muscle. The facial nerve is easily avoided if dissection occurs along the surface of temporal fascia (TF) proper.

Through the temporal incision, the dissection begins with the subcutaneous dissection through the scalp. The thinner, delicate STF is encountered first. Blunt dissection with tenotomy scissors vertically will then reveal the TF. The TF can be scored with a 15 blade to visualize the temporalis muscle and ensure that the plane of dissection is correct. The optical pocket is then created between the STF and TF. Both the endoscope and temporal dissector are then inserted into this temporal pocket.

While viewing the video monitor, the surgeon elevates the STF from the TF taking special care not to injure the STF. The conjoined fascia or temporalis line of fusion is where the STF, TF, and periosteum meet. It must be approached from lateral to medial. Under direct endoscopic visualization, the conjoined fascia is elevated off the superior temporal line. Dissection from the central subperiosteal space toward the temporal zone creates the risk of either entering too deep and disinserting the temporalis muscle or being too superficial and damaging the temporal branch of the facial nerve in STF. The release of the conjoint fascia proceeds from superior to inferior. There exists a continuous optical cavity communicating the temporal zones, the central forehead zone, and the posterior vertex zone. The STF should be preserved for direct fixation to the TF after brow elevation and depressor release is complete.

The sentinel vessels will be visualized when dissection continues inferiorly and laterally from the temporal incisions. They are located roughly 3 cm from the lateral canthus in a line drawn from the nasal ala through the canthus. They should be avoided or cauterized. Some authors have remarked that these vessels are a landmark for the inferior most extent of the dissection. However, if midfacial lift or more extensive lateral canthal lift is desired, the vessels should be cauterized and dissection should be accomplished more inferiorly. It is important to release the lateral canthal attachments of the STF/SMAS to the orbital rim completely.

Release of Periosteum

Release of the periosteum is one of the keys to mobilizing the eyebrow and forehead flap. The flap is elevated along the orbital rim and glabellar region with blunt dissection. The superolateral orbital rim attachments in the region of the conjoined fascia are particularly strong and need to be released. The periosteum and arcus marginalis along the superior orbital rim should be mobilized. Dissection should also be advanced onto the radix of the nose. The entire scalp should now be now mobile.

The periosteum and periorbita after release from the rim must be cut and separated. This incision facilitates repositioning of the forehead periosteum and also allows access to the eyebrow musculature for muscle modification. The periosteum can be cut with endoscopic scissors, monopolar cautery, or the laser. A toe up dissector can also help to separate the periosteum. A gap between layers of periosteum should be visualized. Extreme care must be taken to avoid the supraorbital and supratrochlear neurovascular bundles.

74

Endoscopic Forehead Lifting: Dealing with the Central Brow Depressors

Asa D. Morton

1) Surgical Anatomy
   a) Corrugator Supercilii
      i) Arises from the frontal bone near the medial aspect of the supraorbital rim
      ii) Deep to the frontalis and orbicularis
         (1) Courses immediately adjacent to the periosteum at origin
         (2) Lateral course during which it becomes more superficial and interdigitates with the frontalis and orbicularis muscle
         (3) Fibers reach the skin lateral to the supraorbital nerve
      iii) Innervation
         (1) Temporal branch of the facial nerve
      iv) Pulls the brows together
         (1) Vertical frown lines
         (2) Appearance of anger or frustration
   b) Procerus
      i) Inferiorly the medial portion of the frontalis differentiates into the procerus
      ii) Origin
         (1) Bony attachment to the radix of the nasal bone
      iii) Innervation
         (1) Buccal branch of the facial nerve
      iv) Pulls medial brows inferiorly
         (1) Horizontal worry lines
   c) Depressor supercilii
      i) Superior and medial fibers of the orbital orbicularis oculi
      ii) Depression of the eye brows
2) Surgical Techniques
   a) Corrugator
      i) Periosteum is opened and spread
         (1) Exposes supraorbital and supratrochlear fasicles
      ii) Nerve hook used to gently separate out the fasicles of the supratrochlear

(1) Endograsper or scissors can also be used to spread tissue

iii) Endograspers are then used to reach between the fibers of the supratrochlear nerve to strip the fibers of the corrugator
(1) Fibers are grabbed low and stripped up
(2) Tailor the removal to the amount of overaction, severity of rhytids and patient's concern about an angry look

iv) Cautery
(1) With tumescent anesthesia see very little bleeding, but focal bleeders can be treated with suction cautery or insulated endoscopic grabbers
(2) Diffuse oozing best packed with pledgets and revisited in several minutes
(a) Epinepherine (1:50,000) soaked pledgets helpful
(i) 1 amp 1:1000 epi in 50cc of NS

b) Procerus
i) Periosteum elevated
(1) Exposes muscle
ii) Nerve hook placed just medial to the supratrochlear fasicles can be used to elevate a vertical strip of procerus
iii) Tip of the hook is placed between subcutaneous fat and the muscle and used to strip in a vertical fashion
iv) Strip of muscle can then be excised.
(1) Tailor the removal to the amount of overaction, severity of horizontal rhytids and patients concerns
v) Some use cutting cautery to excise muscle

c) Depressor supercilii
i) Generally do not specifically remove these fibers
ii) They can be significantly weakened during periosteal spreading
iii) With greater overaction muscle can be stripped between the supratrochlear and supraorbital nerves

75

Elevation and Fixation of the Lateral Brow and Canthus

Robert G. Fante

Elevation is accomplished by thorough dissection of the temporal pocket inferiorly to the zygomatic arch and including a subperiosteal dissection at the superolateral orbital rim at least down to the canthus.

Fixation of the released and elevated temporal flaps is thought to be primarily accomplished by re-adherence of the temporoparietal fascia flap to the deep temporal fascia. To ensure that this occurs at the proper height, intraoperative fixation is performed by placement of one or two sutures (2-0 or 3-0) to engage the temporoparietal fascia flap inferiorly and the deep temporal fascia superotemporally.

- A double skin hook can be passed into wound to engage the temporoparietal fascia flap permitting choice of best placement vector for suture. Traction with the hook will facilitate suture placement.
- Avoid superficial passage of the suture resultant skin dimpling.
- A rectangle of deep temporal fascia (exposing the temporalis muscle) can be excised under the temporoparietal fascia flap to enhance tissue readherence.
- Sutures are tied with careful attention to symmetry between the two sides, using surgeons' knots or the fisherman's knot.

Midface extension over malar eminence is accomplished prior to fixation of the temporal flap. Continued subperiosteal dissection inferiorly along the lateral orbital rim will expose the proximal portion of the zygoma and can be continued over the malar eminence until the convex curvature makes visualization impossible. The zygomaticofacial nerve will be encountered and should be safeguarded. Release in this area will enhance the lift in the medial temporal region.

Repositioning of the lateral canthus can be accomplished through the endoscopic approach, but is difficult. Other oculoplastic techniques are better suited for this purpose.

76

Fixation Methods in Endoscopic Browlifting

Andrea N. Hass

Numerous fixation methods are available for endoscopic browlifts. I have used the Bionix screws, Lactosorb screws, the Medtronix bone bridge system to suture through the bone, and currently the Endotine (Coapt Systems, Inc.) fixation system. Of these, I find the Endotine system to be the best, with minimal postoperative slippage of the tissues and minimal stress on the incision, allowing for a minimal scar once the healing is complete.

The Endotine fixation system uses molded absorbable-suture material in a triangular shape. It has up to five prongs pointing upward to grasp the tissues and a tab that anchors into the bone. If the patient wears bangs or has thick tissues, the implant can be placed anterior to the hairline to better hold. The implant is tender to touch for 1–2 months postoperatively and is palpable for 6–9 months. At 1 year's time the implant is no longer palpable.

A remaining frustration with browlifts, particularly endoscopic lifts, is residual laxity of the tissues over the temporal brow. This needs to be addressed with the patient preoperatively to set appropriate expectations. Despite suture anchoring the temporal incisions to the deep temporalis fascia, this "glide" of the tissues allows for a relaxation of the lateral brow. Sometimes this can be addressed with Botox in the subbrow area postoperatively.

Occasionally the browlift needs to be revised. Rarely the implant loses its hold, in which case prompt revision is best. More typically, initially happy patient over time desires more lift. Revising an endoscopic browlift is easier than redoing a coronal-style lift. Patients should be made aware prior to surgery of the increased risk of paralysis and numbness after surgery. When dissecting, care must be taken over the temporalis muscle to avoid paralysis of the muscle. Preoperative Botox is essential. A fresh location to anchor the Endotine is needed, and place the Endotine implants anteriorly.

77

Endosocopic Browlift with Deep Temporal Fixation Only*

Paul S. Nassif

Endoscopic Browlift with Deep Temporal Fixation Only

Endoscopic browlifting techniques have been progressively refined through experience and improvements in equipment. In general, the temporal dissection and temporal fixation have been standardized; however, different options for forehead dissection are available. Subperiosteal dissection with release (elevation, incision, and spread) of periosteum or subgaleal dissection and release of brow depressor musculature to the supraorbital rim are both effective techniques used in endoscopic browlifts. Methods of bony fixation remain a controversial topic since there are numerous methods. Some of these methods include absorbable and nonabsorbable screws, bone tunnels with sutures, fixation to soft tissue using absorbable attachment devices such as Endotine (Coapt Systems, Inc., Palo Alto, CA), and fibrin glue. We advocate deep temporal fixation only (DTFO) without bone fixation.

To maximize brow elevation with the endoscopic technique, the surgeon must release the periosteum from one inferolateral orbit to the other and release the brow depressor musculature (corrugator, procerus, depressor supercilii, and supraorbital orbicularis oculi). Following the browlift, all depressor vector forces should be eliminated to promote the maintenance of the newly elevated brow position since periosteal reattachment to bone takes approximately 6–12 weeks.

Temporal Lift

In patients with adequate medial brow position and ptotic lateral brow and lateral canthal hooding, an endoscopic temporal (temple) lift may be performed. A temporal lift is performed with the same principles and technique as the endoscopic browlift (surgical technique described

*This chapter is slightly modified from Facial Plastic Surgery Clinics of North America, Vol. 14, Nassif PS, Endoscopic brow-life with deep temporal fixation only (DTFO), 203–211, © 2006, with permission from Elsevier.

below) except that the medial border of the periosteal and brow depressor musculature release is the supraorbital neurovascular complex. The supraorbital orbicularis oculi muscle is the only brow depressor treated. The medial brow and glabellar region is not dissected, resulting in elevation of the lateral two thirds of the brow–lateral canthal complex.

Treatment of the Depressor Muscles with Botulinum Toxin

Botulinum toxin may be used synergistically with the surgical brow depressor musculature release in an effort to weaken the inferior vector forces and promote the maintenance of the newly elevated brow. Botulinum toxin is used to block the depressor function of the corrugator, procerus, depressor supercilii, and lateral supraorbital orbicularis oculi muscles.[11] Two weeks prior to surgery, the corrugator, procerus, and depressor supercilii muscles (medial brow depressors) are typically injected with a total of 20 units of botulinum toxin, and the lateral supraorbital orbicularis oculi muscles (lateral brow depressor) are injected with about 4 units of botulinum toxin on each side. No botulinum toxin is injected into the frontalis muscle since it acts as the only brow elevator.

Surgical Technique

Incisions

Most procedures are performed under general anesthesia. The incisions are then marked: one midline and two temporal (two paramedian incisions are made if bone fixation is to be performed). The anteroposterior midline incision is approximately 2 cm posterior to the hairline and is 1 cm in length, just large enough to allow the introduction of periosteal elevators into the subperiosteal space. The temporal incisions are 3 cm in length and are approximately 2 cm posterior to the hairline. The key to obtain a natural looking brow is to create a temporal incision parallel to the tail of the brow with its medial extent at the temporal conjoint fascia (Figure 77.1). The temporal incision orientation will help elevate the lateral half of the brow in a superolateral vector.

Temporal Dissection and Release of the Periosteum and Lateral Supraorbital Orbicularis Oculi Muscle

The temporal incisions are made and extended to the deep temporal fascia. A blunt elevator dissects over the deep temporal fascia inferiorly until a branch of the zygomaticotemporal vein called the "sentinel vein" is encountered (Figure 77.2). This is the inferior limit of the dissection without the use of the endoscope. A facelift scissors is used to connect the temporal incision to the central forehead incision by severing the temporal conjoint fascia (fusion of the galea and the temporoparietal fascia). The conjoint fascia is released with a periosteal elevator in an inferior direction to the level of the supraorbital rim. Adequate release of the conjoint tendon at the lateral supraorbital rim is an essential factor of the periosteal release.

The endoscope is placed into the temporal dissection along with the elevator visualizing the sentinel vein. This vein is a reliable marker for the frontal branch of the facial nerve, which lies superficial to the dissection on the undersurface of the temporoparietal fascia.[16,17] If possible, the sentinel vein is preserved and the dissection is performed medial and inferior to the vein. If the vein is cauterized, the bipolar forceps are placed at the base of the sentinel vein to help prevent a thermal injury to the frontal branch of the facial nerve. Lateral and slightly inferior to the sentinel vein, the zygomaticotemporal sensory nerve is encountered and is usually considered the lateral border of the dissection.

Continuing dissection in a medial diagonal direction towards the malar eminence over the superficial temporal fat pad, the periosteum is penetrated just inferomedial to the lateral canthus over the frontal process of the zygoma and malar eminence. To prevent elevation of the lateral canthus, an assistant places a finger in the interior aspect of the lateral rim at the lateral canthus. If the surgical plan calls for lateral canthal angle elevation, the lateral canthus is released. The periosteal release (elevation, incision and spreading) begins inferior to the lateral canthus onto the medial malar eminence and extends medially to the supraorbital neurovascular complex with care not to injure the nerve. Following the periosteal release, the lateral supraorbital orbicularis oculi muscle is meticulously released from the inferomedial orbit to the supraorbital nerve, exposing the yellow brow fat. This same procedure is performed on the contralateral temporal region.

Release of the Brow Depressor Muscles

For the temporal lift, this portion of the procedure is eliminated. The endoscope remains placed through the temporal incision and the periosteal elevator is placed through the central incision. The dissection is carried to the central supraorbital region and radix of the nose releasing the periosteum, avoiding injury to the supraorbital and supratrochlear nerves. Thorough corrugator, procerus, and depressor supercilii myotomies are performed. To ensure that complete myotomies have been performed, each nerve of the supratrochlear and supraorbital should be easily visualized without obstruction from overlying muscle fibers. Finally, harvested deep temporalis fascia placed at the myotomy site of the corrugator muscles may prevent reanastomosis of muscle fibers.

Brow Elevation and Fixation

Prior to fixation, a 10 French drain is placed and fed from one temporal dissection to the other positioned across the inferior extent of the dissection and exiting a puncture site superior to the right temporal incision. **If a complete release of all periosteum and brow depressor musculature is performed, the entire brow complex will elevate to an unnaturally high**

position without any tension (Figures 77.3 and 77.4). Brow fixation is achieved by securing the superficial temporal fascia medially to the deep temporal fascia in a superolateral vector with two 2-0 PDS horizontal mattress sutures while the brow is lifted laterally and overcorrected. The overcorrected brow will gradually drop to its final position after 3 weeks. The incisions are closed with surgical staples.

Results (Before and After Photographs)

Since January 2000, the author has performed endoscopic browlifts with DTFO in more than 150 patients with good results (Figures 77.5 through Figure 77.7). This procedure has the advantage of addressing the ptotic eyebrow while avoiding bony fixation. The endoscopic browlift with DTFO may be combined with the endoscopic subperiosteal transtemporal transbuccal midface lift to rejuvenate the aging forehead, brow, and midface.

As with any new procedure, thorough knowledge of the current literature and anatomy and observation of this procedure by an experienced surgeon should prelude your attempt in performing the endoscopic browlift with DTFO.

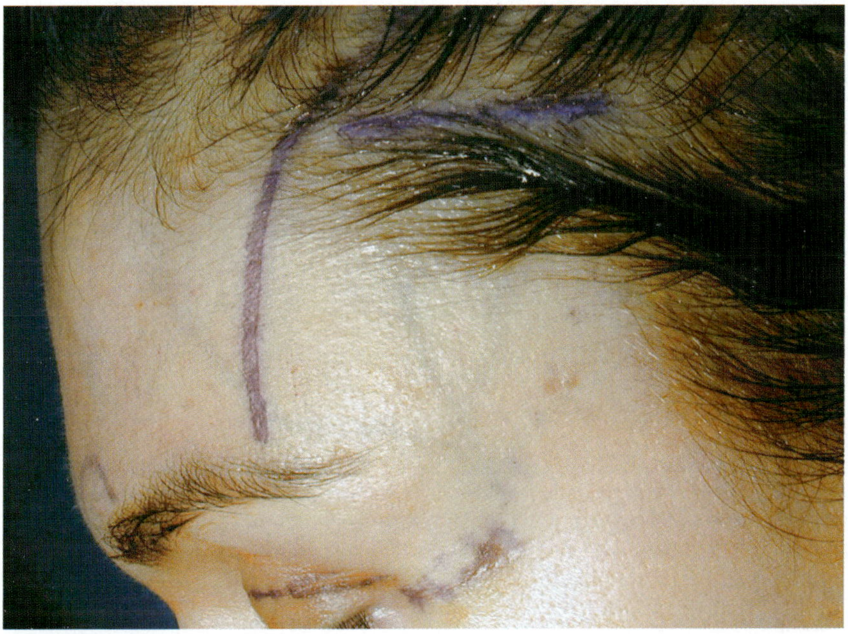

Figure 77.1. Marking of the temporal incision (large arrow) parallel to the tail of the brow with its medial extent at the temporal conjoint fascia (small arrow).

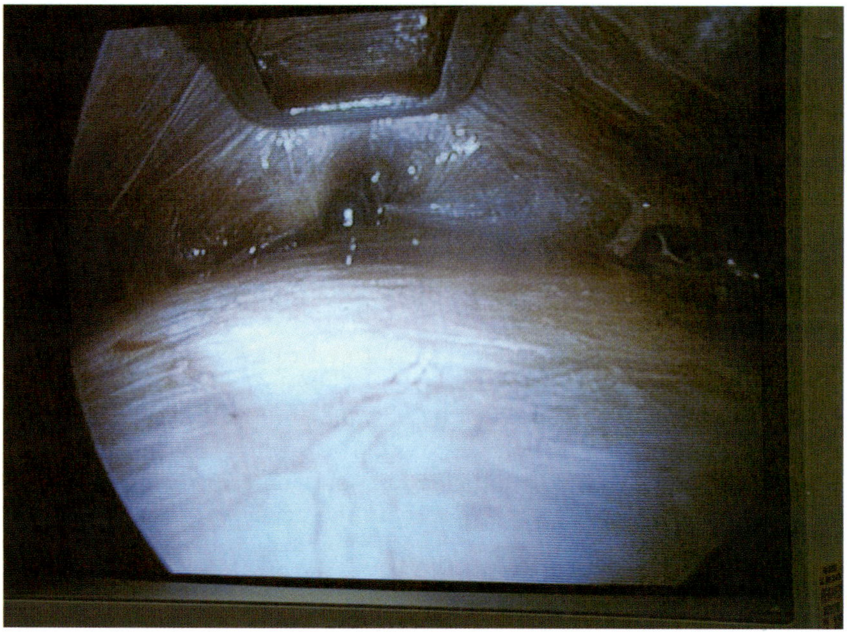

Figure 77.2. The temporal incision has been made and taken down to the deep temporal fascia.

A

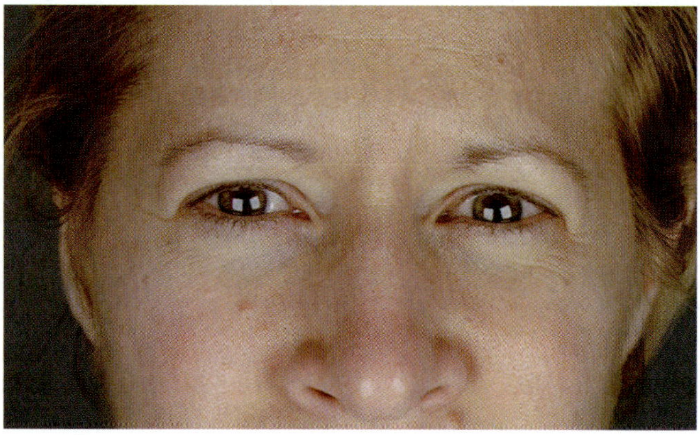

Figure 77.3. Patient before (A) and 1 week after (B) endoscopic browlift with deep temporal fixation only (DTFO). (C) Intraoperative photograph of the patient's elevated brow complex to an unnaturally high position after a complete release of all periosteum and brow depressor musculature prior fixation.

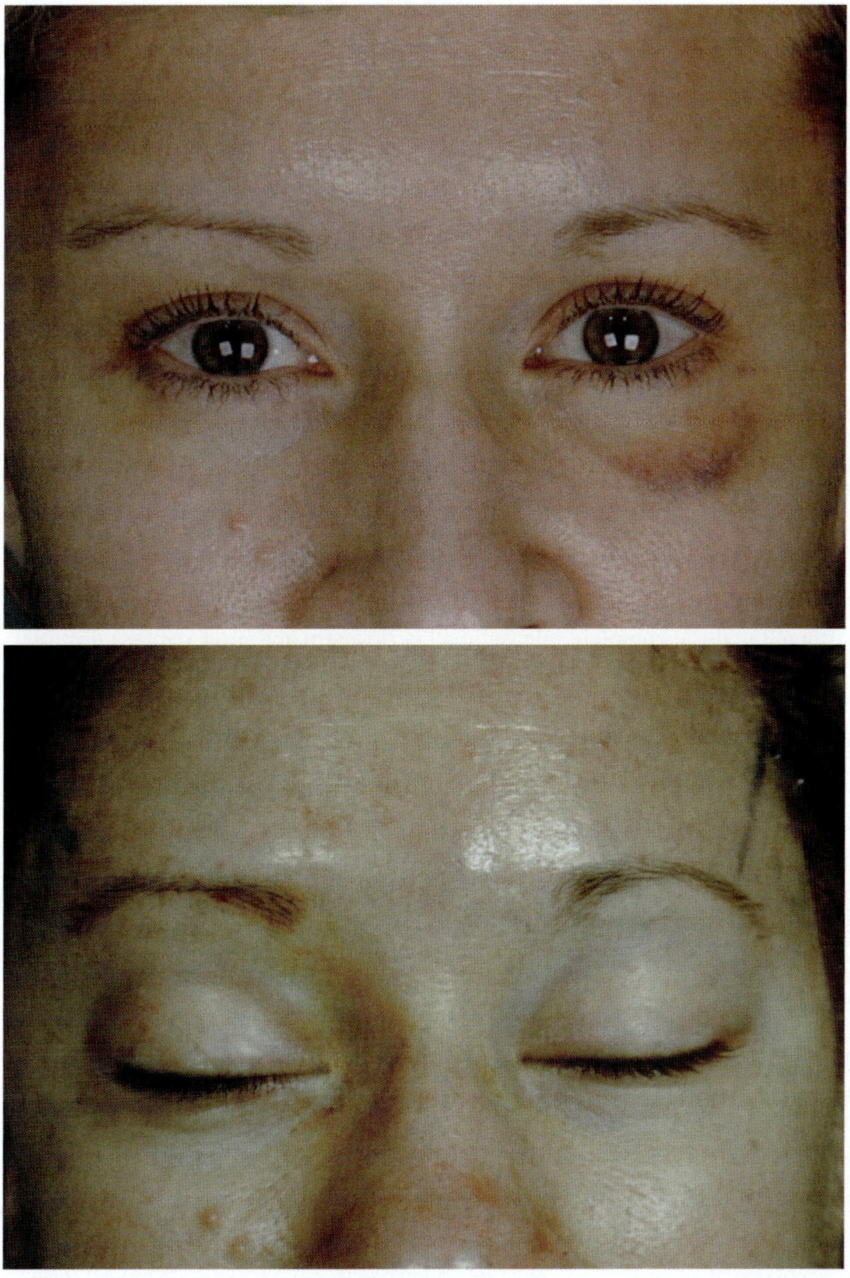

B

C

Figure 77.3. *Continued*

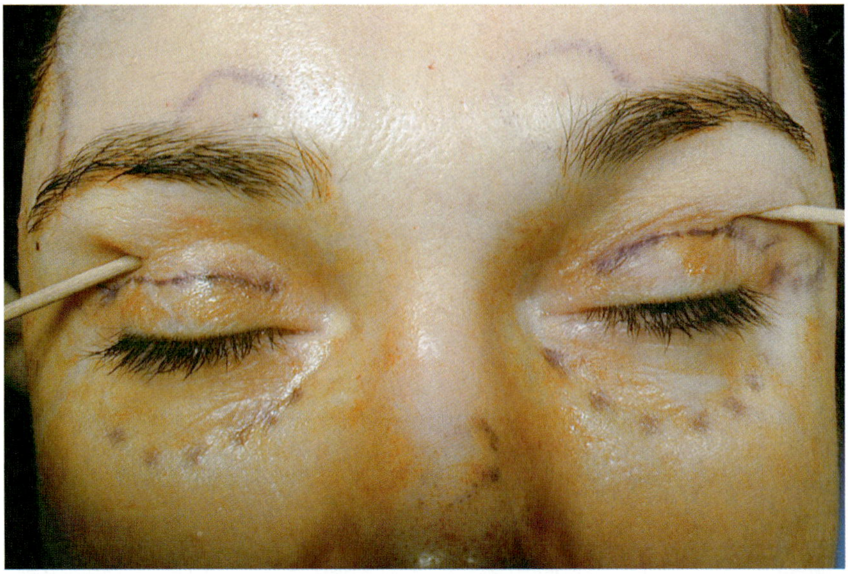

Figure 77.4. Intraoperative photograph of a patient's elevated left brow complex after a unilateral complete release of all periosteum and brow depressor musculature prior to fixation. Q-tips positioned at the inferior border of the supraorbital rim.

A

B

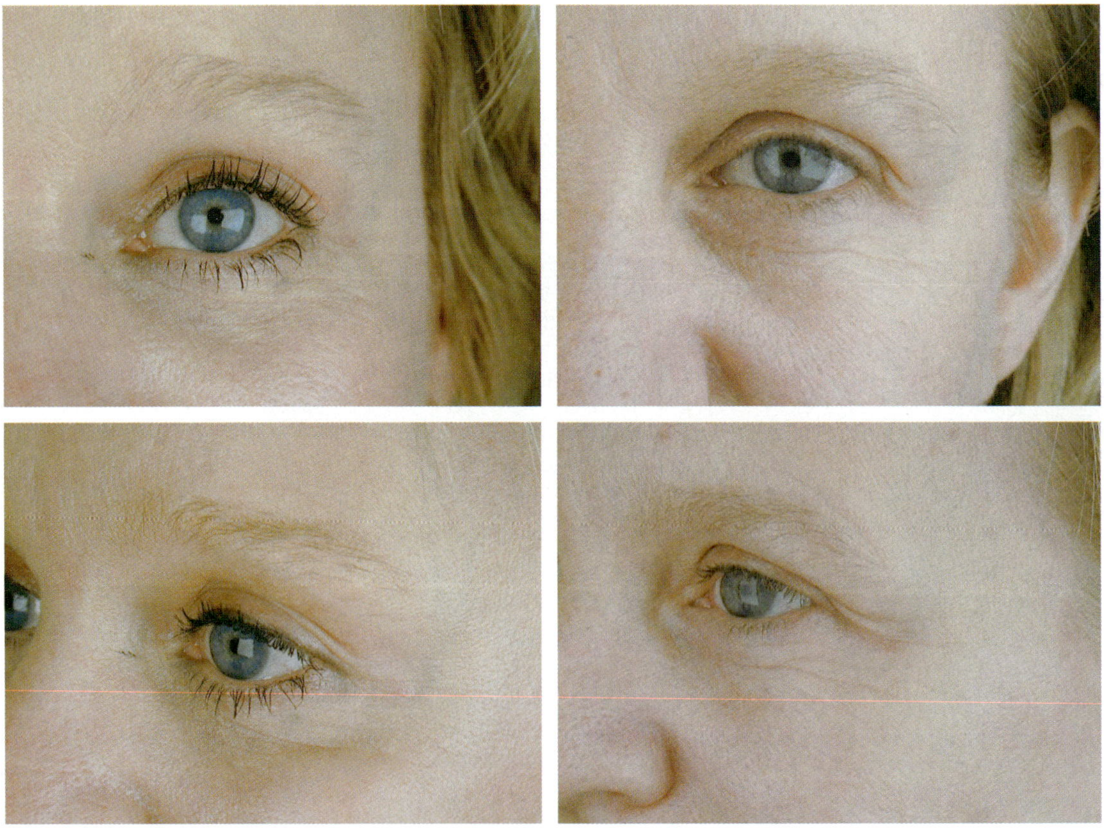

Figure 77.5. Middle-aged patient with brow ptosis and fat herniation of the lower eyelids—before and 20 months postoperatively following DTFO endoscopic browlift and bilateral lower fat repositioning blepharoplasty. Notice the orbital region is rejuvenated with the natural shape of the eyebrow kept intact. (A) Frontal of before (left) and after (right). (B) Left oblique of before (left) and after (right).

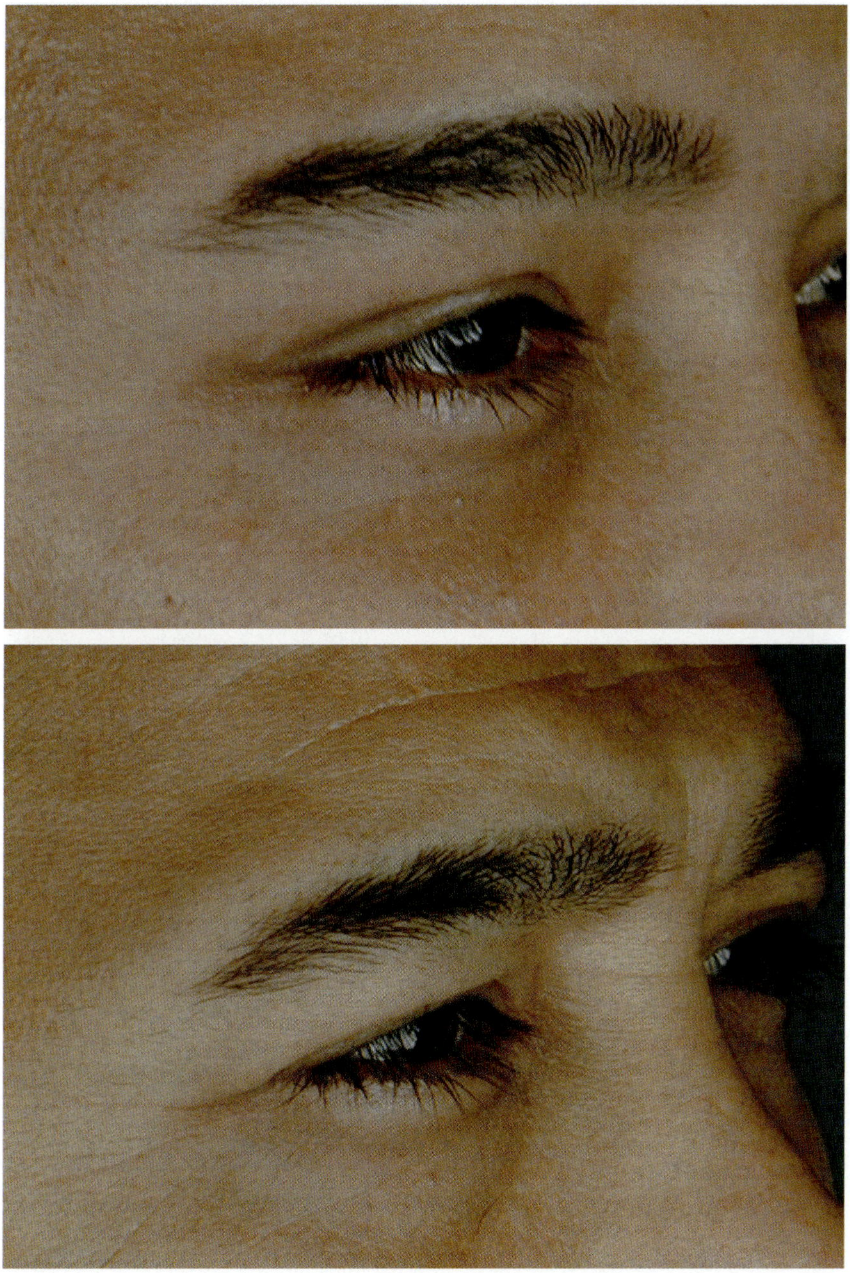

A

B

Figure 77.6. 43-year-old-male status post an upper blepharoplasty four years ago now complaining of a "tired look": right oblique of before (left) and after (right). The brow, especially in the temporal region, descends below the supraorbital rim causing temporal hooding and the supratarsal crease is covered by overhanging ptotic upper eyelid skin. Following a DTFO endoscopic browlift, the patient's brow ptosis is moderately improved.

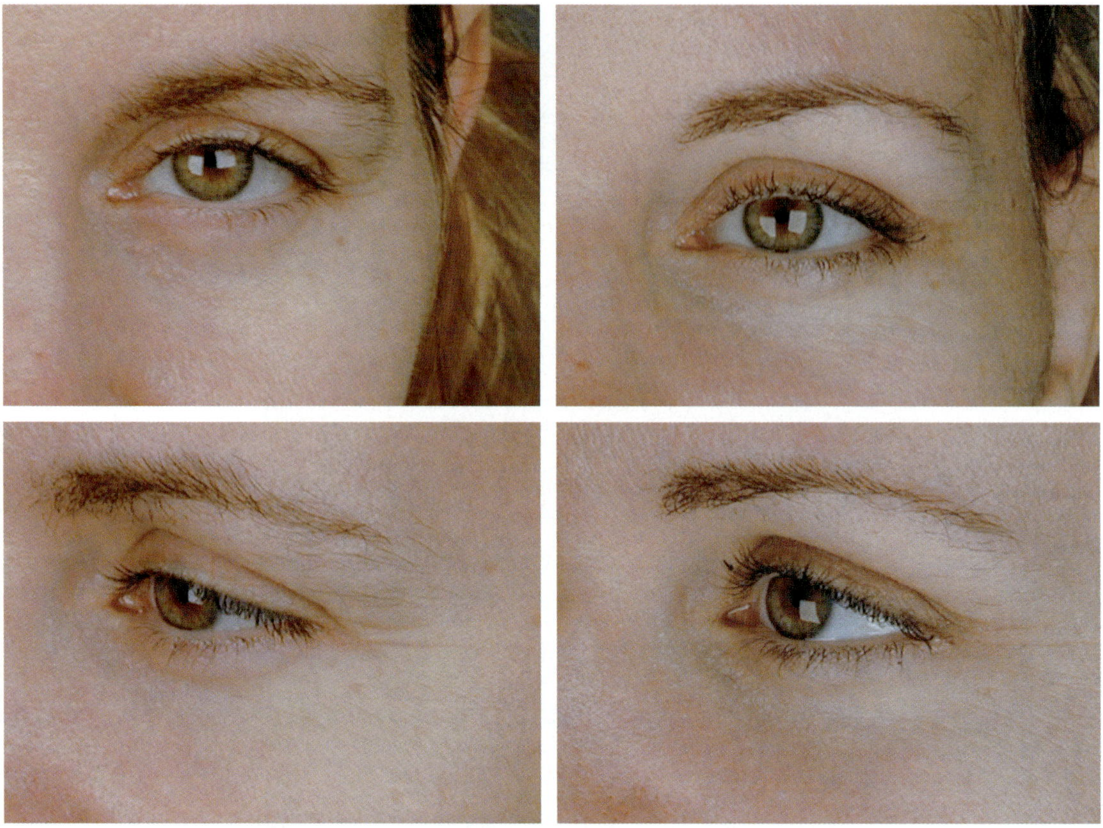

A

B

Figure 77.7. 41-year-old-patient with brow ptosis and fat herniation of the lower eyelids. Following DTFO endoscopic browlift and bilateral lower transconjunctival blepharoplasty, notice the significant medial brow elevation. (A) Frontal of before (left) and after (right). (B) Left oblique of before (left) and after (right).

78

Tridimensional Brow, Glabella, and Temple Enhancement with Micro Fat Injection During Endoscopic Forehead Rejuvenation

Oscar M. Ramirez and Camilo O. Reyes

Introduction

Endoforehead lift is one of the most common endoscopic procedures among the techniques in endoscopic plastic surgery. The endoscopic "browlift" or "forehead lift" is similar to the open procedures where unidimensional or bidimensional stretching of the brow and forehead soft tissues is performed. Since the early pioneering techniques of Dr. Ramirez, I have been gradually introducing several modifications to improve the outcome of the typical endoforehead. One of these modifications is the tridimensional or volumetric restoration of the upper face. Among the several modalities to obtain tridimensionality, We will deal in this chapter with tridimensional enhancement of the brow, glabella, and temple with micro fat injection.

Surgical Technique

The brow glabella and temple augmentation by micro fat injection is done at the completion of the endoforehead and after the fixation of the temporal and frontal flaps have been performed. The fat is obtained from the upper abdomen using 10 cc syringes and 2. 1-mm harvesting cannula of the "Cell Friendly" system of Tulip Biomedical Company (San Diego, CA). The fat is spun on a manual centrifuge at about 500 rpm/m. The water as well the oily elements are decanted and the fat is mixed with triamcinolone acetonide (Kenalog) in a ratio of 10 mg per each 30 cc of injectable fat. This mixture is then transferred to 1 cc Luer-Lock syringes for injection.

The injection is done using 0.9- and 1.2-mm diameter Ramirez type of microcannula of the Tulip "Cell Friendly" system. These cannulae are atraumatic to the fat cell as well as to the recipient tissues.*

---

*Dr. Ramirez is an unpaid member of the Medical Advisory Board of Tulip Biomedical. He does not receive any royalties for these canulas.

The micro stab wound incisions are done using an 18-gauge needle. The pearls of fat are injected in different parallel layers in the brow area, from the infrabrow to the suprabrow areas in the vertical plane, from the head to the tail of the brow in the horizontal plane, and from the subdermal to the galeal layer in the anteroposterior plane (Figure 78.1). An average of 2 cc (1–4 cc) of fat is injected to each brow. In the glabellar area the creases are injected first using the 0.9-mm cannula then using the 1.2-mm cannula fat is injected to the entire glabellar area including the area toward the medial infrabrow and under the head of the brow

The fat is crisscrossed in different directions and different planes from the subdermal to the subcutaneous layer (Figure 78.2). An average of 4 cc of fat is injected in the whole glabellar area. If the glabellar augmentation creates a deep nasoglabellar angle or if the patient has a preexistent deep angle, additional fat is injected to fill in this area. Fat also can be extended to the proximal nasal dorsum.

Fat also can be injected into the temporal areas. The temples become wasted with development of a concavity during aging. Injection can be done through the tail of the brow. The fat is injected in multiple layers starting deep into the temporal fascia proper, then into the intermediate temporal fascia, into the temporalis fascia proper, and then in between the temporoparietalis fascia and subgaleal fascia. I do not recommend the injection into the subcutaneous or subdermal plane because there are large veins in this area that can be easily traumatized and also because contour irregularities can be produced very easily. The amount of fat injection will depend on the depth and surface that needs to be augmented. I have injected as little as 3 cc and as much as 15 cc to each temporal area.

Each one of the puncture wounds used for the fat injection is closed with single 6-0 Prolene sutures. This prevents the irritation of the point of entrance by the free oil, which can mimic an acne pimple and also the potential of extravasation of the fat.

Fat harvesting is done by the assistant and preparation by the scrub technicians while the surgeon is performing the endoforehead. So, the actual increase in time for the fat injection part of the procedure is very minimal. It will take as little as 5 minutes and as much as 15 minutes depending on the amount fat to be injected.

The aim of the volumetric enhancement of the temple, glabella, and brow areas with micro fat injection was to enhance the esthetic results obtained with the typical endoforehead (Figures 78.3 to 78.8). It will not only give you a tridimensional volumetric augmentation, but also prevent the skeletonized or depressed look on those areas; this is commonly present after brow/forehead lift. The procedure does not add on significant morbidity or recovery time to the basic operation. It can be done as an isolated procedure or as a secondary surgery following the standard endoforehead operation. It can also be used as an isolated procedure for patients who do not wish to have the endoscopic brow and forehead lift. However, the muscle action in the glabellar areas will prevent a good take of the fat, and there will be recurrence of the glabellar creases very quickly. The brow may also tend to become too heavy if they are not lifted prior to the fat injection. The temple areas will get the benefit in either of those situations (operated or nonoperated cases).

Conclusions

Fat injection techniques provide a tridimensional or volumetric augmentation to the forehead area; this restores the volume lost as a consequence of the aging process. It also prevents some of the undesirable sequela of the standard brow/ forehead lift. The volumetric enhancement obtained provides to the patient the impression of vitality and youth. This gives a true rejuvenation to the brow and forehead areas. Representative views of patients with brow augmentation with microfat injection are included.

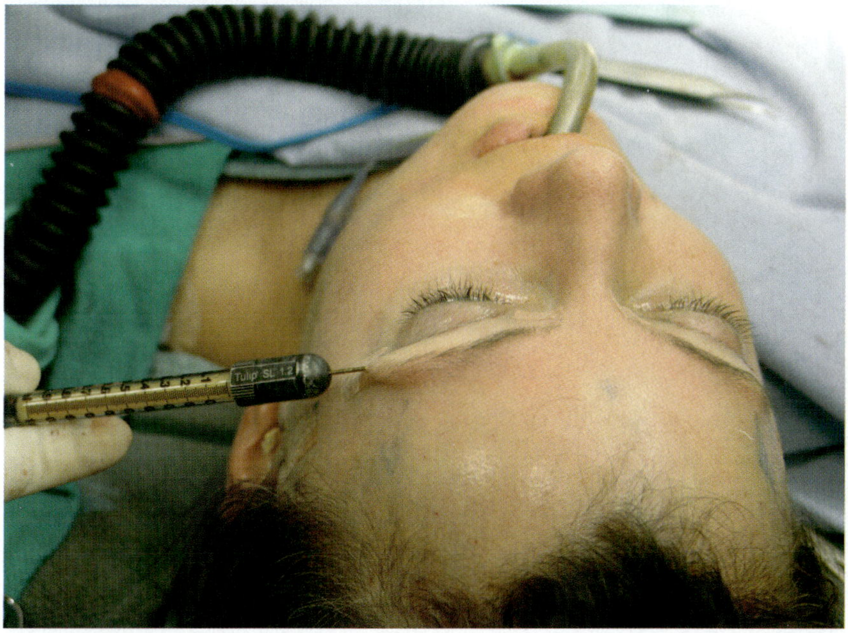

Figure 78.1. Fat is injected into the brow using the Ramirez "Cell Friendly" cannula of Tulip.

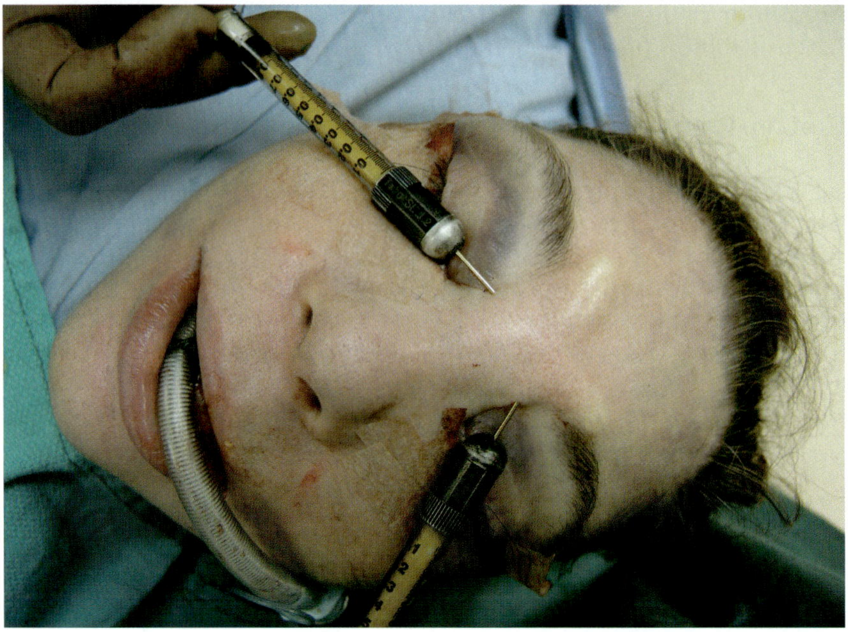

Figure 78.2. The crisscrossing technique for fat injection into the glabella.

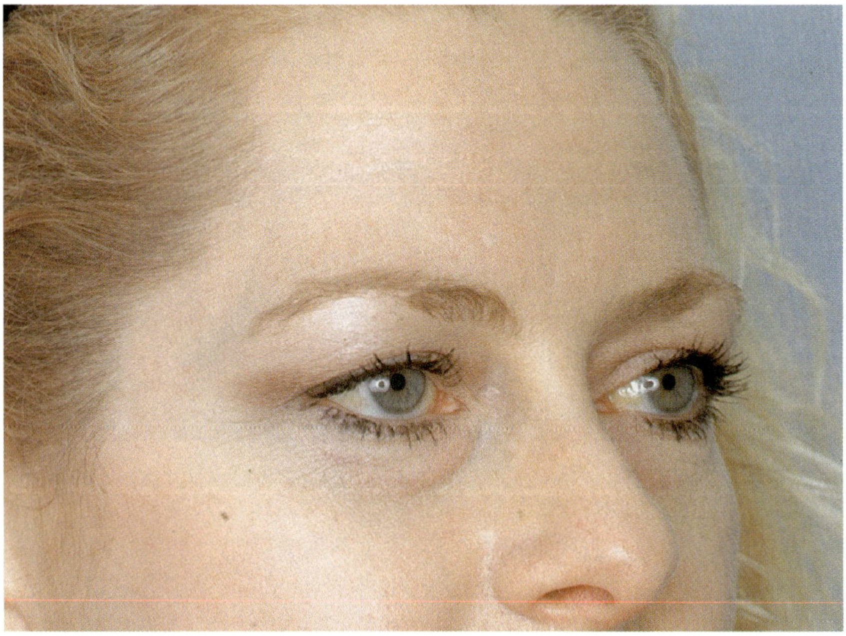

Figure 78.3. Preoperative frontal view. Observe the early sagging of the brow as well as a deflation process.

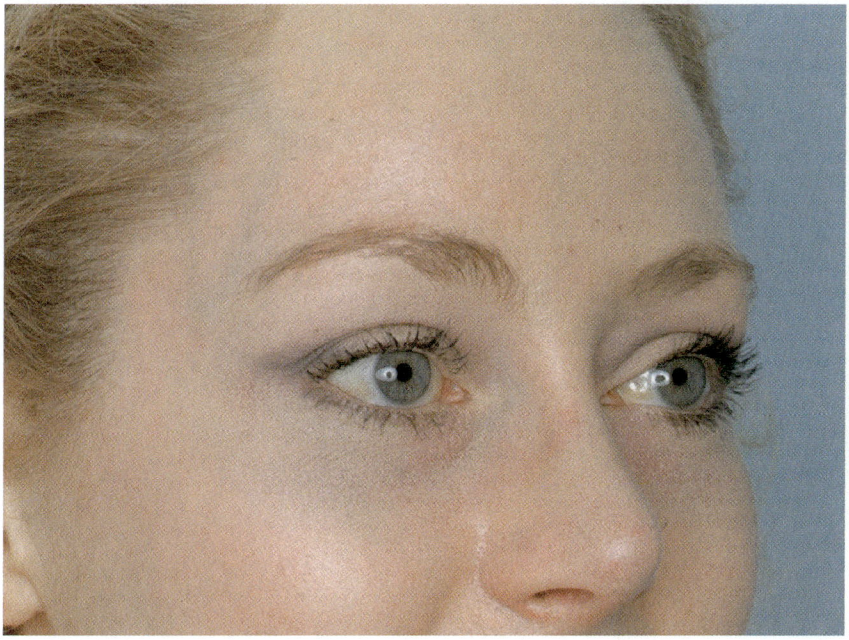

Figure 78.4. Postoperative frontal view of same patient. Notice the plump look of the brow and glabella.

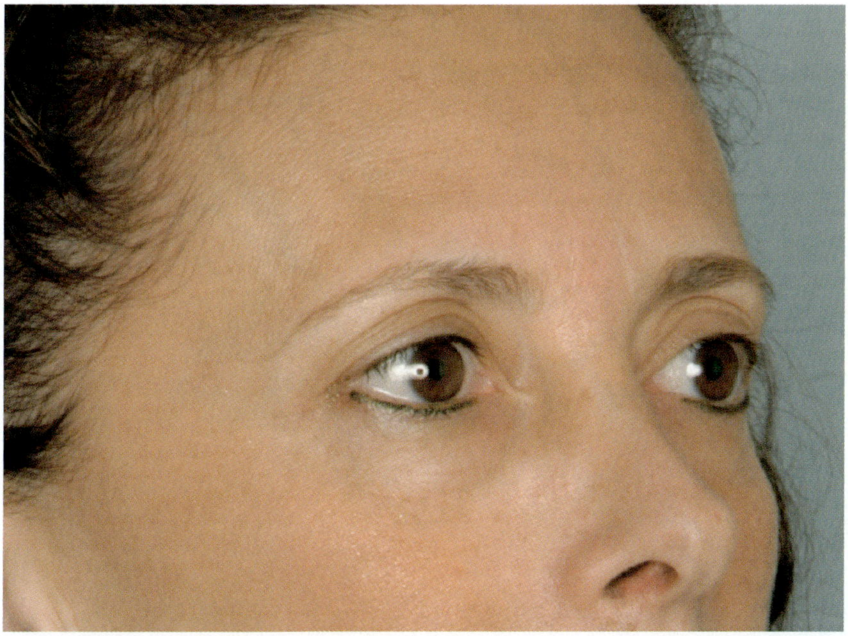

Figure 78.5. Preoperative $^3/_4$ view of a middle-age woman. Notice the thin deflated brow with orbital skeletonization.

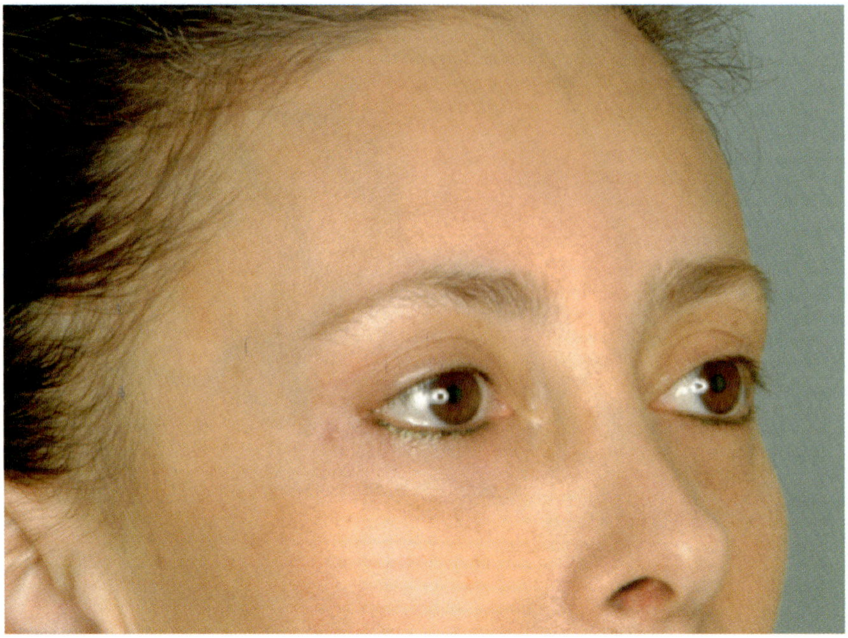

Figure 78.6. Postoperative $^{3}/_{4}$ view of same patient. Brow and orbital are full. No skeletonization. Also notice the volumetric augmentation of glabella.

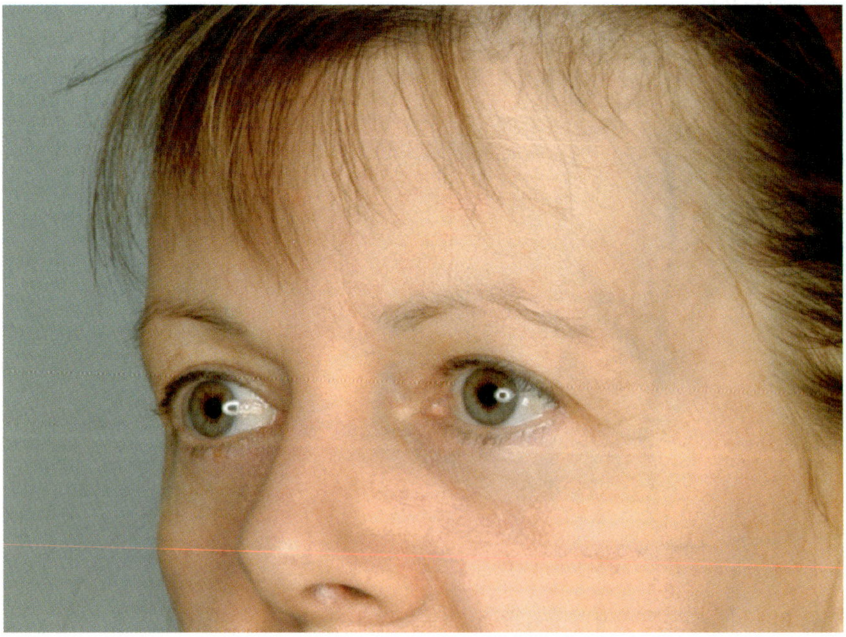

Figure 78.7. Preoperative $^{3}/_{4}$ view in another middle-age woman. Notice the deflated brow and loose infrabrow skin. Also notice the glabellar crease.

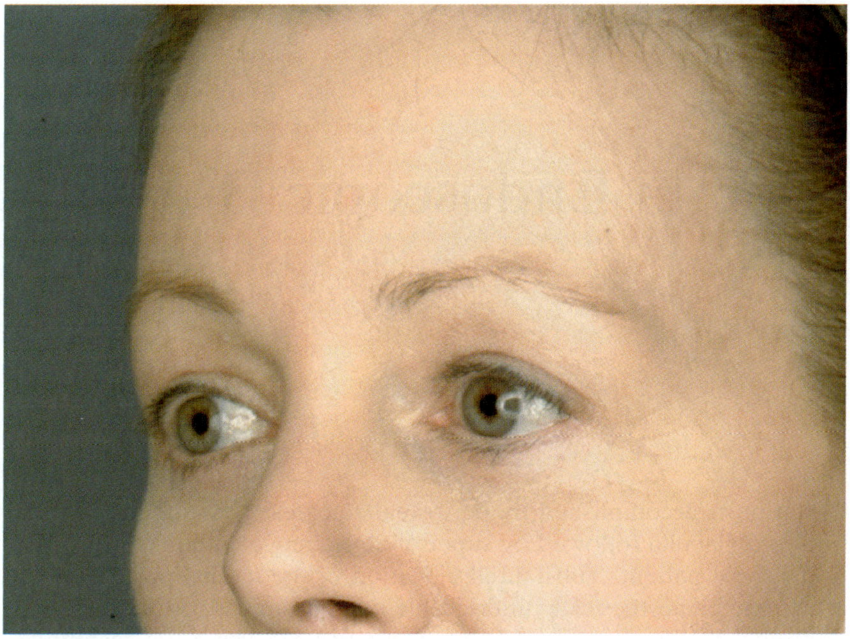

Figure 78.8. Postoperative $^3/_4$ view. Observe the plump and convex glabella as well as the subtle fullness of the brows.

References

1. Ramirez OM. Anchor subperiosteal forehead lift: from open to endoscopic lift. Endoscop Plast Reconstr Surg 2001;107:868–873.
2. Ramirez OM. Why I prefer the endoscopic forehead fift. 1997; Plast Reconstr Surg 100:1033–1039.
3. Ramirez OM. Classification of facial rejuvenation techniques based on the subperiosteal approach and ancillary procedures.Plast Reconstr Surg 1996;97:45–55.
4. Ramirez OM. Endoscopic forehead and face lift: step by step. Plast Reconstr Surg 1995;2:129–136.
5. Ramirez OM. Endoscopic full facelift. Aesth Plast Surg 1994;18:363–371.

79

Scalp Fixation in Endoscopic Browlift

Robert G. Fante

Elevation is accomplished by periosteal release at the superior orbital rims and glabella followed by superior stretching at orbital rim.

For some patients, substantial elevation of the medial portion of the brow may be aesthetically undesirable or undesired. For these patients, periosteal release is still performed but fixation using the techniques below may be unnecessary. Instead, a pressure dressing using Reston self-adhering foam (3M) will prevent hematoma and encourage early periosteal re-adherence. Mild superior traction can be applied with Coban or Kerlix wrap (see below).

Fixation of the released and elevated forehead flap is thought to be primarily accomplished by re-adherence of the periosteal flap to the frontal bone. To ensure that it re-adheres at the proper height, intraoperative fixation can be accomplished using several techniques:

- Endotine Forehead Bioabsorbable Implant (Coapt Systems, Inc.).
  - Holes drilled in outer cranial table with special bit provided with device. Holes are placed at desired elevation and through parasagittal scalp incisions to achieve eyebrow contour improvement.
  - Easier than suture techniques with saving in OR time, but additional expense of implants.
  - Fixation tines engage frontal periosteum while scalp flap is elevated to desired height. Flap can be lifted from tines and adjusted intraoperatively or within 2 weeks postoperatively in offices.
  - 3.0-mm device for women and men with male pattern baldness, 3.5-mm device for most men and women with thick, heavy scalp.
  - Carefully wash hair early postoperatively to avoid loss of fixation
  - Inform patient that implant will absorb in approximately 6 months and will be palpable and/or visible until that time.
- Percutaneous titanium screws and staples.
  - 12- to 15-mm-long screws, 1.2–2 mm in diameter (Leibinger, W. Lorenz, etc.).
  - Placed in outer cranial table at the parasagittal incisions in holes 2–3 mm deep using stopped drill bit.
  - Forehead flap is retracted posteriorly while drill hole is made so that the screw passes through the incision with the forehead elevated.

  - Staples bridging the sagittal wounds are placed behind the screw thereby fixating the forehead flap at the desired height.
  - Screws are removed in the office at 8–14 days.
  - Advantages include ease of use and intraoperative adjustment.
  - Disadvantages include risk of scalp necrosis, unsightly scarring, and possibility that periosteal re-adherence will not have taken place by the time of screw removal.
- Permanent titanium screws and galeal/periosteal suture.
  - 5-mm-long screws 1.5 or 2 mm diameter (Leibinger, W. Lorenz, etc.).
  - Placed in outer cranial table at the parasagittal incisions (avoid sagittal sinus in midline) in holes 3–4 mm deep using stopped drill bit.
  - Forehead flap is retracted posteriorly while drill hole is made.
  - At anterior end of incision, the periosteum and galea are engaged with long-lasting 2-0 or 3-0 suture on a cutting needle using a buried horizontal mattress technique. Avoid superficial placement.
  - Screw can be tied to the suture prior to placement in the bone, or the suture can be tied into a knot over an instrument and then placed over the screw head before it is completely tightened.
  - Advantages include long period of suspension and no need to remove the screw.
  - Disadvantages include difficulty of placing and tying the suture.
- Mitek® (Mitek Surgical Products) anchors and galeal/periosteal suture.
  - 4-mm countersunk screw anchor with preattached suture.
  - Placed in outer cranial table at the parasagittal incisions in holes 3–4 mm deep using stopped drill bit.
  - Forehead flap is retracted posteriorly while drill hole is made so that the screw is passed through the incision with the forehead elevated.
  - At anterior end of incision, the periosteum and galea are engaged using buried horizontal mattress technique. Avoid superficial placement.
  - Advantages include relative ease of use, lack of potentially permanently palpable screw head.
  - Disadvantages include increased cost of Mitek anchor.
- Lactosorb (W. Lorenz) screws and galeal/periosteal suture.
  - 5-mm absorbable screw 2 mm in diameter with eyelet for suture
  - Placed in outer cranial table through the parasagittal incisions in holes 3–4 mm deep using stopped drill bit and then a tap
  - Forehead flap is retracted posteriorly while drill hole is made so that the screw is placed within the incision when the forehead is elevated.
  - At anterior end of incision, the periosteum and galea are engaged with long-lasting 2-0 or 3-0 suture using a buried horizontal mattress technique. Avoid superficial placement.
  - The suture is passed through the eyelet prior to placement of the screw.

  - Advantages include relative ease of use, lack of potentially permanently palpable screw head.
  - Disadvantages include possibility of premature release of the suture, possible tissue reaction, and bone loss.
- Bone tunnel and galeal/periosteal suture.
  - Tunnel created in outer cranial table through which suture is passed to elevate the forehead flap.
  - Medtronics/Xomed Browlift Bone Bridge System assists in creation of bone tunnel.
  - Forehead flap is retracted posteriorly while bone tunnel is made so that the flap can be elevated.
  - At anterior end of incision, the periosteum and galea are engaged with long-lasting 2-0 or 3-0 suture using a buried horizontal mattress technique. Avoid superficial placement.
  - The suture is passed through the bone tunnel prior to tying.
  - Advantages include relative ease of use, lack of potentially permanently palpable screw head.
  - Disadvantages include relative difficulty of technique, possibility of diploic bleeding.
- K-wire suspension.
  - Flap is fixated using cutaneous K-wires passed into predrilled holes in the outer cranial table.
  - K-wires are removed with staples/sutures at 7–10 days.
- Occipitalis suspension.
  - Extra incision(s) created at posterior scalp.
  - Sutures engage the galea and periosteum at the anterior end of the incision and are tunneled to engage the occipitalis or simply the scalp using a curved suture carrier.
  - Advantages include lack of potentially permanently palpable screw head.
  - Disadvantages include relative difficulty of technique, possibility of creating scalp contour deformity.

Suggested Reading

Gallaher T, et al. An outer-table suspension technique for endoscopic browlift. Aesth Plast Surg 1997;21:262–264.

Hoenig JF. Rigid anchoring of the forehead to the frontal bone in endoscopic facelifting: a new technique. Aesth Plast Surg 1996;20:213–215.

Kim SK. Endoscopic forehead-scalp-fixation with K-wire. Aesth Plast Surg 1996;20:217–220.

Loomis MG. Endoscopic brow fixation without bolsters or miniscrews. Plast Reconstr Surg 1996;98:373–374.

Muller G. Endoscopic forehead lift: the subperiosteal pulling stitch. Aesth Plast Surg 1996:20:297–301.

Newman JP, et al. Transcalvarial suture fixation for endoscopic brow and forehead lifts. Arch Otolaryngol Head Neck Surg 1997;123:313–317.

Pakkanen M, et al. Biodegradable positive fixation for the endoscopic brow lift. Plast Reconstr Surg 1996;98:1087–1091.

Smith DS. A simple method for forehead fixation following endoscopy. Plast Reconstr Surg 1996;98:1117.

80

Closing and Dressing the Wounds in Endoscopic Browlift

Robert G. Fante

Closing the Wounds

As with any wound under tension, layered closure will provide better scar appearance. It is easy to place several buried interrupted dermal absorbable sutures (e.g., 4-0 or 5-0 Monocryl, Vicryl) at each of the incisions prior to placement of skin staples. For highly visible incisions in men with male pattern baldness, consider meticulous skin closure with 5-0 or 6-0 polypropylene instead of staples.

In patients with moderate to severe skin laxity, consider excision of an ellipse of temporal scalp prior to closure. This will contribute to the appearance and stability of the temporal browlift as the skin laxity will otherwise tend to neutralize the temporoparietal fascia lift.

Dressing the Head

Following skin closure, rinse the hair with warm saline and peroxide mix (1 liter saline to 8 oz. peroxide) to which baby shampoo may also be added. Ask the nurses for help to avoid making a mess. Consider use of the 3M 1016 drape, which has a built-in fluid collection pouch with suction drain. (This drape can be placed under the patient's head prior to the prep and will catch all fluids during the entire case.) Towel-dry the hair, consider detangling spray (e.g., Johnson & Johnson's for the kids), and loosely comb out any bad snarls. Bacitracin or Neosporin ointment is applied to the wounds.

Compression over the dissected areas prevents hematoma and the need for placement of a drain. It also encourages rapid readherence of the periosteum and temporal fascial layers. Smooth tape can be applied to the forehead, if desired. A typical compression wrap includes fluffs over the incisions, then an axial/coronal wrapping with Coban or Kerlix. Reston foam may also be applied to the forehead skin prior to the compression wrap. Watch the height and curvature of the brows as any dressing is applied to avoid altering the operative outcome.

The patient is instructed to keep the compression dressing in place for 2 days and then to wear a tennis-type headband for 1 week afterward. If Reston foam dressing/compression wrap is the only method used for central suspension, it is left in place for 5 days. Hair may be washed once the original dressing is removed.

81

Endoscopic Forehead Rejuvenation: Avoiding and Managing Complications

Asa D. Morton

1) Alopecia
   a) Avoid elecrocautery
      i) Incisions
         (1) 15 blade, one pass through all layers down to outer table of the skull (or through dermis in temporal area)
         (2) Tumescent anesthesia of scalp, forehead, and temporal pocket, as well as infiltration of the dermis around incision, minimize need for any cautery
         (3) Bipolar better if needed
         (4) Attempt to parallel follicles with incision
2) Depressed incisions
   a) Ensure good eversion of tissue edges when stapling
   b) Incisions in balding patients should be closed with sutures
   c) Consider periosteal buried stitch to close deeper layers before closing surface
3) Lagophthalmos
   a) Convervative brow elevation in patient with previous blepharoplasty
   b) Avoid damage to facial nerve motor fibers to eyelid protractors
4) Scalp itching
   a) Less than with coronal incision
   b) Associated with nerve regeneration around the incisions or downstream from stretched nerve branches
   c) Can be intense and last for several months following surgery
   d) Cool compresses may be helpful
5) Neurosensory
   a) Most patients experience transient numbness of the forehead and scalp in the distribution of supraorbital and suprarochlear nerves (branches of V1). May also have patchy numbness over temporal area following transection or stretch of the zygomaticotemporal nerve (branch of V2)
   b) Facial nerve injury
      i) Weakened protractors of eyelid (orbicularis oculii)
      ii) Facial nerve at risk in dissecting temporal pocket

            (1) Ensure dissection is directly on top of temporalis fascia proper (superficial layer of the deep temporal fascia).
                (a) Novice surgeons should verify by making small incision in the fascia, looking for the red muscle fibers
                (b) Dissection must be deep to superficial temporal fascia which is layer that facial nerve travels in
            (2) More inferiorly it is best to approach the zygoma from within the intermediate fat pad[1]
                (a) Ensures you are deep to the facial nerve

6) Asymmetry
   a) Contour and height differences possible
      i) Parasagital fixation defines brow arch position
         (1) Cautious measurement and preop assessment
   b) Vigilance for slipped fixation early postoperatively
7) Infection
   a) Usual precautions minimize risk
   b) Scalp very vascular, hence low risk
   c) Some use prophylactic antibiotics, I do not
8) Hematoma
   a) Oozing patients should have drain for 24 hours
      i) Rarely necessary in my experience
   b) May require aspiration or exploration
   c) Meticulous head wrap following surgery very important
9) Bleeding
   a) Patients, especially early in the surgeon's learning curve, should be counseled on the possibility of converting to an open procedure should significant bleeding be encountered
      i) Very unlikely
      ii) Insulated endocautery and grabbers very effective
      iii) Packing for 5 minutes with epi-soaked pledgets useful
   b) Careful preop counseling about medicines that can cause bleeding crucial
      i) Don't forget to ask about vitamin and supplement use
      ii) Vitamin E must be stopped
10) Cerebrospinal fluid leak
   a) Case report in a patient with previous neurosurgical procedure—don't forget to ask![2]
      i) Oculocardiac reflex—anesthesia beware![3]

References

1. Benvenuti D. Endoscopic brow lifts with injury to the supraorbital nerve and neuroma formation. Plast Reconstr Surg 1999;104(1):297–298.
2. Hwang IP, Pratt DV, Jordan DR. Cerebrospinal fluid leakage during endscopic forehead lifting. Am J Ophthalmol 1999;128(4):531–532.
3. Slade CS, Cohen SP. Elicitation of the oculocardiac reflex during endoscopic forehead lift. Plast Reconstr Surg 1999;104(6):1828–1830.

Section Three

Nonendoscopic Browlifting

82

The Direct Browlift: Focus on the Tail

John B. Holds

Described by Passot in 1919, the direct browlift is often reviled as a cosmetically unacceptable or inappropriate procedure. Nonetheless, this procedure may be employed alone or as an adjunct to blepharoplasty surgery with excellent functional and cosmetic results. The direct browlift provides the most predictable and effective (on a millimeter-for-millimeter basis) lift available.

The direct browlift employs a suprabrow incision, which may extend variably across the brow. When extended medially over the head of the brow, the incision is more visible, with questionable value as a cosmetic procedure.

Over the years I have shortened the incision and avoid the head of the brow. With age the tail of the brow tends to become more ptotic, lending an antimongoloid slant to the brow. Often the medial brow has little of no involutional descent. The absence of the frontalis muscle as an elevating structure in the temporal brow and deflational descent due to soft tissue thinning in the temporal fossa area contribute to this change.

If a direct browlift incision is limited to 3 cm or less in overall length and the incision is beveled medially paralleling the brow cilia, it will heal almost imperceptibly. It is important to utilize a meticulous layered skin closure to achieve ideal wound construction and avoid a permanently visible scar.

Patient Selection

Temporal brow ptosis with limited medial brow ptosis
Temporal hairline sufficient distance from brow to allow lift
Patient without history of scarring problems (keloid, etc.)
More acceptable in older patients with bushy brow and prominent forehead rhytids
Patient willing to accept possibility of visible surgical scar (incision readily apparent long-term in 5% of patients)

Procedure

Mark temporal brow over area of expected lift
In upright position, lift brow to determine amount of excision (Figure 82.1)
After anesthesia, incise skin, beveling medially to parallel brow cilia
Excise skin and subcutaneous fat, stopping at frontalis muscle
After hemostasis, layered closure:

1. subcutaneous layer inverted 5-0 Vicryl
2. deep dermis inverted 5-0 Vicryl
3. skin 5-0 nylon (prefer running vertical mattress medially, simple running laterally) (Figure 82.2)

Postoperative

Antibiotic ointment three times daily
Suture removal 6 days
Incision generally imperceptible once erythema fades at 3–6 months (Figure 82.3)

Complications

Cosmetically objectionable scar or contour abnormality usually responds to waiting 3–6 months for scar maturation. Occasional incisional revision required.
Medial undercorrection suggests the selection of an inappropriate procedure and may be improved with Botox therapy or further surgery.
Forehead hypesthesia may result from damage to the supraorbital or supratrochlear neurovascular bundles from inappropriate deep medial excision.

Conclusion

The direct browlift is an effective cosmetic technique for the limited correction of temporal brow ptosis. Patient selection and appropriate surgical technique are key in achieving an adequate surgical result.

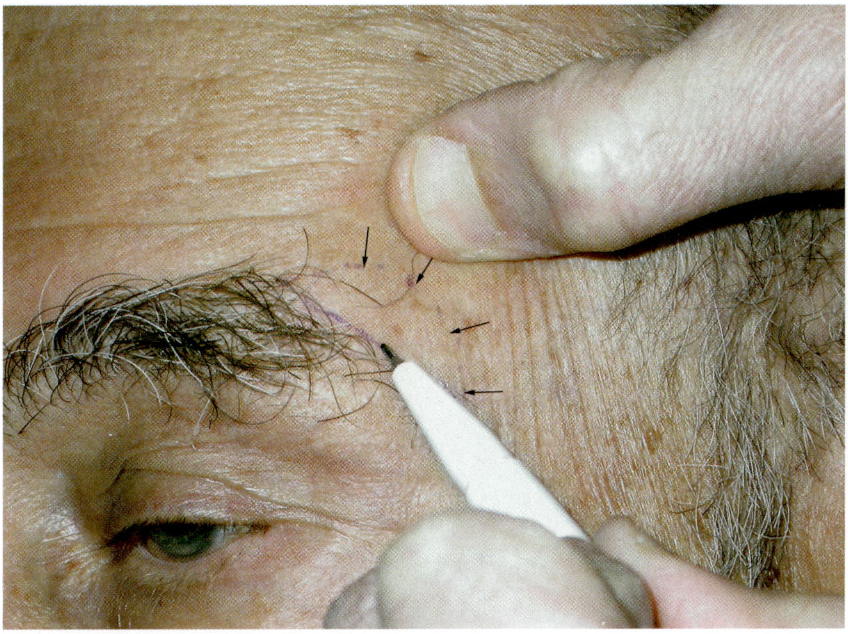

Figure 82.1. Demonstration of brow marking in the upright position to determine amount of temporal suprabrow tissue for excision.

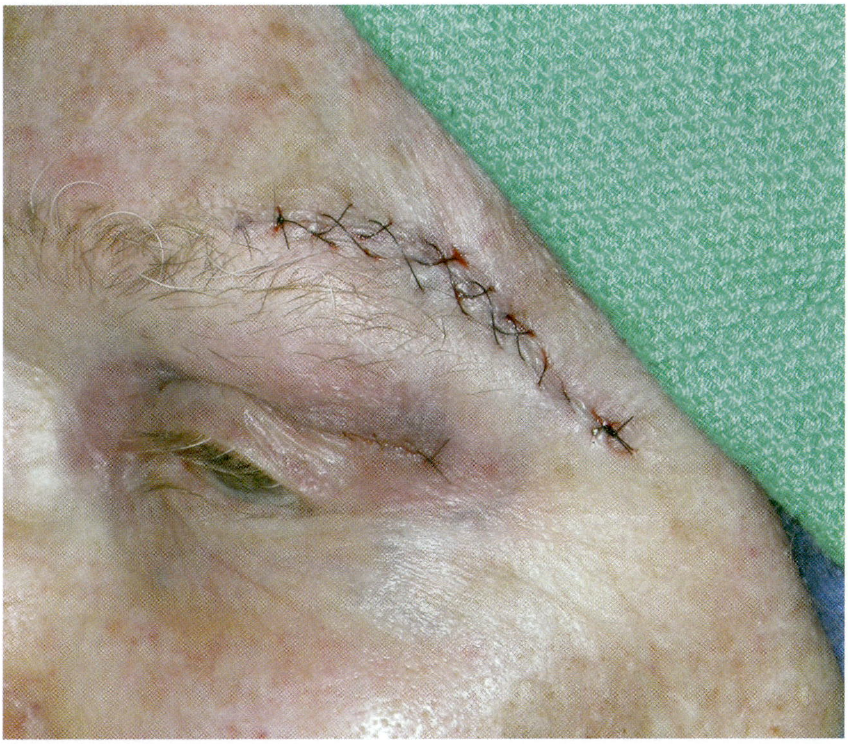

Figure 82.2. Vertical running closure that provides excellent eversion while breaking up line of closure.

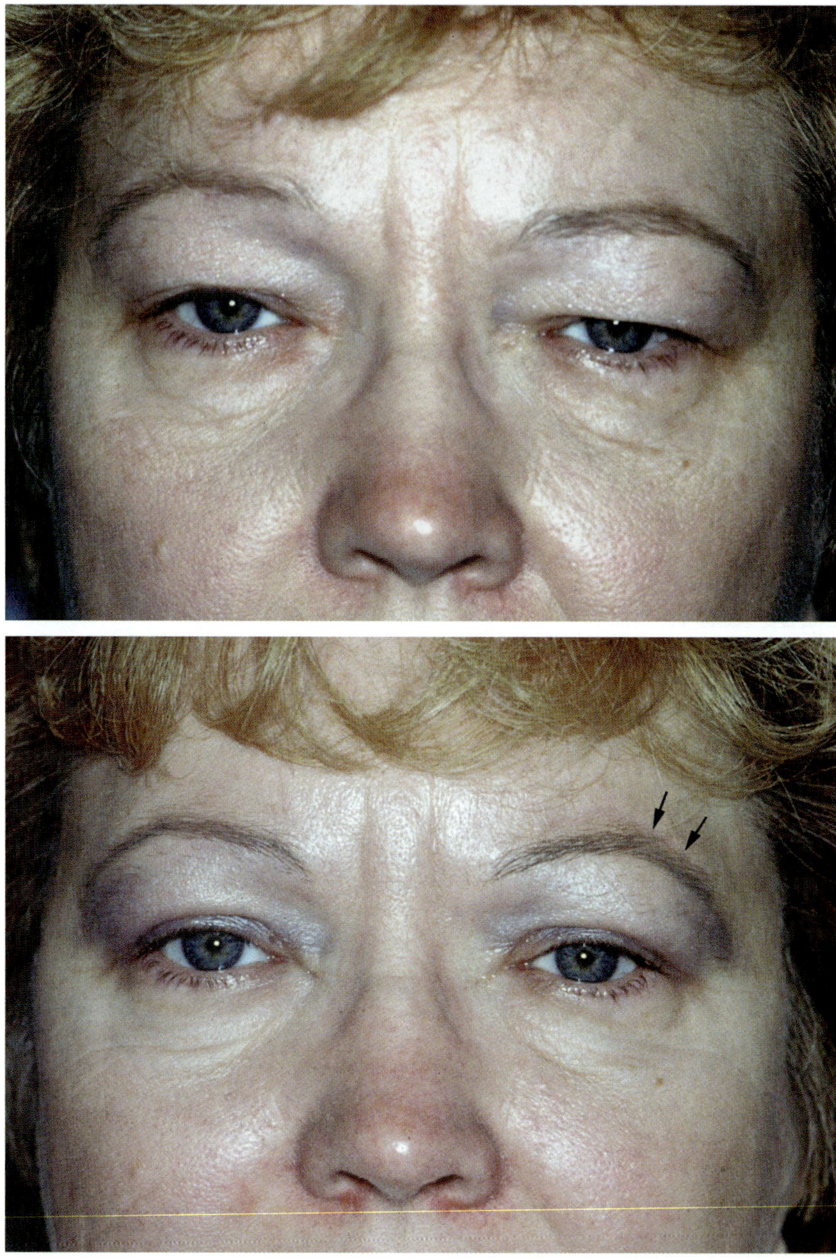

A

B

Figure 82.3. Patient (A) preoperatively and (B) 3 months postoperatively after limited upper blepharoplasty bilaterally with left direct browlift to correct congenital brow asymmetry. Note barely visible incision line.

83

Soft Tissue Augmentation of the Temporal Brow in Browlifting Surgery

David E.E. Holck, Jill A. Foster, Manuel A. Lopez, and Kevin A. Kalwerisky

Introduction

Over the past decade, improved appreciation of facial aging changes have modified management considerations for facial rejuvenation. In the brow region, traditional changes of soft tissue descent due to loss of skin elasticity and gravitational effect have been updated to include soft tissue and bony volume loss (deflation).[1,2] Thus, optimal management of age-related brow ptosis should address these changes.

Brow descent may be appropriately addressed using open (coronal, pretrichial, midforehead, direct) or endoscopic techniques, as well as less invasive transblepharoplasty techniques (transblepharoplasty internal browpexy, release of orbicularis retaining ligaments as well as weakening the brow depressors).[3–7] However, techniques describing aggressive resection of the retro-orbicularis oculus fat (ROOF) pads for aesthetic brow rejuvenation must be reconsidered.[7,8] Excess resection may only exacerbate the soft tissue deflation. Indeed, brow volume augmentation in conjunction with ROOF resuspension should be considered in lieu of soft tissue resection.

Several reports have described augmenting the temporal brow region utilizing soft tissue fillers and bony onlay implant techniques.[9,10] Soft tissue augmentation of this region is usually accomplished using temporary fillers (collagen and hyaluronic acids) as well as autologous fat injections. Bony volume augmentation may be facilitated through the use of a superior lateral orbital rim onlay implant to aid in the rejuvenation of the supero-temporal orbital area (MEDPOR, Porex Surgical Inc., Newnan, GA). We describe using the patient's own dermal/subcutaneous soft tissue obtained at the time of open or endoscopic brow elevation surgery to augment the temporal brow region to facilitate both brow elevation as well as to enhance the soft tissue volume in this area.

Procedure

At time of coronal or pretrichial browlifting, excised segments of scalp are taken (Figure 83.1). In the endoscopic technique, a crescent-shaped segment of temporal hair-bearing scalp is excised to augment the temporal lift. These excised tissues are used for the brow volume augmentation. The optimal segments are trimmed to approximately 10 mm × 30 mm. A no. 10 blade scalpel is used to excise the epidermis from the dermis and subcutaneous tissue, leaving a 3- to 4-mm-thick remnant (Figure 83.2). The subcutaneous tissue is placed along the temporal superior orbital rim. In an open technique, the graft may be sutured to underlying periosteum (Figure 83.3). In the endoscopic technique, the graft may be fixed to the ROOF using a percutaneous suture. The graft material is placed below the inferior row of brow hair and above the inferior portion of the superior orbital rim. This allows the soft tissue graft to act as a support for the brow as well as augment soft tissue volume.

The same material may also be used after extirpation of the corrugator muscles. In this setting, strips approximately 8 mm × 5 mm are sutured to the cut ends of the corrugator muscles (Figure 83.4). This prevents the muscle edges from reapproximating, further weakening the corrugators. Additionally, the augmented volume prevents subcutaneous depressions and dimpling in the area of corrugator extirpation.

With follow-up approaching 1 year, the soft tissue augmentation appears to persist (Figure 83.5). Indeed, magnetic resonance imaging at 9 months postoperatively demonstrates persistence of the graft.

Conclusions

In the management of brow ptosis, elevation and volume augmentation may provide the optimal rejuvenation. Injectable fillers placed at the lateral two thirds of the brow in the subdermal plane have been shown to elevate and augment brow soft tissue volume.[10] However, these materials offer a temporary result. The technique described above provides long-lasting volume augmentation as well as maximizes the brow lift. Managing both descent and deflation may provide the optimal rejuvenation of the brow region.

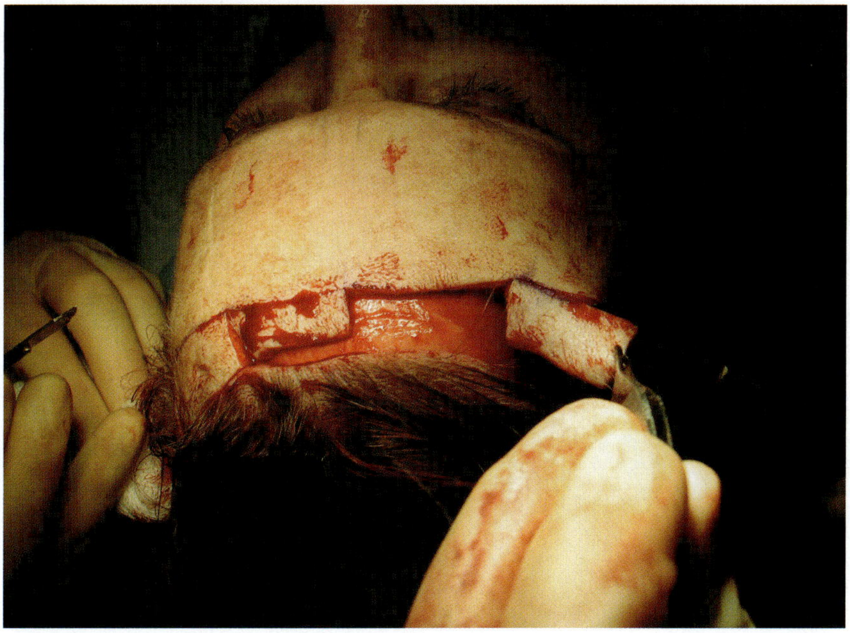

Figure 83.1. Scalp segments are excised in a pretrichial browlift. The segments are approximately 10 mm × 30 mm.

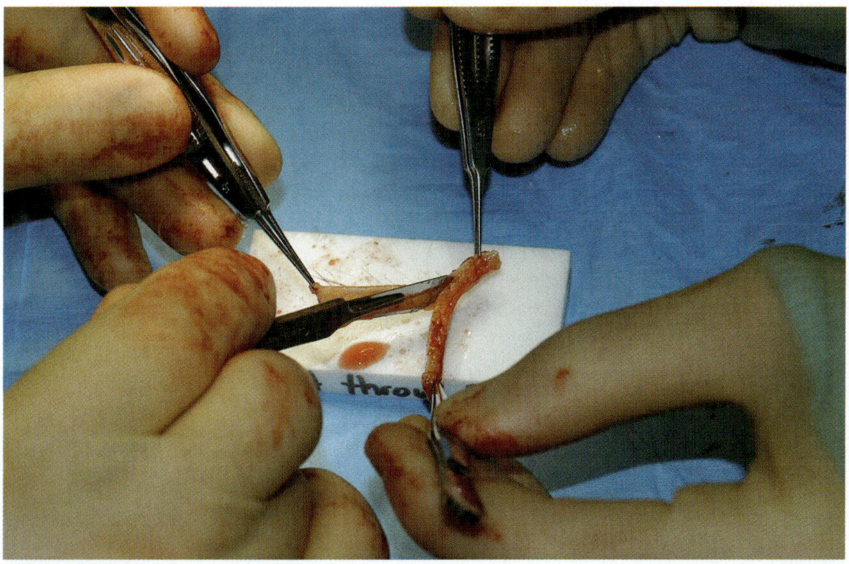

Figure 83.2. The epidermis (with care taken to remove all hair follicles) is removed, leaving the dermis and subcutaneous tissue.

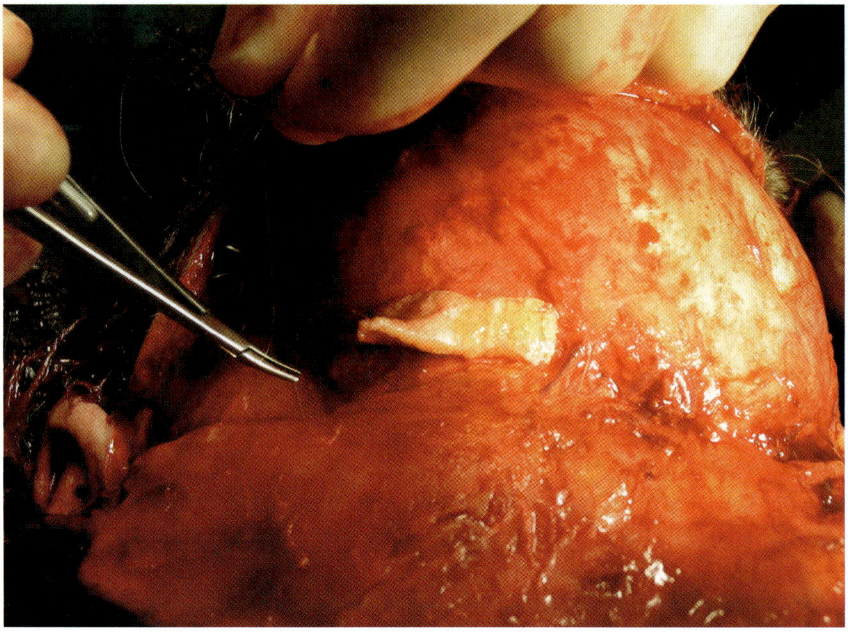

Figure 83.3. The graft is sutured to the underlying periosteum along the superior orbital rim on the lateral two thirds of the rim. The supraorbital neurovascular bundle is visible just nasal to the graft.

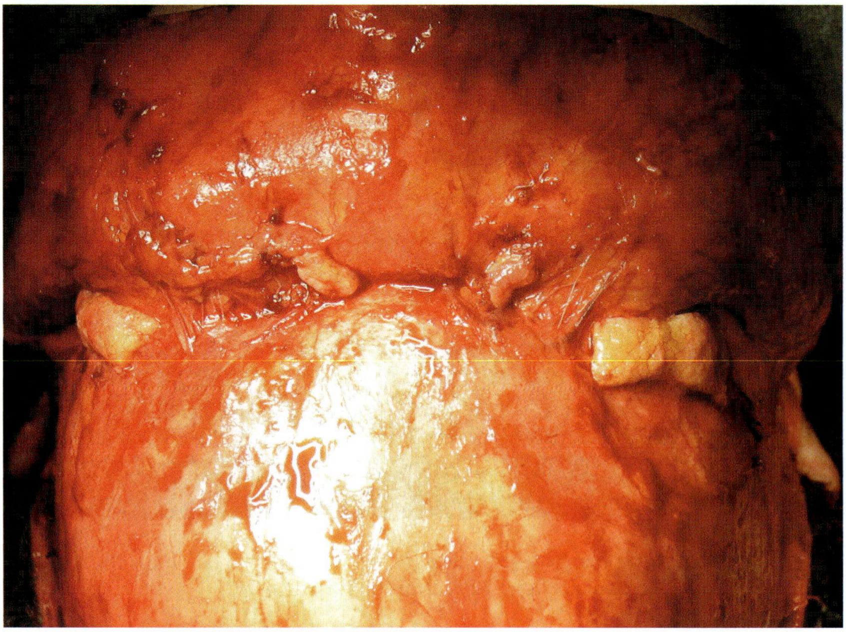

Figure 83.4. Graft segments of approximately 8 mm × 5 mm are sutured to the cut ends of the corrugator muscle to avoid soft tissue depression and prevent the cut ends from rejoining.

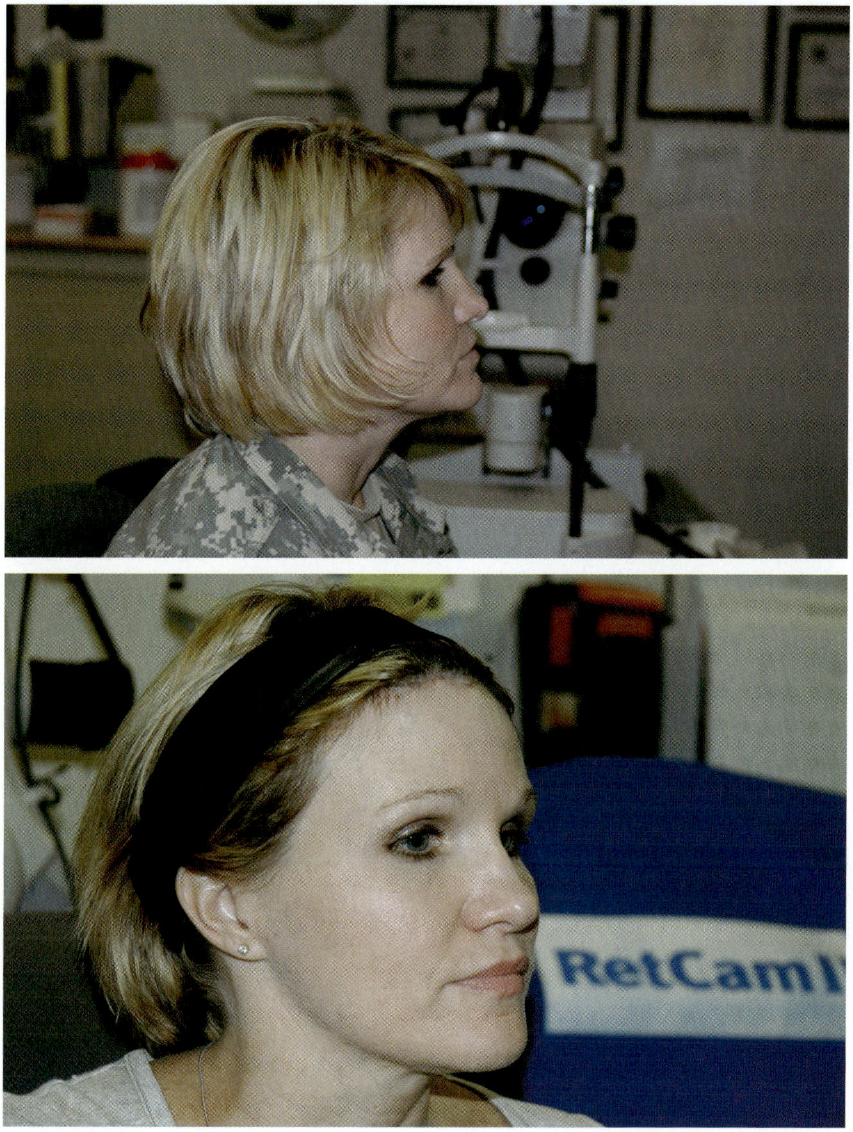

A

B

Figure 83.5. Pre- and 6-month postoperative view demonstrating elevation of the temporal brow with soft tissue volume augmentation.

References

1. Whitaker LA, Bartlett SP. Skeletal alterations as a basis for facial rejuvenation. Clin Plast Surg 1991;18(1):197–203.
2. Pessa JE, Chen Y. Curve analysis of the aging orbital aperature. Plast Reconstr Surg 2002;111(2):751–755.
3. Kerth JD, Toriumi DM. Management of the aging forehead. Arch Otolaryngol Head Neck Surg 1990;116(10):1137–1142.
4. Holck DE, Ng JD, Wiseman JB, Foster JA. The endoscopic browlift for forehead rejuvenation. Semin Ophthalmol 1998;13(3):149–157.

5. Burroughs JR, Bearden WH, Anderson RL, McCann JD. Internal brow elevation at blepharoplasty. Arch Facial Plast Surg 2006;8(1):36–41.
6. Muzaffar AR, Mendelson BC, Adams WP Jr. Surgical anatomy of the ligamentous attachments of the lower lid and lateral canthus. Plast Reconstr Surg 2002;110(3):873–884.
7. McCord CD, Doxanas MT. Browplasty and browpexy: an adjunct to blepharoplasty. Plast Reconstr Surg 1990;86(2):248–254.
8. May JW Jr, Fearon J, Zingarelli P. Retro-orbicularis oculus fat (ROOF) resection in aesthetic blepharoplasty: a 6-year study in 63 patients. Plast Reconstr Surg 1990;86(4):682–689.
9. Ramirez OM. High-tech facelift. Aesthetic Plast Surg 1998;22(5):318–328.
10. Carruthers JD, Carruthers A. Facial sculpting and tissue augmentation. Dermatol Surg 2005;31(11 Pt 2):1604–1612.

Part VI

Mid-Face Lift

84

Mid-Face Lift: General Considerations and How I Do It

Guy G. Massry

The endoscopic mid-face lift is a great volumizing procedure, but a poor lifting procedure:

- It can be done with or without browlift.
- Standard temporal posthairline incisions—like browlift.
- Dissect over white glistening surface of deep temporal fascia (DTF) to lateral canthus.
- Stay subperiosteal over zygomatic arch. Dissect over the medial third of the arch to reduce incidence of damage to the fascial nerve branch.
- Avoid sacrificing sentinel vein (potential arborization of new vessels—lower lids).
- This can all be done blindly in most patients. It helps to use bimanual technique (one hand guiding elevator, the other applying external guidance over arch), especially when there is thick tissue or in redo cases.
- Remove scope, advance with elevator while feeling and guiding with other hand over skin. Make sure tip of elevator rubs on bone to stay subperiosteal. When entering mid-face will feel a "pop." Advance radially over the face of the maxilla.
- Place a 4×4 gauze deeply into the temporal pocket for hemostasis before continuing with oral dissection. This also elevates tissue over zygoma so that there is less chance of entering wrong plane when connecting subperiosteal maxillary dissection with temporal pocket.
- Infiltrate gingivobuccal sulcus with same 1% anesthetic.
- Make a small 1/2-inch vertical incision over 2nd premolar (in line with infraorbital nerve).
- Use a small, hooked retractor to elevate all tissue off of the maxilla and begin subperiosteal dissection.
- Dissect all the way to the arcus marginalis of orbital rim—around infraorbital neurovascular bundle. Visualize inrafraorbital foramen and nerve. I use a small Freer elevator medial to nerve to get to arcus and then release it. Temporal to nerve I use any one of a number of larger elevators to release arcus to canthus.

- At canthus I connect to temporal pocket subperiosteally.
- Important to continue dissection over zygoma to insertion of masseter muscle (visualize origin of fibers). This is necessary for proper mobilization
- Equally as important is lysing the arcus marginalis. This breaks the fixed attachments and allows elevation. If this is not done we will only achieve the tissue-folding effect and volume augmentation. Also, if this is not done the tear trough may become deeper.
- Place a long $1^1/_2$-inch 25-gauge needle at my suture placement site from skin to subperiosteal space. The higher the placement, the more lift achieved—the lower, the more volume (differences are dramatic).
- Engage the superficial tissue at the suture demarcation site (get a good bite). I use a long tonsil through the temporal pocket to the gingivobuccal opening to engage the suture (grab ends of suture) and pull it through.
- Retract the temporal wound and engage suture (double bite) to DTF as low as you can. I cinch up in a slip knot. I then check mid-face volume and lift and adjust as necessary before securing knot.
- I then use a tonsil to guide a 10-French drain from temple to mouth and fix it with externalized suture.
- Irrigate temple wound to mouth with antibiotic/saline solution, and then mouth with same.

85

Ten Rules for Mid-Face Lifting for the Repair of Lid Retraction

Morris E. Hartstein and Guy G. Massry

1. Get real: Counsel the patient preoperatively as to the difficulty in fixing this problem—both doctor and patient need realistic expectations.
2. What is the culprit? Septal scar will tether the lid on upgaze. Anterior lamellar shortage will limit a mobile lid in upgaze. There may be components of both.
3. Stay clean: Dissect in a virgin plane so as not to disturb previous scar tissue. The subperiosteal plane is often undisturbed.
4. Deglove: Complete release and mobilization of the mid-face through the lid and/or mouth.
5. Take a load off: Elevating the mid-face, in addition to augmenting the skin, will take the gravitational burden off the eyelid and reduce the negative vector.
6. Avoid the poor man's mid-face lift: An orbicularis strap, while useful in routine blepharoplasty, is not helpful in this situation and may cause more cicatrization.
7. Aim high: The cheek flap should be secured higher than just the inferior orbital rim. Consider multiple point cheek flap fixation in a vertical direction to the orbital rim, ZF suture, and DTF.
8. Don't go it alone: For cicatricial lid retraction, elevation of the mid-face alone will not suffice—a spacer graft is usually required to support the lid. Choices of spacer grafts include hard palate, dermis fat, and processed collagen.
9. What goes up, must come down: No matter how high the fixation, all cheek flaps will fall postoperatively. Frost sutures, keeping the lid on upward stretch for 5–7 days, are crucial.
10. Wait to exhale: There are many forces influencing the healing and position of the lid. It may be several months before the lid settles to its final position. Wait at least 1 month postoperatively before even thinking that the procedure was successful.

86

The Subperiosteal Mid-Face Lift Using Bioabsorbable Implants for Fixation*

David E.E. Holck, Jill A. Foster, Kevin A. Kalwerisky, and Manuel A. Lopez

In recent years, the mid-face has received significant attention in the management of lower eyelid and facial reconstruction as well as rejuvenation. The transtemporal subperiosteal approach descriptions by Ramirez provide excellent vertical lift to mid-face soft tissue and allows redraping or volume redistribution without aggressive preperiosteal soft tissue dissection.[1,2] This approach may be continued as an extension of an endoscopic or open browlift procedure as well as combined with lower third facial rhytidectomy surgery to optimize entire facial rejuvenation (facial harmony).[3] This technique also allows for fat graft injection, orbital fat pedicle repositioning, malar augmentation, and/ or lateral retinacular suspension of the lower eyelid if desired, in a safe fashion. Using a resorbable midface elevation device on a leash allows predictable reliable midface elevation with improved surgical efficiency (Figure 86.1).

Standard endoscopic browlift or open coronal temporal hairline incisions may be used. A dissection plane is established on the surface of the deep temporalis fascia and carried toward the lateral canthus. Within a few millimeters of approaching the superior border of the zygomatic arch, the superficial layer of the deep temporalis fascia overlying the intermediate temporal fat pad is incised (avoiding excessive trauma to the underlying fat pad to avoid fat atrophy) to traverse the arch and body of the zygoma in the subperiosteal plane (Figure 86.2). Under endoscopic or direct visualization (in the open approach), care is take to avoid direct trauma to the sentinel vessels, the zygomaticotemporal/zygomaticofacial neurovascular bundles, and the temporal branch of the facial nerve. The dissection is carried over the anterior two thirds of the zygoma

*The authors have no financial interest in the products mentioned herein.

and continued subperiosteally into the midface beyond the zygomatico-maxillary buttress. A straight periosteal dissector is useful in the proximal portion of the dissection to the prominence of the zygoma. Further inferior, a gently curved dissector is useful to approach the anterior face of the maxilla. Medially the dissection exposes the piriform aperture and anterior nasal spine. Laterally the dissection degloves the zygoma, and exposes approximately 5–6 mm of the medial edge of the masseter muscle. As needed, dissection may be continued to the frontal processes of the maxilla medially (Figure 86.3A). From a temporal approach, the dissection is accomplished with minimal risk of injury to the infraorbital neurovascular bundle.[4] The dissection releases the origin of the zygomaticus major and minor muscles, which some authors feel may contribute to an unnatural appearance postoperatively (we have not found this to be the case).[5] At the level of the gingivobuccal sulcus (LeFort I level), the periosteum is incised using an up-biting periosteal elevator to optimally open the periosteum. The midface soft tissue envelope is then stretched (using a periosteal elevator or digitally) for maximal mobilization (Figure 86.3B).

As needed, an intraoral gingival buccal incision may be created to allow subperiosteal midface dissection under direct visualization. This is useful for surgeons beginning to perform subperiosteal mid-face lifting or as a route for placement of malar implants. The incision is begun high in the region of the zygomatic buttress at the level of the first molar tooth, 10–15 mm above the mucogingival junction. Care is taken to avoid the orifice of Stenson's duct. As the incision proceeds anteriorly, it is directed more inferiorly as it approaches the pyriform rim adjacent to the canine tooth, staying approximately 5 mm superior to the mucogingival junction. This avoids trauma to the alar portion of the nasalis muscles. The resulting cuff of mucosa facilitates closure and prevents contraction of the sulcus postoperatively. Under direct visualization, the subperiosteal dissection continues superiorly to the inferior orbital rim, exposing the infraorbital neurovascular bundle. The intraoral dissection is easily connected to the previously created temporal dissection.

Upon completion of the dissection cavity, malar implants may be placed as indicated in the subperiosteal pocket. The orbital septum may be approached and opened through the intraoral approach. The fat pads may be draped over the orbital rims and secured to the undersurface of the periosteal release.

With adequate release, the midface is then advanced superiorly. Using a bird's-eye view, the power of the mid-face lift is apparent. Fixation is accomplished using bioabsorbable implants that may be placed through a temporal approach or retrograde through a sublabial approach. The Endotine Midface ST bioabsorbable implant (Coapt Systems, Inc., Palo Alto, CA) has tines to fix the midface soft tissue envelope (Figure 86.1). The leash allows fixation to the deep temporalis fascia. Advantages of the midface implant include more rapid placement than sutures as well as the ability to elevate the midface without necessarily having to make a gingivobuccal incision. The device is typically nonpalpable and asymptomatic, resorbs over a period of 6 months. The mid-face soft tissue and periosteum at the level of the malar fat pad is pushed onto the prongs until they are engaged (Figure 86.4). The leash is pulled from the temporal incision until the desired elevation is achieved (Figure 86.5). The leash is fixed to the deep temporalis fascia using multiple 3-0 PDS or Vicryl sutures, with excess leash trimmed after suture fixation (Figure 86.6).

Alternatively, fixation of the midface is accomplished by suturing midface periosteum to the deep temporalis fascia from the temporal hairline dissection. We place two to three sutures (typically 2-0 ePTFE, or PDS sutures) in the mid-face periosteum: one at the level of the suborbicularis oculi fat pad, one more inferior at the periosteum of the low alar groove in proximity to the buccal sulcus incision, and possibly a third in the maximal projection of the malar fat pad. These fixation points may be somewhat tenuous and take some effort and multiple passes to fixate. The fixation sutures may be modified based upon the degree of lift desired.

If opened, the gingivobuccal incision is closed with a running 4-0 chromic gut suture. Care is taken to avoid tension. The temporal hairline incision is closed with 35R staples. Postoperatively, the patient gently rinses their mouth with antiseptic. The scalp is covered with a cotton mesh dressing for 24–48 hours. The staples are removed at 7–10 days postoperatively.

We have found that this resorbable midface lifting device has reliably and predictably elevated the midface in a vertical vector of pull (Figure 86.7). The device allows increased surgical efficiency, allowing predictable symmetric mid-face lifting with minimal increase in operative duration using an endoscopic or open browlift approach. An additional observation is elevation of the lateral canthal angle without a lower eyelid surgical approach. We have found that the resorbable fixation device is neither palpable nor uncomfortable for the patient. Keys to success using this technique includes wide surgical undermining, adequate stretching of the mid-face soft tissue envelope after periosteal release at the Le Fort 1 level, judging symmetry upon placement of both fixation devices, and multiple point fixation of the leash to the deep temporalis fascia.

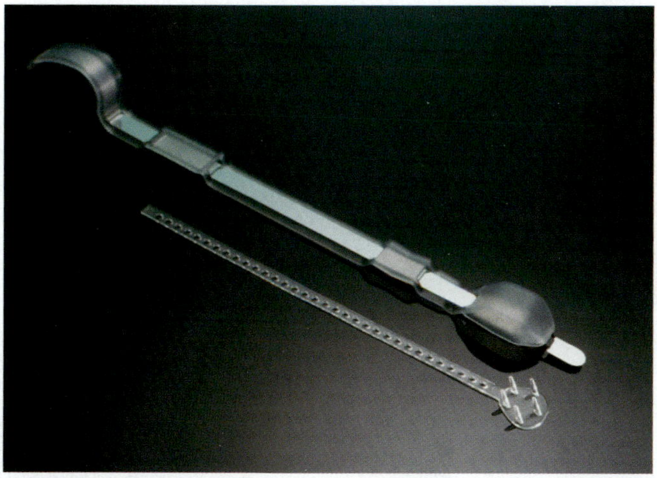

Figure 86.1. The Endotine Midface ST bioabsorbable implant (Coapt Systems, Inc. Palo Alto, CA) has a 4.5-mm-length five-point tine to fix the mid-face soft tissue envelope through a subperiosteal approach. The implant has an 11.5-cm leash with fixation holes that allows fixation to the deep temporalis fascia. Shown alongside is the introducer with a rounded hub to prevent soft tissue capture of the tines before adequate positioning.

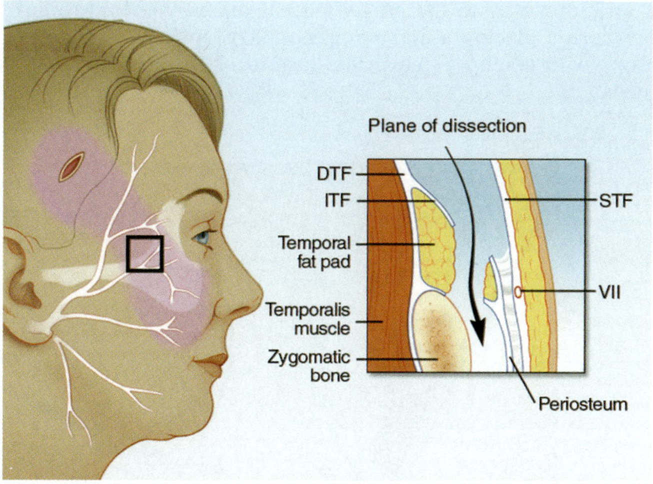

Figure 86.2. Area of subperiosteal dissection and transition zone from deep temporalis fascia of the temporal region to the subperiosteal plane of the zygoma and midface. DTF, deep temporalis fascia; STF, superficial temporalis fascia; ITF, intermediate temporalis fascia; VII, frontal branch of facial nerve, cranial nerve VII.

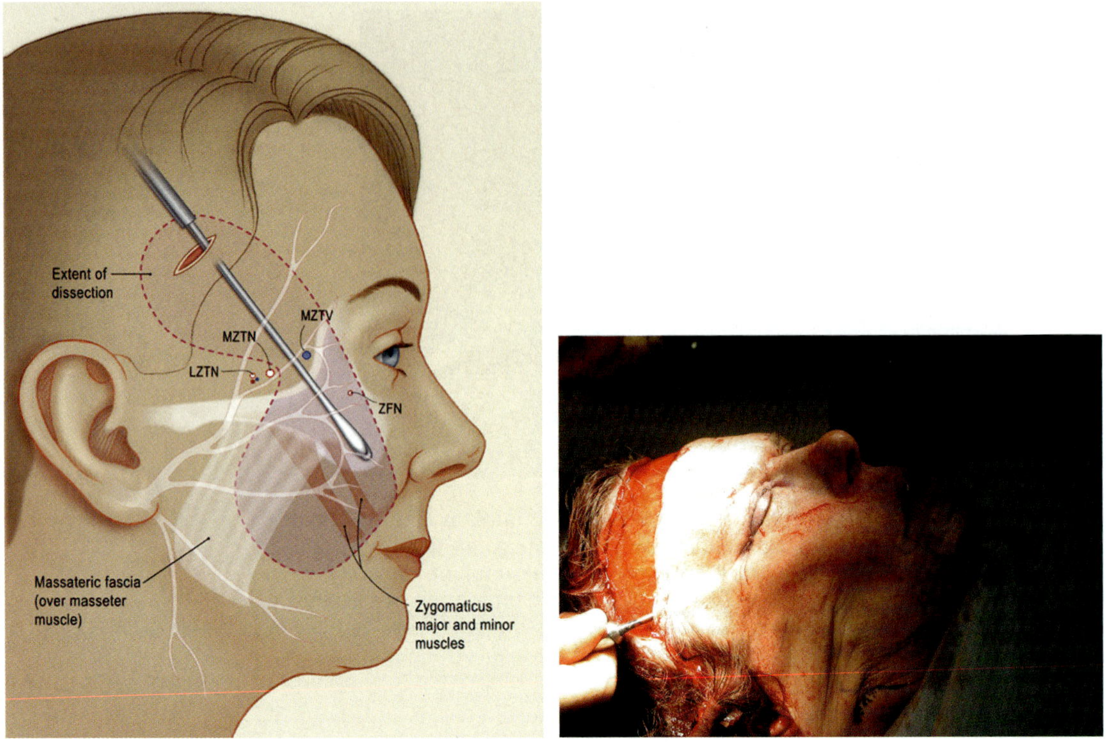

Figure 86.3. (A) Subperiosteal dissection is continued nasally to the pyriform aperture, laterally over ~5 mm of medial masseteric fibers, and inferiorly to the gingivobuccal sulcus. We do not make a gingivobuccal incision unless we are considering placing a malar implant. (B) Operative photo of a patient undergoing a pretrichial browlift along with a subperiosteal mid-face lift. Not the periosteal elevator is at the level of the gingivobuccal sulcus.

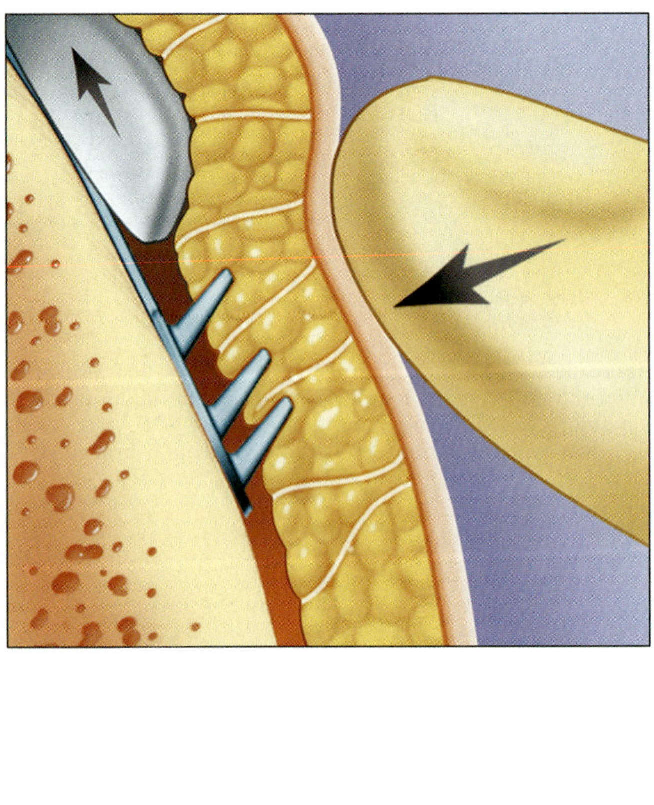

Figure 86.4. After removal of the introducer, the mid-face soft tissue at the level of the malar fat pad is pressed to engage the head of the leash containing the 4.5-mm tines.

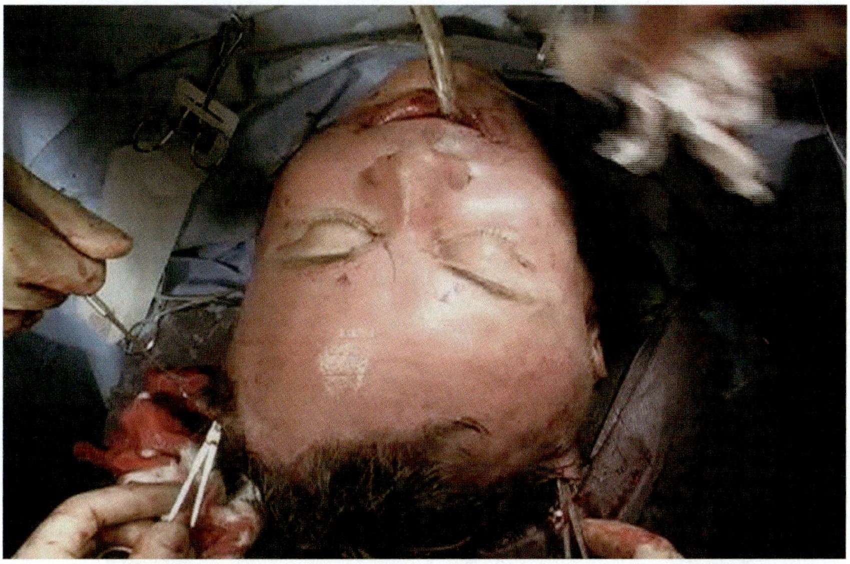

Figure 86.5. Pulling on the right leash demonstrates right midface elevation compared to the unelevated left side.

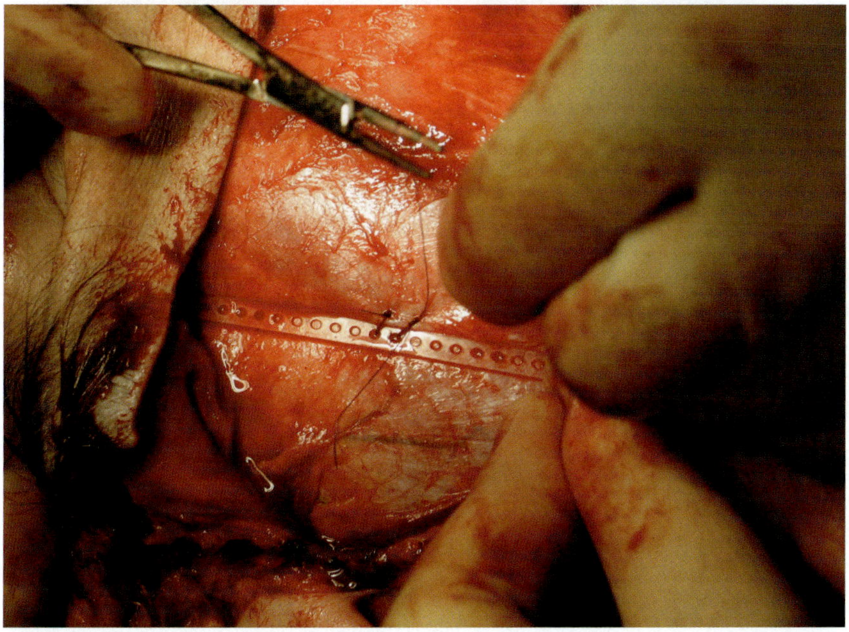

Figure 86.6. After adequate positioning is found, the leash is fixed to deep temporalis fascia using multiple 2-0 or 3-0 Vicryl or PDS sutures. Excess leash material may be trimmed.

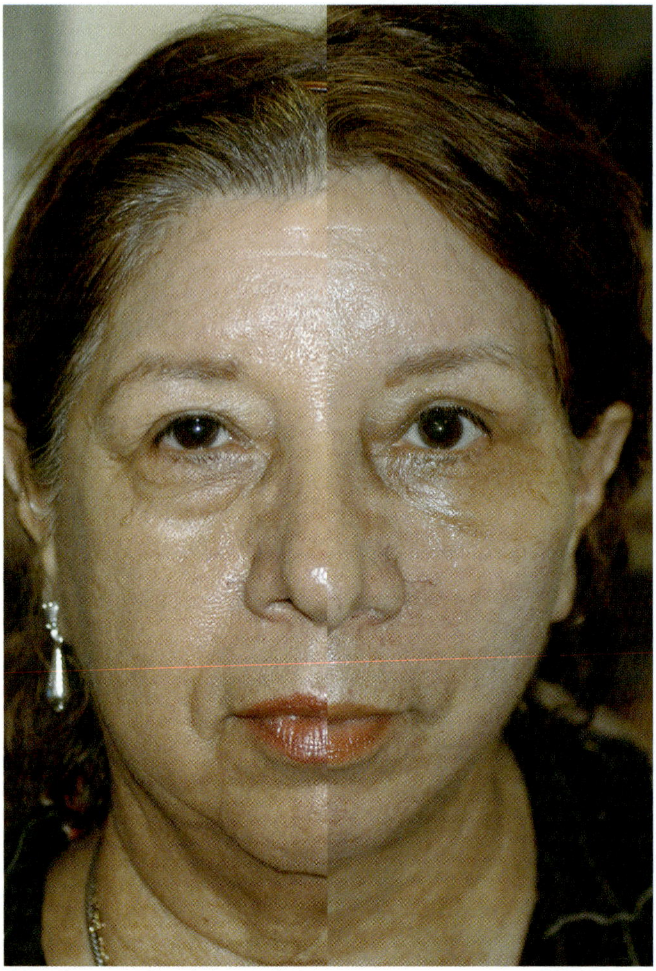

Figure 86.7. Preoperative and 1-month postoperative mid-face elevation using the device. This patient also underwent endoscopic browlifting.

References

1. Ramirez OM. The subperiosteal rhytidectomy: The third generation facelift. Ann Plast Surg 1992;28:218.
2. Ramirez OM. Three-dimensional endoscopic midface enhancement: A personal quest for the ideal cheek rejuvenation. Plast Reconstr Surg 2002; 109(1):329–340.
3. Little JW. Discussion: three dimensional endoscopic midface enhancement: a personal quest for the ideal cheek rejuvenation. Plast Reconstr Surg 2002;109(1):341–343.
4. Holck DEE, Robertson OB. Expert commentary, the midface lift. In: Joseph Mauriello (ed.). Techniques of Cosmetic Eyelid Surgery: A Case Study Approach. Philadelphia: Lipppincott, Williams & Wilkins, 2004:173–179.
5. Hamra ST. Prevention and correction of the "face-lifted" appearance. Fac Plast Surg 2000;16(3):215–230.

87

Cheeklifting Pearls

Clinton D. McCord, Jr.*

The lower eyelid should not be viewed as an isolated structure apart from the tissues beneath it, namely the mid-face, which can undergo significant ptosis. Lower blepharoplasty can be viewed as one part of midface rejuvenation and can be performed during a cheeklift. The cheeklift relates to the area between the nasolabial folds and the eyelid, namely:

- Eyelid fat
- Laxity and/or sagging of midface skin
- Ptosis of midface structures

Traditional facelifting techniques really address the neck and with a more oblique vector; in contrast, the cheeklift restores contour by operating in the vertical vector. The mid-face area can be approached subperiosteally through the lower lid. The two crucial steps to the cheek lift are:

- Controlling the shape of the lid by canthal fixation. Adjustments should be made according to if the eye is deep-set or prominent. With mild prominence, release of the lower retractors can help. With increasing prominence, a spacer graft is placed.
- Supporting the lower lid and cheek by anchoring the cheek flap/orbicularis. The orbicularis is doubly anchored: the base at the orbital rim near the lateral canthus and the tip at different areas of the deep temporal fascia. For nonprominent eyes, a more horizontal vector is used. For more prominent eyes, a more vertical vector is used.

Complications usually arise from problems in canthal fixation leading to eyelid fissure abnormalities, and sagging of the lid and cheek from problems in orbicularis anchoring. Further delineation of cheeklift complications can be categorized as follows:

- Primary fixation problem—correct with canthoplasty
- Primary skin shortage—correct with additional skin recruitment via secondary cheeklift
- Eye prominence—correct with spacer grafts

---

* Originally published in: Chen WPD. Khan JA, McCord, Jr, CD. Color Atlas of Cosmetic Oculofacial Sugery. Philadelphia: Butterworth Heinemann/ Elsevier. 2004.

For postoperative complications of the cheeklift, recall the mneumonic A-V-IS, as any climber knows:

- Anchoring
- Vertical recruitment
- Insertion of spacer

88

Mid-Face Implants

Joseph Niamtu, III*

Cheek implants are anatomic and come in many sizes and shapes. Submalar implants are used to fill the anterior submalar void, malar shells are used to augment the lateral malar region, and the combined submalar implant (Implantech, Inc., Ventura, CA) is a versatile implant that augments both the anterior and lateral cheek regions (Figure 88.1).

Cheek implants are placed in the subperiosteal plane. Local anesthesia is injected intraorally or transcutaneously across the anterior maxilla, the infraorbital area, and over the medial portion of the zygomatic arch. A 1-cm incision is made over the canine tooth about 5 mm above the attached gingiva. The incision is made through the periosteum and subperiosteal dissection is made over the anterior maxilla with care to protect the infraorbital nerve. The dissection is extended over the malar area and tapers out over the media portion of the zygomatic arch (Figure 88.2). The superiomedial origin of the massetter muscle is often seen, and larger implants may rest over this part of the massetter muscle. The subperiosteal dissection should be just slightly larger in all dimensions that the actual implant to be placed. Too small a pocket causes the implant to buck; too large and the implant might be mobile and migrate.

The pocket is irrigated with antibiotic solution and the implant is placed through the incision. A long, narrow tonsil clamp facilitates positioning the tail of the flexible implant into the pocket (Figure 88.3). It is imperative to make sure that the implant lies passive in the pocket and that the tail is not folded. After the implant is placed, the upper lip is pulled down and gentle pressure is placed on the cheek skin. If the implants are displaced from this maneuver, then the pockets are widened to passively accommodate the implants. It is imperative to obtain hemostasis prior to closing, otherwise hematoma formation can be problematic. The incision is closed with interrupted 4-0 gut suture. Patients are placed on a cephalosporin 24 hours preoperatively and for one week postoperatively. Appropriate analgesics and a tapering dose of steroids are also prescribed. Patients are asked to refrain from significant animation for several days.

Swelling from mid-face implants can be formidable and must be explained to the patient in advance. The disruption of the lip elevators will produce compromised animation in smiling and puckering, which will typically return to normal within 2 weeks. Altered sensation is common for the first week or two but is rarely a persistent problem.

Dr. Niamtu has received lecture honoraria from Implantec.

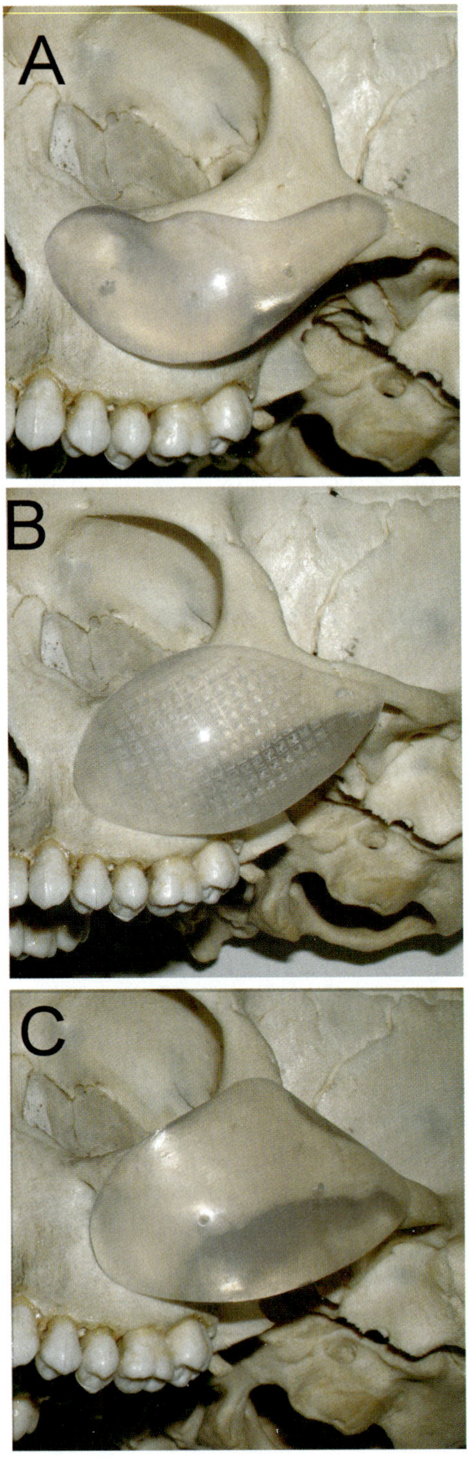

Figure 88.1. Implantech, Inc. offers a wide selection of silicone implants to augment various areas of the midface.

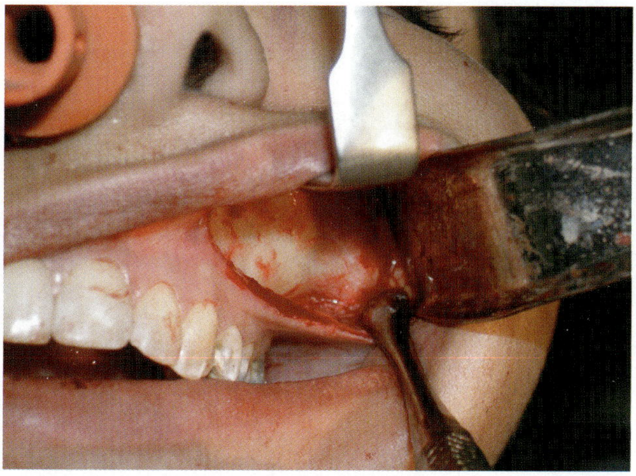

Figure 88.2. The incision needs only be 1 cm. and the mucosa will stretch. This figure also illustrates the required dissection for the larger implants.

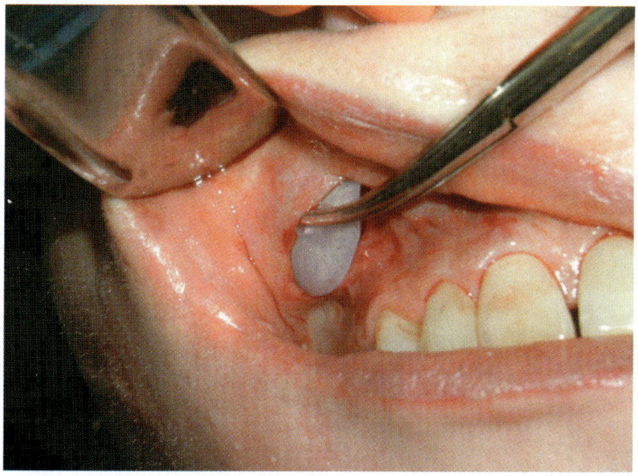

Figure 88.3. The implant is placed into the dissection pocket with a tonsil clamp.

Part VII

Botox

89

Introduction to Botox

John R. Burroughs and Richard L. Anderson

Botulinum toxin type A (Botox®) interferes with acetylcholine release from nerve terminals causing temporary paralysis of the injected muscles. The pioneering work of Scott[1] over 25 years ago was for strabismus. In 1989 it was approved for blepharospasm, hemifacial spasm, torticollis, and strabismus. Since then it has been approved for cosmetic treatment of the glabellar furrows and axillary hyperhydrosis. Botox has become the number one cosmetic procedure and is widely used to treat rhytids of the glabella, forehead, eyelids; nasal; cervical; and perioral areas. Off-label oculofacial uses include: hyperkinetic wrinkles of the face; hyper-lacrimation; eyelid retraction; spastic entropion; blepharoptosis; migraine/stress headaches; and improving symmetry for facial palsy.

Reference

1. Scott AB. Development of botulinum toxin therapy. Dermctol Clin 2004; 22(2):131–133.

90

Evaluating Potential Botox Patients

Samuel M. Lam

Understanding the clinical benefits and limitations of Botox (BTX) therapy is important; these must be effectively communicated to every patient in order to ensure uniform satisfaction. As almost every practitioner of cosmetic enhancement, surgeon and physician alike, use Botox in his or her clinical practice, it is important to differentiate the quality of one's Botox therapy from competitors. This chapter will recount how to attain consistently excellent results and to minimize patient discomfort so as to increase patient loyalty and repeat visits. Botox injection is easy to perform but must be undertaken with care and attention for optimal results.

Evaluation of the Potential Botox Patient

Botox therapy provides excellent and safe periocular cosmetic enhancement when applied in a deliberate and conscientious method. During the initial consultation, the physician should ask what experiences the patient may have had with Botox in the past and what expectations he or she should hold. Review of the patient's prior experiences is informative as to what pitfalls the physician can avoid in the current session. For example, if the patient says that the brow position descended excessively with prior usage, the physician should pay particular attention to how to treat the frontalis. Excessive ecchymosis from a previous treatment may reflect careless or inadvertent venopuncture or a patient's excessive usage of a nonsteroidal antiinflammatory medication. Counseling a patient during the initial phone encounter to avoid aspirin, herbal therapies, or other blood-thinning medications is important as is avoiding treatment 1–2 weeks before an important professional or social engagement in case ecchymosis arises and cannot be entirely camouflaged.

It is helpful during the discussion to study the patient's habits of animation and particular anatomic features before injection is undertaken. During discussion with a patient, the physician may glean clues that can be very informative. For example, the patient may constantly raise or hold the eyebrows skyward to compensate for brow ptosis. Treatment of these frontalis rhytids with Botox will compromise the patient's ability to lift the brows and be quite devastating for the patient. Having the patient close the eyes tightly and then slowly open them, concentrating all the while on not using the brow muscles, will prove conclusively to the patient that the frontalis is being used to alleviate brow ptosis and therefore should not be injected. Also, the surgeon may observe that the patient constantly frowns during pensive moments. Therefore, the surgeon can advise that therapy of the glabellar musculature may prove beneficial to break this undesirable habit. In fact, treatment of this unintended habitual action over a period of a year may actually break the habit, as the patient unconsciously unlearns this behavior over time. These clinical clues can only be effectively discerned when the patient is unwittingly observed, so the initial cosmetic consultation can be invaluable in many respects for the physician.

Any anatomic differences like brow asymmetry and wrinkle distribution can be pointed out to the patient at this time or during the injection session itself. Unlike many other attempts at correcting asymmetry, Botox can provide a noticeable improvement in asymmetry since it goes to the root of the problem (i.e., muscular pull). The correction of brow asymmetry with a browlift ultimately fails over time as muscular contraction returns the position of the brows back to their native asymmetry.

Prejudices about Botox usage can be unearthed and dispelled during the initial encounter as well. The words "poison" and "toxin" are bandied about as if they were contaminants that would cause ineluctable harm for the body. I usually counter these concerns by explaining that Botox has been perhaps one of the most studied products in the cosmetic industry with the longest history of safety than any product in the cosmetic market, emphasizing that I use only the FDA-approved version made by Allergan, which has been unequivocally safe. I substitute the word "purified protein" for "toxin" when discussing Botox to allay fears and to deliver the proper message.

Reviewing with the patient the precise aesthetic objectives is very important. As BTX only treats wrinkles in animation, a patient who presents with deeply set static wrinkles would most likely gain very little benefit from therapy. I emphasize that BTX serves two major objectives: to prevent wrinkles from setting in *if a consistent regimen is maintained* and to make the patient look better during animation so that deep wrinkles do not manifest. For patients who undergo skin therapies like phenol or TCA peels, I stress the importance of Botox in maintaining the durability of that result, like a shirt that is ironed flat (chemical peel) should keep its form if it is never worn (Botox therapy). Establishing realistic objectives underscores every cosmetic endeavor to minimize patient dissatisfaction and physician headaches thereafter. Finally, patients who express concern that emotion will be restricted, I explain that Botox limits so-called negative expressions (surprise, anger, worry) but does not limit positive expressions (happiness and joy). Obviously, patients who have careers that require emotive display like actors and screen personalities may not be acceptable candidates for Botox therapy.

91

Botox: General Principles of Treatment

Samuel M. Lam

Review with the patient the exact aesthetic goals and whether the patient is abstinent from all blood thinners for a week. The physician wipes all makeup off the patient with an alcohol pad before starting, ensuring that the alcohol has time to evaporate before Botox (BTX) injection (alcohol can deactivate the toxin). With the makeup removed, the physician should carefully study the patient's anatomy in repose and in animation. Proper illumination is used to determine the presence of major vessels around the eyes that could be punctured, which would lead to massive and sustained ecchymosis. Preoperative asymmetry and wrinkle distribution are determined. A permanent marker or eyebrow crayon can be used to mark out the injection sites. Gentian violet should never be used due to its persistence. One should not inject through a skin marking to avoid permanent tattooing of the skin.

At the end of the session, the patient is reminded not to disturb the treated area for a minimum of 2–3 hours. It is not necessary to actively contract the muscles, but there is no harm in doing so. The patient should not lie down for the prescribed 2–3 hours for fear that pressure applied to the treated areas might cause unwanted migration of the toxin.

Meticulously record all patient concerns, anatomy, and injection points on a treatment record. Document that the patient had all questions answered and give written instructions. The lot number and expiration on the Botox bottle may be recorded.

There are two principal methods to charge for Botox: per treatment area or per unit. I prefer the former method for two reasons. First, I charge slightly more for the first treatment area and less for subsequent areas if performed the same day so as to encourage more complete treatment. I also like to give touch-up treatments without a charge to promote good will and patient rapport. The reader is encouraged to follow the standards of one's community when deciding on pricing preferences.

I undertake a referral program that rewards patients who refer their friends and family to have BTX therapy. That has proven to be a helpful method in promoting my practice. I also give patients the option of either scheduling their next treatment session or electing to receive a postcard, which they fill out themselves to remind them of their next appointment.

BTX therapy has become a valuable and effective method of periocular rejuvenation and a mainstay of a youthful maintenance regimen. Often patients who are the best candidates think they do not need it because they are too young. Dissemination of knowledge that BTX is intended to prevent or minimize the onset of static wrinkles will help in achieving increased patient satisfaction.

92

Botox: Where It Works Best

Jemshed A. Khan

Botox injection works well and reliably in crow's-feet, glabella, and forehead.

With experience, the eyebrows may be repositioned through treatment of the adjacent orbicularis oculi, procerus, corrugator supercilii, and depressor supercilii.

Dose is often individualized and may be related to muscle mass such that relatively smaller doses are sometimes used in females and Asians.

Glogau wrinkle classification scale.

- Type I: no wrinkles
- Type II: wrinkles in motion
- Type III: wrinkles at rest
- Type IV: only wrinkles

Table 92.1. General Guidelines for Typical Botox Cosmetic Doses

Site	Dose per site (units)	No. of injections/ side	Total dose per side (units)	Spacing of ipsilateral injection (cm)	Recommended initial dose (units) per side/no. injection sites per side/ distance between injections (cm)
Forehead	**2.5–5**	**2–5**	**10–15**	**1–3**	**2.5/2/3**
Glabella	**5–10**	**1–2**	**10–20**	**1–2**	**5/2/1+**
Crow's-feet	**3–10**	**1–5**	**10–15**	**1–2.5**	**5/2/1+**
Upper lip	**1–1.5**	**1–2**	**1–2**	**1.5**	**1/1/na**
Lower lip	**1–1.5**	**1–2**	**1–2**	**1.5**	**1/1/na**
Lateral Commisure	**5–10**	**1–2**	**5–10**	**1–1.5**	**5/1/na**
Platysma	**5**	**Variable**	**15–50+**	**1–3**	**5/ variable/ 1.5+**

Reprinted with permission from Chen WPD et al. [ref. 1].

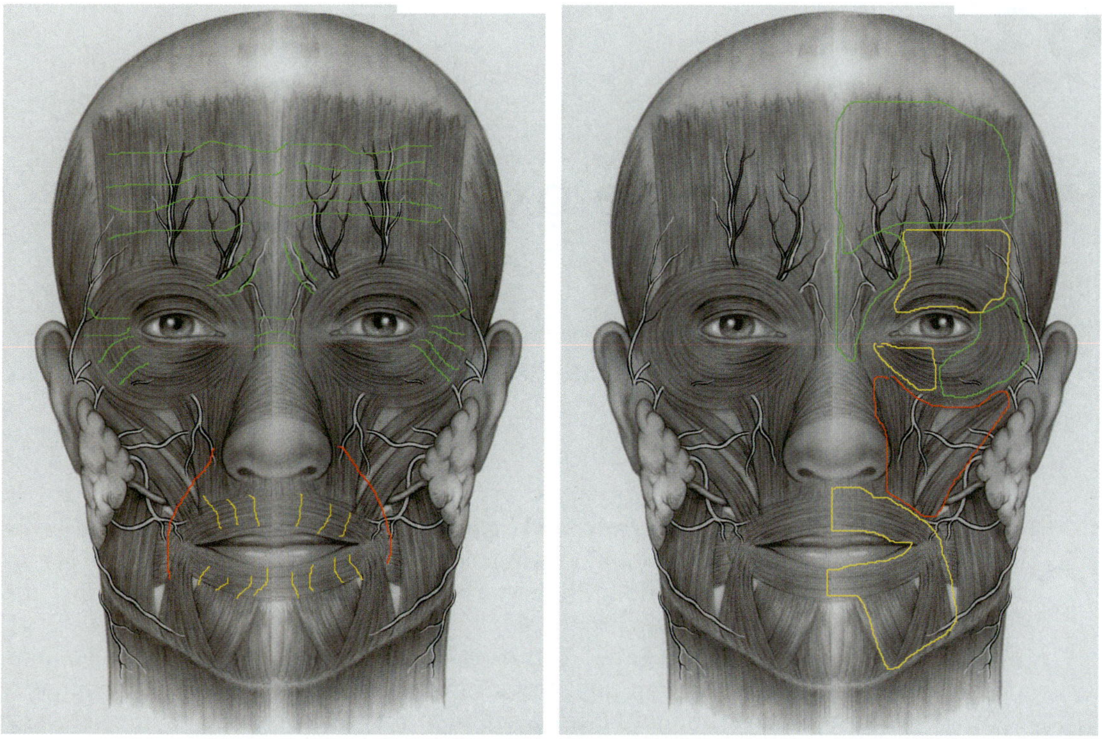

A B

Figure 92.1. (A) Wrinkles indicated for Botox treatment: green, wrinkles that respond well; yellow, wrinkles that should be treated cautiously; red, lines that should not be treated. (B) Facial zones and underlying muscle groups. Green areas respond predictably and well. Caution is used in yellow areas because of unwanted effects such as adynamic and ptotic eyebrow. Red areas will produce unwanted effects such as drooping cheek and mouth. (Reprinted from ref. [1]).

Reference

1. Chen WPD, Khan JA, McCord CD Jr. Color Atlas of Cosmetic Oculofacial Surgery. Philadelphia: Elsever; 2004.

93

Preparation of Botox

Jemshed A. Khan

Botox is an extremely labile lyophilized albumin and neurotoxin cryoprecipitate that should be reconstituted without agitation in order to prevent inactivation. Preserved (bacteriostatic) saline may be used for its mild anesthetic properties.

I use 2.2 ml of saline as diluent because approximately 0.1 ml remains in the vial through capillary attraction to the glass surface. The reconstituted drug should be used within 4 hours according to manufacturer's recommendation, although studies suggest it is stable for a week or more refrigerated (stopped removed) or 7 d (stopper in place). A fine 30-gauge needle is used for administration.

Bullet Points

- Store in freezer prior to use
- (optional step) Break seal and remove stopper
- Drip in nonpreserved saline slowly, 2.2 ml
- 2.2 ml nonpreserved saline = approx. 5 units/0.1 ml
- Roll gently to mix—do not shake or stir
- Withdraw required amount via insulin syringe without dulling tip
- Refrigerate unused portion and use within 4 hours

Originally published in: Chen WPD Khan JA, McCord, Jr. CD. Color Atlas of Cosmetic Oculofacial Sugery. Philadelphia Butterworth Heinemann/Elsevier. 2004.

94

Documentation of Treatment: Botox

Jemshed A. Khan

Anatomic documentation of treatment sites creates a historical record upon which further treatment modifications may be individualized. For example, if a patient has inadequate lateral forehead wrinkle reduction, one may refer to the treatment diagram and use this as a basis for adding new lateral treatment sites.

While botulinum toxin A appears to be a safe and effective drug, the very long-term consequences of neurotoxin injection are unknown. Therefore, informed consent is important despite the relative simplicity of the procedure. Informed consent discussion should include both the known side effects as well as a discussion of unknown risks related to the use of human albumin in botulinum toxin A.

LIFETIME CONSENT FOR ADMINISTRATION OF BOTOX

1. I, ___________ ___________ (first name, last name), request that Dr. ___________, or whomever he designates, administer botulinum toxin to me for either medical or cosmetic purposes. Botox is not FDA approved for headache treatment, tarsorrhaphy, or muscle twitching. Photos of me may be taken and used for educational, scientific, or marketing purposes.
2. If botulinum is given for medical purposes, such as involuntary muscle spasm, tarsorrhaphy, blepharospasm, hemifacial spasm, muscle twitch or tick, etc, I hereby acknowledge that I understand that there may be alternative treatments for this condition, including, but not limited to, medical therapy including the administration of oral medicines, muscle stripping or other operations, removal of motor nerves, or procedures to release pressure on involved nerves.
3. I acknowledge that I understand that Botox A includes human albumin. Albumin is a protein, similar to the white of a chicken egg, that is derived from human blood products. While it is not believed that there has been any transmission of diseases from Botox A, I

Originally published in: Chen WPD, Khan JA, McCord, Jr. CD. Color Atlas of Cosmetic Oculofacial Sugery. Philadelphia: Butterworth Heinemann/Elsevier. 2004.

understand that this is very unlikely but possible. I accept the risk of the possibility of acquiring an infection, including viral or other types of infections from Botox administration and accept the risk of unknown future complications from Botox use. I understand that botulinum B can also be used for my condition and does not contain albumin.

4. Botulinum toxin usually works well in 95% of patients. There is a 5% chance that it will not have an adequate effect. It is not always possible to predict the effect, and it may work too well or not well enough. Some of the side effects may include flu symptoms, headache, temporary droopiness of one or both eyelids or double vision. Permanent muscle weakness is very unlikely.
5. By signing this document, I agree that it includes all botulinum toxin injections already provided by Dr. Khan or whomever he designates, as well as all future Botox treatments.
6. I understand that the effects of botulinum toxin use with pregnancy or breast-feeding are not known and that I should not take Botox if the possibility of pregnancy or nursing exists.
7. In summary, the risks, consequences, benefits, and alternatives of treatment, including no treatment, have been explained to me.

Signed (Patient) ____________ Date ____/____/03

Witnessed By ____________ Date ____/____/03

Reproduced with permission from:

Patient name: Dx: BEB / Hemifacial spasm / Cosmetic/ _____.

Date
Pt comments:

CC: Spasms returning
Cosmetic

U Given Discard Share
Notes:

RTC
Signed:

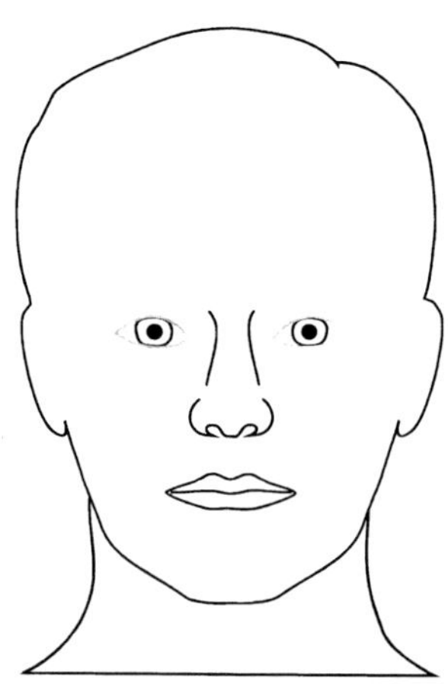

Figure 94.1. Sample chart note and diagram for Botox therapy.

95

Botox Injection Technique

John R. Burroughs and Richard L. Anderson

A half-inch 32-gauge needle (Air-Tite Products) minimizes injection discomfort. In the periorbital areas we inject in an oblique manner to the skin to lessen the chance of deep injections or even injury should a patient suddenly move. Pinching upward or gently rubbing the adjacent skin during injection minimizes patient discomfort by distracting the patient during the injection and "confusing" the sensory sensation of the injection (Figure 95.1). We recommend premarking the areas to be injected, and utilizing bright lighting and wearing magnification to avoid injury to eyelid vessels. We seldom use topical anesthetics, and some suggest a reduced duration of effect in patients treated with topical anesthetic prior to injection.[1] We inject into the subcutaneous tissue planes to avoid the underlying muscle and neurovascular structures. This reduces patient discomfort and lessens the risks of bruising and deep dissemination. In general the injections can be given obliquely or perpendicular to the skin, but in the orbicularis areas it is critical to inject at as flat an angle as possible because of the thinness of the eyelid skin and to point away from the eye. It is also helpful when injecting the lower orbicularis areas to put the skin on stretch, which helps with placing the Botox in the subcutaneous plane. Botox must be avoided in the central upper eyelid to prevent ptosis and over the inferior oblique in the lower eyelid to avoid diplopia.

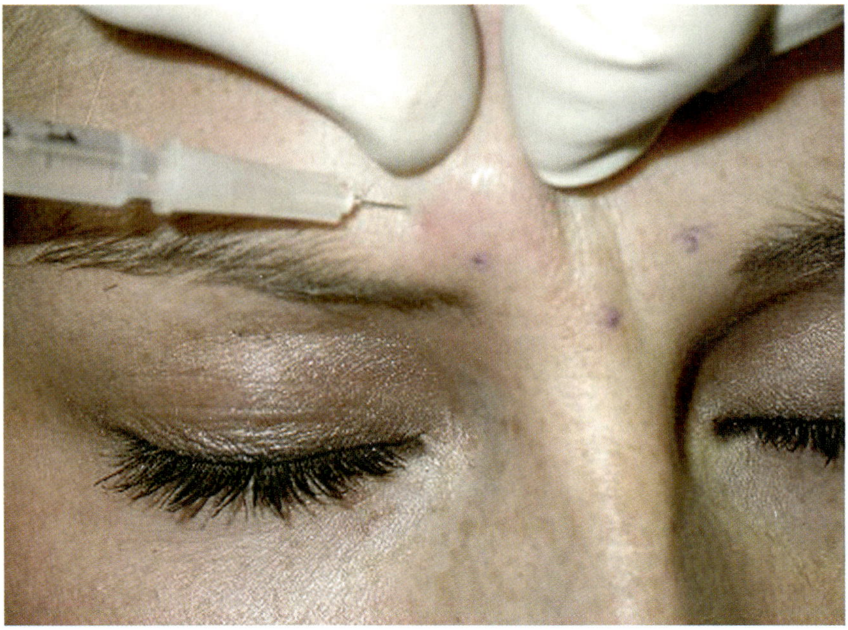

Figure 95.1. Pinch technique during oblique injection of corrugator. This descreases discomfort and avoids neurovascular structures and bleeding.

Reference

1. Sami MS, Soparkar CN, Patrinely JR, Miller LM, Hollier LH. Efficacy of botulinum toxin type a after topical anesthesia. Ophth Plast Reconstr Surg 2006;22:448–452.

96

Cosmetic Botox Applications: General Considerations and Dosing

John R. Burroughs and Richard L. Anderson

Cosmetic applications of Botox continue to expand beyond the FDA-approved use for glabellar furrows. Patients should sign informed consent for off-label cosmetic uses. Treatment of eyelid and facial rhytids is gratifying for the patients and physicians. Not only do the eyelid injections improve current rhytids, but the future development of mimetic rhytids is prevented. It is paramount to understand the anatomy of the eyelid and facial muscles and that the rhytid-inducing musculature is the injection site rather than the actual wrinkles. Patient desires and expectations must be clearly defined as some patients may want to be smooth and adynamic, whereas others prefer a natural youthful appearance. We strongly encourage the latter. Aesthetic appreciation and training is essential in obtaining excellent cosmetic results.

Nearly all patients have facial asymmetry, and this must be evaluated similar to preoperative surgical evaluation prior to injections. Facial asymmetry can be greatly improved by tailoring Botox injections or worsened by a "cookbook" approach. Therefore, we recommend injections by physicians. Preexistent brow ptosis must be noted and excessive frontalis paralysis avoided to prevent worsening. Browlifting and contouring is possible by careful placement of Botox to either the medial brow depressors and/or the lateral orbicularis oculi. Botox injections to highly dynamic areas, such as the crow's feet and lips, may last 3 months, and in less dynamic areas, such as the forehead or glabella, up to 5–6 months with good dosing. Our typical dosages for cosmetic Botox use are shown in Table 96.1.

Table 96.1. Typical Botox Dosages for Cosmetic Applications

Forehead	15–35 units in 3–8 sites
Glabella	25–45 units in 5–8 sites
Crow's feet	15–30 units in 4–6 sites
Nasal scrunch lines	2–5 units in 2 sites
Upper lip	2–4 units in 2 sites
Lower lip	2–4 units in 2 sites
Melolabial lines	4–8 units in 2 sites
Mentalis lines	4–10 units in 2 sites
Platysmal bands	20–60 units in multiple sites (variable)

97

Botox: Avoiding Pitfalls

John R. Burroughs and Richard L. Anderson

Botox is extremely safe, with an LD_{50} of 3500 units in humans. Despite a high safety profile, non-life-threatening complications can be frequent and frustrating to both the patient and the physician. Proper understanding of oculofacial anatomy is paramount to correctly understanding the indications and proper administration of Botox. Botox will not address skin pigmentation/quality, excess skin, contour deformities, volume loss/deformities, or tissue drop. Botox therapy is ideal for initiating cosmetic surgery to patients into practice.

We reconstitute Botox with preserved saline to maximize patient comfort and dilute each vial with 1 ml (10 units/0.1 ml) for eyelid use in blepharospasm and hemifacial spasm and 2.5 ml (4 units/0.1 ml) for cosmetic use and injections in other parts of the face and neck. Dilution increases tissue spread, which is useful in large areas as the forehead, but may increase diplopia or blepharoptosis risk in critical areas of the eyelids. Higher dilutions also have quicker onset and more even distribution of effect. We avoid injection of Botox near operative sites when combined with surgical procedures such as blepharoplasty or facelifts as postoperative edema may cause toxin diffusion to undesired locations.

Ophthalmic complications of Botox can include ptosis, eyebrow ptosis, eyebrow widening, lower eyelid retraction, diplopia, and dry eye. We utilize pressure to injection sites if any hematoma is noted. We recommend blood thinner avoidance if not medically necessary for several days prior to planned treatments.

Botox effect is usually seen 2–3 days following injection with maximal effect at approximately 2 weeks. We therefore do not recommend any touchups until 2 weeks have passed. Ocular complications are fortunately transient and of shorter duration than the intended use but can last up to 3 months. Induced blepharoptosis can be improved by the application of an α-adrenergic agonist (Alphagan or Iopidine) or Naphcon. Diplopia is more problematic. Dry eye syndrome will generally respond well to ocular lubricants. Displeasing induced brow elevation can be managed by giving small dosages to the protagonist areas. For instance, an overarched lateral brow "Spock or Elvira" effect can be managed by placing a few units into the peaked frontalis area. Brow ptosis is more problematic.

In general, men and older patients generally require higher doses for cosmetic and functional injections that often last a shorter duration. Higher doses frequently provide better and longer-lasting results. Many of our referred patients, who have "failed" prior Botox treatment, respond more favorably to higher doses and in optimally placed injection sites. Caution is required if the lower eyelids are lax and only very small amounts can be used in the mid-face to avoid lid droop or altered facial expressions.

98

Botox Injection Techniques: Minimizing Bruising and Discomfort

Jemshed A. Khan

The goal of Botox injection is to deliver an appropriate intramuscular drug dose while minimizing bruising and pain. Ecchymosis is easily visible in the thin skin when it arises from the orbicularis oculi muscle.

- Inject subcutaneously over the orbicularis oculi muscle. Avoid direct intramuscular injection and visible ecchymosis.
- Ecchymosis may also result from transection of fine subcutaneous vessels; look for and avoid such vessels when injecting in the crow's feet area.
- Superficial injection may be delivered by perpendicular or tangential placement of subdermal Botox to relax the frontalis muscle.
- Application of pressure immediately and directly to the injection site will minimize bruising. In the areas of thicker dermis overlying the orbicularis oris, mouth depressors, and corrugator supercilii muscles, intramuscular injection may be OK as the thick overlying tissue will obscure ecchymosis.

Gently pinching the skin overlying the procerus, corrugator, and frontalis muscles may help reduce discomfort and ensure superficial placement of drug. One may also reduce discomfort with topical anesthesia techniques including ice, EMLA, Betacaine LA, etc.

Originally published in: Chen WPD, Khan JA, McCord, Jr. CD. Color Atlas of Cosmetic Oculofacial Sugery. Philadelphia: Butterworth Heinemann/Elsevier. 2004.

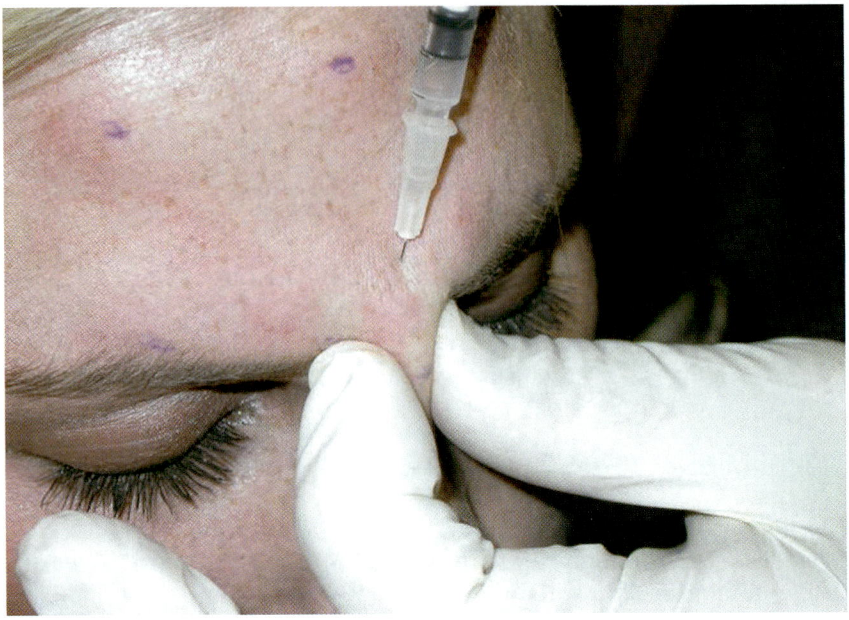

Figure 98.1. The pinch technique is used to ensure correct anatomic placement of the needle tip over the procerus muscle and to reduce discomfort. (Figure courtesy of Richard L. Anderson, MD.)

99

Botulinum Toxin Injections Pearls

Rona Z. Silkiss

For patients undergoing Botox injections in the area of the procerus and glabellar region who are not undergoing filler injection simultaneously, it is often advantageous not only to inject into the origin and insertion of the muscle, but to use part of the Botox volume to "fill" the vertical glabellar rhytids. This provides for an appreciated, albeit short-term, improvement in the rhytids appearance prior to the onset of the Botox effect.

100

Botox Complications

Jemshed A. Khan

Complications may be minimized with appropriate refinement and adjustment of injection sites and doses on subsequent visits.

Botox may be used to reduce the perioral rhytids and to improve the lateral angle of the mouth. However, the risk of perioral treatment includes the possibility of inducing a neurolytic incompetence of the oral sphinter resulting in temporary drooling or inability to whistle. Botox is not helpful in the treatment of the nasiolabial and marionette lines because such treatment results in facial ptosis.

Avoidance of complications includes:

- Appropriate dosing.
- Appropriate anatomic technique.
- Facial ptosis—Limiting injection into mid-face resolves spontaneously.
- Eyelid ptosis—Avoid deep or inferior glabellar treatment, with Iopidine drops or Naphcon-A drops.
- Perioral complications—drooling, inability to whistle.
- Diplopia, dry eyes, exposure keratitis, and lagophthalmos are unusual with cosmetic injections.
- Can sometimes treat antagnoist muscle with additional botox to correct complication.

Originally published in: Chen WPD Khan JA, McCord, Jr. CD. Color Atlas of Cosmetic Oculofacial Sugery. Philadelphia Butterworth Heinemann/Elsevier. 2004.

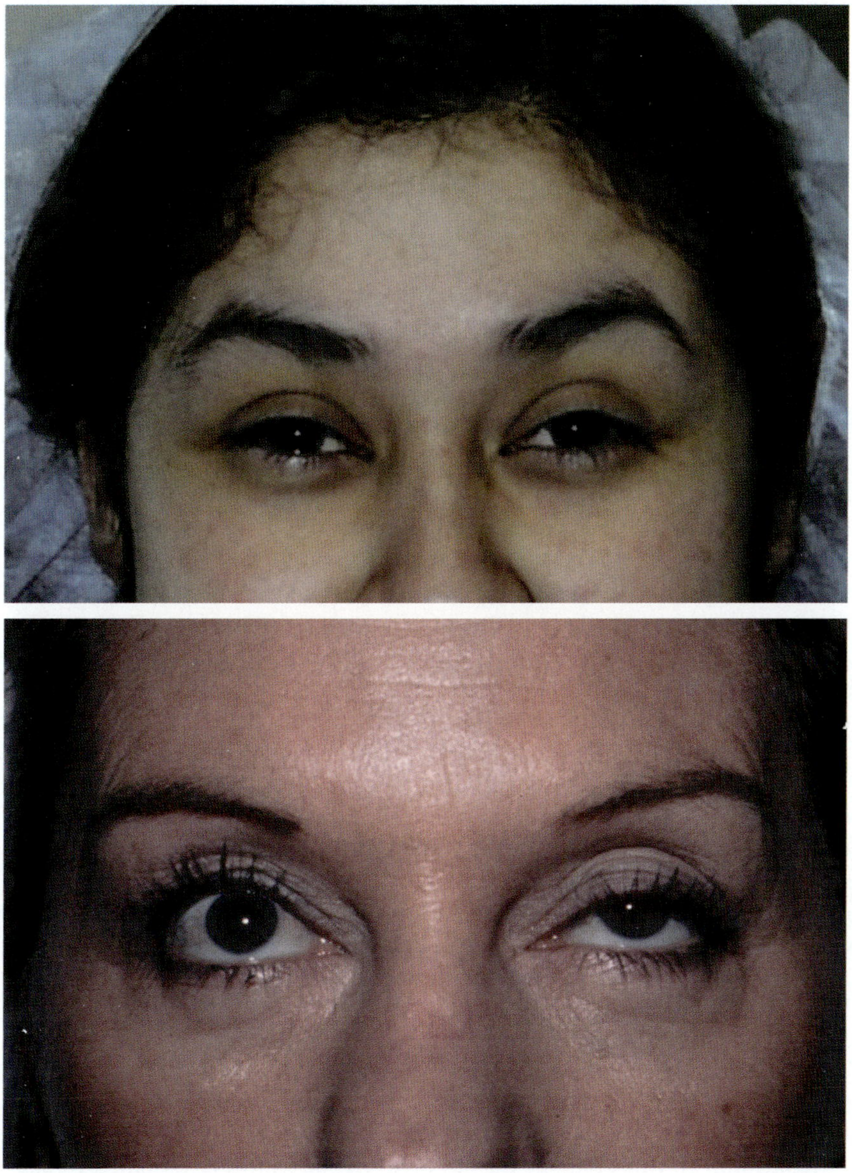

A

B

Figure 100.1. (A) Patient complained of temporal eyebrow tenting following forehead Botulinum type A injections. Placement of additional doses of 5 u in to each lateral frontalis muscle corrected the eyebrow contour deformity. (B) Temporary eyelid ptosis following Botox treatment of forehead and glabella, resolved over 4 weeks.

101

Glabella Treatment with Botox

Samuel M. Lam

I treat the glabella after the forehead, as I do not want the pressure from the ice pack to push the Botox (BTX) over the orbital rim and into the levator complex. The corrugator is the principal muscle to paralyze, but the procerus should almost always be treated in tandem. Even if the corrugator muscle appears to be the only muscle active, treatment of the corrugator alone will often cause recruitment of the procerus, leading to undesirable observation of procerus movement. Routinely, I treat the procerus with 2.5 units and each corrugator with 6.5 units. With more pronounced activity, I will increase this dosage. Although this initial dosage may seem low, proper injection into the correct plane can provide remarkable and enduring aesthetic benefit. If the procerus demonstrates significant activity, I may use two injections of 2.5 units down the length of the procerus as needed. When treating the glabella and at times when combining treatment with the orbicularis,, other neighboring muscles may be recruited after paralysis treatment (i.e., when certain muscles are blocked the unblocked muscles begin to manifest movement and wrinkling to compensate for the lack of movement elsewhere). This phenomenon is observed in the so-called "bunny lines" that extend down the sides of the nasal dorsum are related to nasalis activity. The physician can inject these lines with 1–2 units of BTX per side as needed.

Treatment of the glabella should progress as follows. A small ice pack is placed over the midline radix of the nose for about 20 seconds to anesthetize the procerus. The midline skin is then pinched in the nondominant hand to create neural distraction, and the Botox is injected into the procerus with the prescribed 2.5 units. The left corrugator is then treated. With the nondominant hand, the index finger is placed into the supraorbital notch and the thumb circumscribes the superior limit of the corrugator. (The references to the fingers used refer to a right-handed injector.) The belly of the corrugator is then pinched firmly with the nondominant hand while at the same time gently vibrating the tissues and rubbing the supraorbital notch with the index finger (Figure 101.1). This maneuver accomplishes three important objectives. First, the acupressure movements virtually eliminate all discomfort. Second, the skin is tented upward to allow passage of the needle deeply just above the bone where the corrugator resides. Third, the index finger protects the orbital rim from spreading of the toxin over the rim and onto the levator. The dominant hand injects the Botox in a superolateral direction in a prescribed deep plane. Injecting the Botox upward rather than downward protects any spreading of the toxin over the orbital rim and onto the levator complex. The same technique is applied to the other side. Before injection, the physician should trace out the extent of the corrugator, which may be more readily observed during animation and also in repose by looking at the contour of the muscle over the bone. Additional dosage and injections may be needed more laterally to capture the full extent of the muscle. There is really no need to inject the midline at the level of the corrugator since there is no muscle in this area to address. If any bleeding is noted in this area, it is best to use almost no pressure with the gauze to avoid the Botox being pushed over the orbital rim. It is also wise to flash the Botox syringe back to ensure that no intra-arterial injection has been accidentally committed.

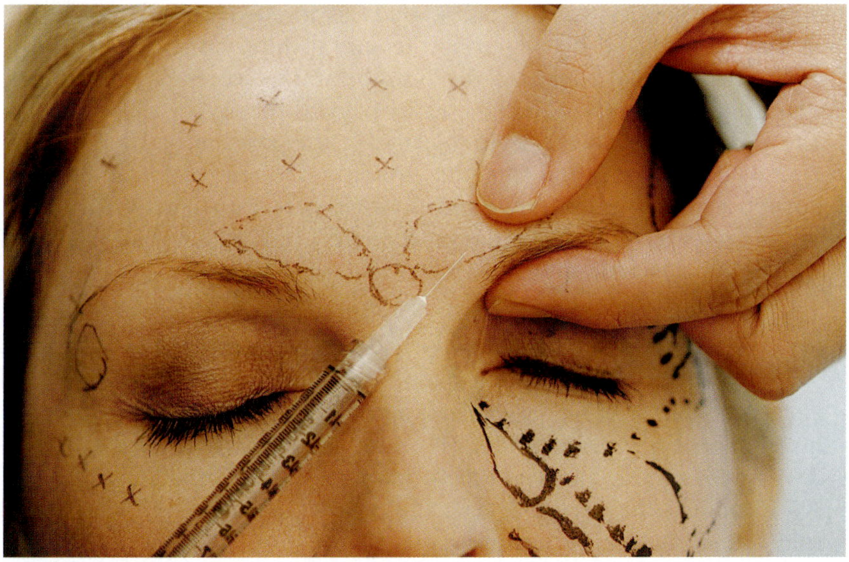

Figure 101.1. The left corrugator muscle is shown being treated. With the nondominant hand, the index finger is placed into the supraorbital notch and the thumb circumscribes the superior limit of the corrugator. (The references to the fingers used refer to a right-handed injector.) The belly of the corrugator is then pinched firmly with the nondominant hand while at the same time gently vibrating the tissues and rubbing the supraorbital notch with the index finger. Typically, a total of 6.5 units is used for each corrugator.

102

Corrugator and Procerus Rhytid Treatment with Botox

Jemshed A. Khan

Cosmetic injection of Botox for glabellar rhytids was approved by the FDA in April 2002. To reduce pain and avoid blunting the needle tip during injection, avoid injecting too shallow or too deep: stay deep enough to be subdermal, but not so deep as to engage the periosteum. Pain may be reduced by palpating the supraorbital notch and thereby avoiding the vertical course of the supraorbital nerve. Stay 5 mm superior to the eyebrow to reduce the risk of eyelid ptosis.

The procerus muscle may be injected in the midline or by pinching the nasal bridge and entering the procerus tangentially. The drug is deposited in the midline. Generally, a single procerus injection is place over the upper nasal bridge either at or up to 7 mm higher than the level of the medial canthal tendon.

Corrugator Treatment Keys

- Perpendicular or tangential injections
- Insulin syringe with integrated 30-gauge needle
- Avoid supraorbital neurovascular bundles
- Avoid dulling the needle against the periosteum
- Inject at subdermal or intramuscular depth
- Deeper injection is more painful
- Injection sites placed at least 5 mm superior to the upper eyebrow border
- Injection sites placed at least 5 mm medial and lateral to the path of the supraorbital nerve
- Two injections of 5 units each delivered to each corrugator muscle and 5 units into the procerus
- Apply pressure after each injection

Originally published in: Chen WPD, Khan JA, McCord, Jr. CD. Color Atlas of Cosmetic Oculofacial Sugery. Philadelphia: Butterworth Heinemann/Elsevier. 2004.

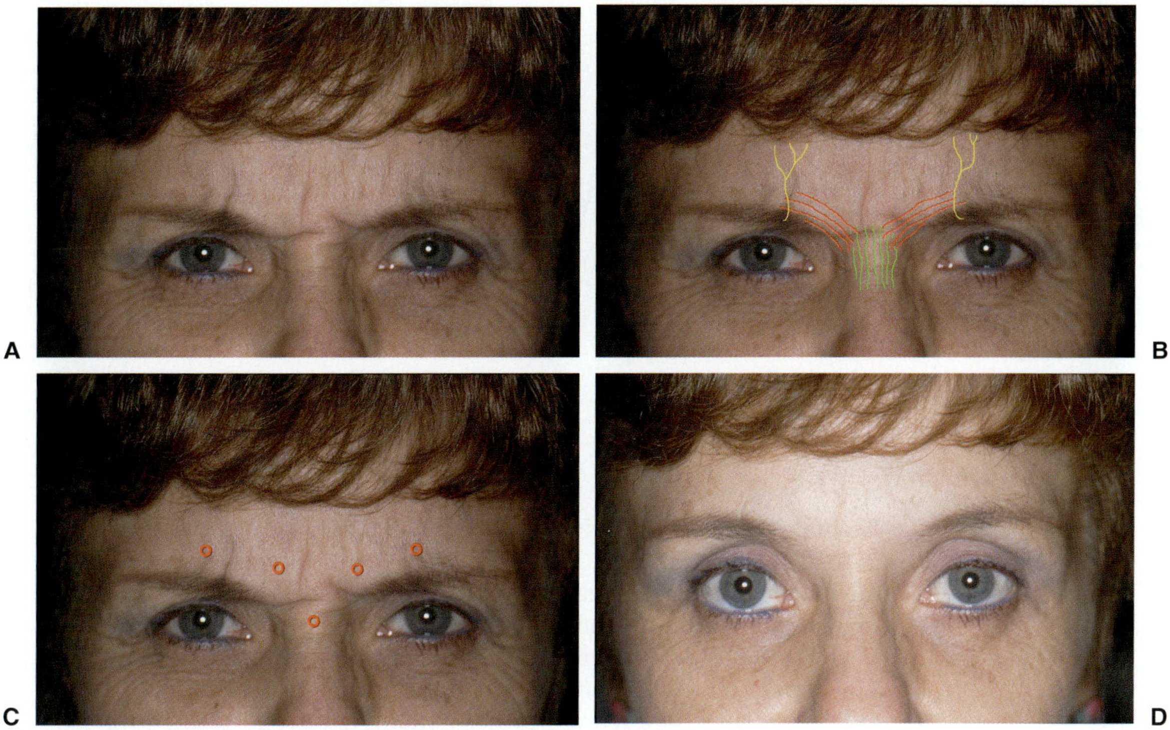

Figure 102.1. (A) Hyperkinetic glabellar zone pre-Botox therapy. (B) The corrugator muscles are represented by red lines; the procerus muscle by green lines. Note the course of the supraorbital nerve (yellow) located 2.5 cm lateral to the midline. The inferior portion of the nerve should be avoided because of postoperative pain or ecchymosis. (C) Five injection sites of 5 units each are typically used. The lateral site is never placed directly superior to the supraorbital notch. (D) Improvement in rhytids following Botox injection. Note the smoother appearance to the glabellar area. (Images courtesy of Joan Kaestner, MD.)

Procerus Treatment Keys

- Procerus muscle is midline structure
- Procerus action creates horizontal furrows
- Emotional signal created by procerus action is aggression
- Inject 5 units into the midline procerus

103

Frontalis Injection with Botox

Jemshed A. Khan

Frontalis injection is useful in treated horizontal forehead wrinkles.

Injection sites: at least 2.0 cm above the eyebrows to avoid a ptotic or adynamic and expressionless eyebrow. Injection is delivered across the medial and lateral frontalis to avoid segmental eyebrow elevation. Two injections per side is usually a good starting point, which may be increased to 10 sites depending upon patient response.

Prior to injection, search for any underlying eyelid ptosis with compensatory eyebrow elevation. Forehead injection and the resulting eyebrow depression may worsen an underlying eyelid ptosis such patients.

Frontalis Treatment Keys

- Frontalis is a paired muscle.
- Connected to the occipitalis muscle.
- Frontalis action raises the eyebrows and furrows the forehead.
- Emotional signal created by frontalis action is surprise.
- Usual injection dose is 1.5–4.0 units per site.
- Usually 4–10 injections sites per patient depending upon frontalis activity.
- Use proper technique to avoid brow ptosis.
- Use proper technique to avoid adynamic eyebrows.

Originally published in: Chen WPD, Khan JA, McCord, Jr. CD. Color Atlas of Cosmetic Oculofacial Sugery. Philadelphia: Butterworth Heinemann/Elsevier. 2004.

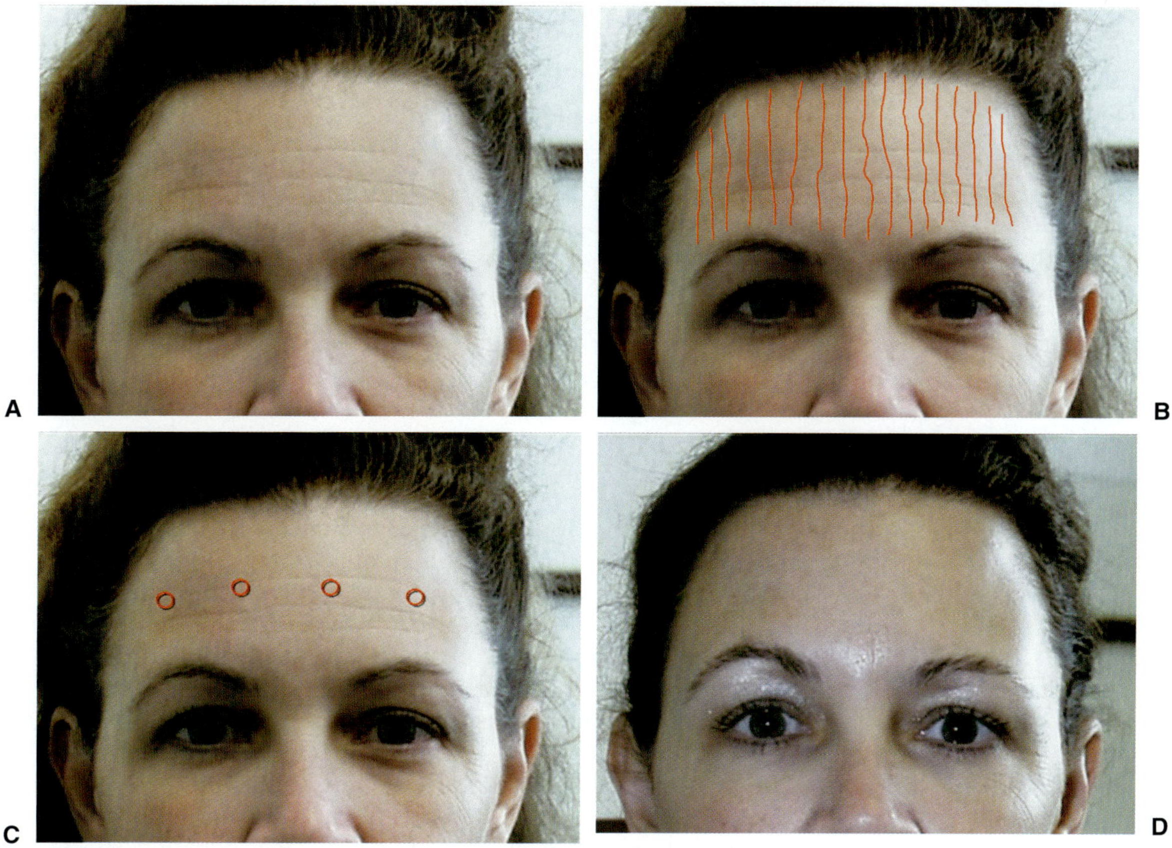

Figure 103.1. (A) Note horizontal forehead furrows prior to injection. (B) Red lines depict the frontalis muscle location. (C) Four injection sites of 1.5–4.0 units per site is a safe beginning dose. (D) Smooth forehead appearance 2 weeks following injection.

104

Frontalis Treatment with Botox

Samuel M. Lam

The only elevator of the forehead is the frontalis muscle, so chemical paralysis of the frontalis without treatment of the three depressors (orbicularis oculi, corrugator, and procerus) may lead to brow descent. This outcome is more commonly observed in the older individual and should be discussed with every patient, especially if the depressors are not simultaneously treated. Foreheads come in all shapes and sizes, and dosage is dependent on the physical size of the exposed forehead as well as patient gender (Figure 104.1). Men tend to have very active frontalis muscles that require larger doses (20–25 units) compared with women (15–20 units) in order to attain an effective and lasting result. I have often exceeded these dosages, depending on the patient's specific anatomy and aesthetic desires.

When treating a forehead, avoid the areas immediately above the lateral tail of the hairy eyebrow (about one fingerbreadth distance above the eyebrow) as injection of the attenuated fibers of the frontalis in this region may lead to brow ptosis. If I see excessive activity in this area, I caution the patient that I will most likely need to do a "touch-up" (approximately 1 unit of Botox) in this area after a week, and I schedule to see the patient at this later date if I think it will be necessary. For men, I tend to inject this area during the initial session. Men need treatment of the entire brow (unless they are exhibiting brow ptosis already laterally) and can tolerate mild brow ptosis in many cases as long they are forewarned about it. If concerned about the patient's reaction, the physician can avoid this area during the initial session. Women cannot tolerate any degree of brow ptosis for two reasons. First, lateral brow ptosis can masculinize the face. Second, women notice even a millimeter of brow ptosis since they use magnifying mirrors and put mascara in the eyelid crease.

As a general rule, the maximal activity of the frontalis muscle occurs between the rhytids. However, I tend to achieve excellent results whether I inject immediately over a rhytid or between them. Also, many practitioners of Botox advocate not injecting the vertical midline of the forehead where the frontalis is either nonexistent or extremely attenuated. I believe that the midline need not be injected when there is an absence of rhytids in that area but should be addressed when rhytids prominently cross the midline.

I tend to distribute the Botox across the forehead in multiple depots (12–20 sites) to achieve the most uniform results. I think treating the entire forehead with only a limited number of injections (no matter how large the total dose) fails to attain a smooth and durable result. I also do not like injecting the Botox deep past the galea, as doing so elicits discomfort and creates a crunching noise that is disconcerting to the patient. I have also noticed that the forehead can cause the most discomfort compared to treatment of the glabella and the orbicularis due to the multiple injection sites. Limiting the depth of penetration reduces discomfort. I also use ice liberally to reduce the pain of injection, but excessive ice can also cause pain when applied to the forehead. In the rare patient, I may have to rely on topical anesthetic application beforehand. When applying ice on the forehead, I use a small ice pack that extends over no more than half of the forehead for approximately 30 seconds or until the patient claims any discomfort. I then have my assistant precede my injection site with a tiny ice pack that extends only about 2 cm in diameter to precool each site immediately prior to my injection. I follow my assistant's small ice pack as I progress across the forehead. At the midway point, I apply another larger ice pack across the second half of the forehead and repeat the above sequence. I also use acupressure and vibration immediately prior to injection. With all these techniques, my patients have expressed great satisfaction and very little discomfort.

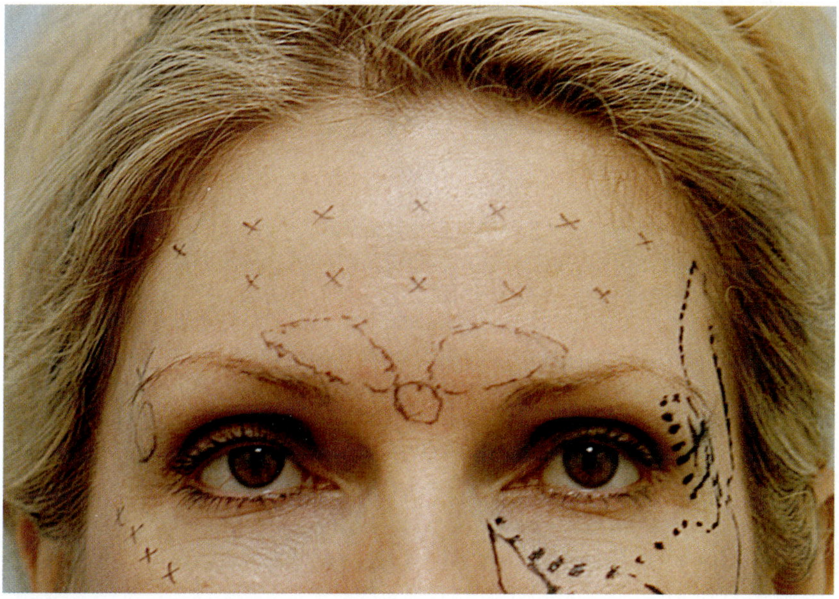

Figure 104.1. Xs on the forehead demonstrate the typical female distribution of injection points for Botox treatment of the frontalis muscle. Each injection point is treated with 2.5 units.

105

Shaping of the Eyebrows with Botox

David F. Horne and Thomas E. Rohrer

By rebalancing the forehead and periocular muscles, Botox injections can improve the shape and position of the eyebrows. It is even possible to induce a modest "chemical brow lift" and help correct intrinsic or iatrogenic asymmetry of the eyebrows. Reports by Carruthers[1] as well as Frankel and Kamer[2] have shown that the majority of patients experience a modest elevation of the brow.

A thorough understanding of the functional anatomy of the upper face is essential to obtain optimal cosmetic outcomes and to avoid undesirable side effects. The muscles involved in modifying the eyebrows may be functionally divided into the elevator (the frontalis), the medial depressors (the medial portion of the orbicularis oculi, the corrugator supercilii, and the procerus), and the lateral depressors (the lateral portion of the orbicularis oculi).

Modifying the Position of the Medial Eyebrows

Treatment of the medial depressors can result in cosmetic improvement of the glabella by elevating the medial aspect of the eyebrow and diminishing dynamic and static "scowl lines" created by contraction of the corrugator supercilii and the procerus. Many patients contract or maintain resting tone in these muscles, causing the medial eyebrows to move inferomedially. This creates vertical rhytides in the glabella, resulting in a tired or angry expression. Chemical paralysis of these muscles results in a decrease in their resting tone, maintenance of the medial eyebrows in a more superolateral position, and an "opening of the glabella" that is cosmetically desirable.

Modifying the Position of the Lateral Eyebrows

The isolated treatment of the medial depressors consistently results in elevation of the lateral eyebrows as well. This may be the result of diffusion of Botox from the medial depressors into the inferomedial portion of the frontalis. Partial paralysis of the medial frontalis triggers a compensatory increase in the resting tone of the lateral frontalis, resulting in an elevation of the lateral and central eyebrow. This effect may be exaggerated in cases where only the medial frontalis is injected with Botox, resulting in marked ptasis of the medial portions of the eyebrows and superolateral movement of the lateral portions. A characteristic and usually undesirable appearance described as a "Jack Nicholson," "Spock," or "quizzical" effect may result. This side effect is treated or prevented by injecting a small amount of Botox into the lateral frontalis muscle. Caution should be taken not to inject too inferior in this area or a ototic lateral eyebrow may ensue. Small injections laterally near the temporal fusion lines above the midway point of the eyebrow and hairline will release the compensatory increase in tone of the frontalis muscle and lower the corresponding lateral eyebrow.

Arching and Lifting the Eyebrows

If the inferomedial and lateral aspects of the frontalis are treated as described above, the compensatory increase in tone of the untreated frontalis overlying the midpupillary area can result in an aesthetically desirable arching of the central portion of the eyebrow. This lifting of the brow can be further supplemented by treating the lateral depressors of the eyebrows, the lateral portions of the orbicularis oculi. In properly selected patients, 1–3 mm of elevation of the eyebrows can be obtained with this technique. Cosmetically unacceptable lifting or arching can be corrected by injecting small amounts of Botox into the portion of the frontalis that has increased in tone. It is important to keep these correcting doses small and located relatively superior to avoid overcorrection and brow ptosis. This chemical brow lift is eliminated if the bulk of the frontalis is treated for dynamic forehead rhytides.

Lowering and Flattening the Eyebrows

An eyebrow that is too high or too arched may be lowered by focally weakening the frontalis that lies superior to it. To avoid overcorrection and ptosis, it is prudent to start with small doses relatively superior (>3 cm above the orbital rim). Reassessment after 10–14 days, with supplemental injections as needed, will minimize the risk of brow ptosis.

Treating Eyebrow Asymmetry

The experienced clinician can use the above principles to improve intrinsic or iatrogenic brow asymmetry in a variety of situations. The patient should be warned that while asymmetric treatment may result in improvement of eyebrow symmetry at rest, dynamic rhytides and functional expression with the eyebrows may be uneven.

Pitfalls

As with any cutaneous injection, pain and small areas of bruising are usually minimal, but sometimes unavoidable. Injecting superificially into thin periorbital skin, using high gauge needles, avoiding obvious underlying blood vessels, and applying pressure for several minutes after injection will minimize these complications.

An unanticipated increase in the resting tone of untreated frontalis is relatively easily treated, as discussed. Overtreatment of the frontalis with resulting brow ptosis is much less acceptable and may persist for weeks to months. Particular caution should be used if treating large portions of the frontalis for reduction of horizontal forehead rhytides at the same time as the glabellar or periocular regions. Using small doses in relatively superior locations in the frontalis or treating the forehead 10–14 days after treating the glabella may avoid this complication.

Inadvertent introduction of Botox into the levator palpebrae superioris will result in eyelid ptosis. Ptosis of the brow or eyelid is cosmetically unacceptable and may partially obstruct the visual field. Fortunately, this is extremely rare. Injections should be placed at least 1 cm above the bony rim of the orbit to reduce the likelihood of this complication. Apraclonidine 0.5% drops three times daily will cause contraction of Müller's muscle. This will partially correct the ptosis until the effect of the Botox has resolved.

Conclusion

With proper technique and understanding of underlying anatomy, intramuscular Botox is a safe and effective way to temporarily modify the shape and position of the eyebrows.

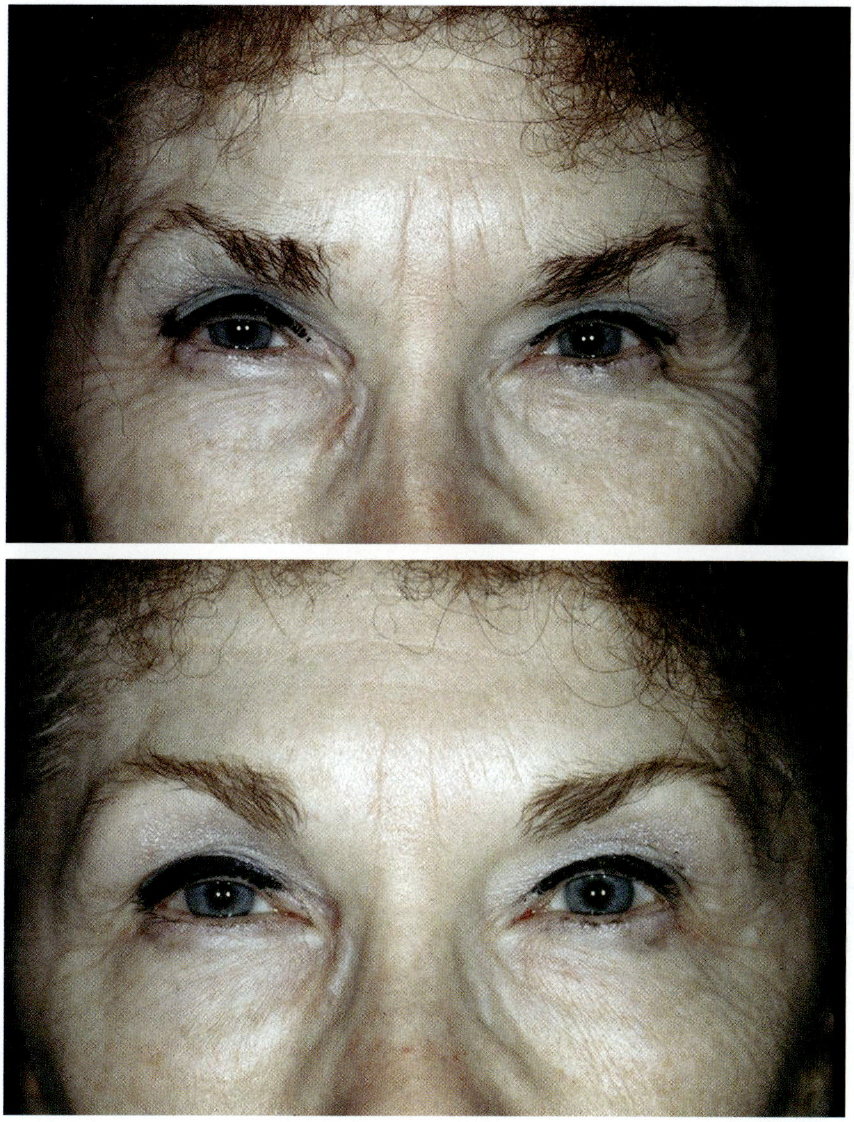

A

B

Figure 105.1. (A) Prebrow and (B) Postbrow shaping with Botox.

References

1. Carruthers A, Carruthers J. Botulinum Toxin. Philadelphia: Elsevier, 2005.
2. Frankel AS, Kamer FM. Chemical browlift. Arch Otolaryngol Head Neck Surg 1998;124:312–323.

106

Botox Injection Techniques: Crow's Feet

Jemshed A. Khan

Crow's feet injection is one of the simplest and most satisfying applications of Botox.

The radiating dermal crow's feet lines result from the concentric constriction of the underlying orbital and preseptal orbicularis oculi muscle. Orbicularis oculi injections of Botox diminshes both active and static crow's feet rhytids, may prophylactically delay the onset and progression of such wrinkles, and improves final outcome following ablative periocular resurfacing (Figure 106.1). Since the thin periocular skin is prone to visible bruising, injection should be in the subdermal plane while avoiding actual intramuscular injection. The loose periocular subdermal plane in the area of crow's feet rhytids should visibly balloon up when the injection is delivered at the proper depth. Following injection, the patient may apply pressure for 1–2 minutes over the injection sites to minimize bruising.

Crow's Feet Treatment Keys

- Avoid visible vessels
- Insulin syringe with integrated 30-gauge needle
- Injection sites 1–2 cm lateral to lateral canthal angle
- 10–15 units total dose per side divided into 2–5 injections per side
- Injections 1–5 cm apart
- Apply pressure after each injection

Originally published in: Chen WPD, Khan JA, McCord, Jr. CD. Color Atlas of Cosmetic Oculofacial Sugery. Philadelphia: Butterworth Heinemann/Elsevier. 2004.

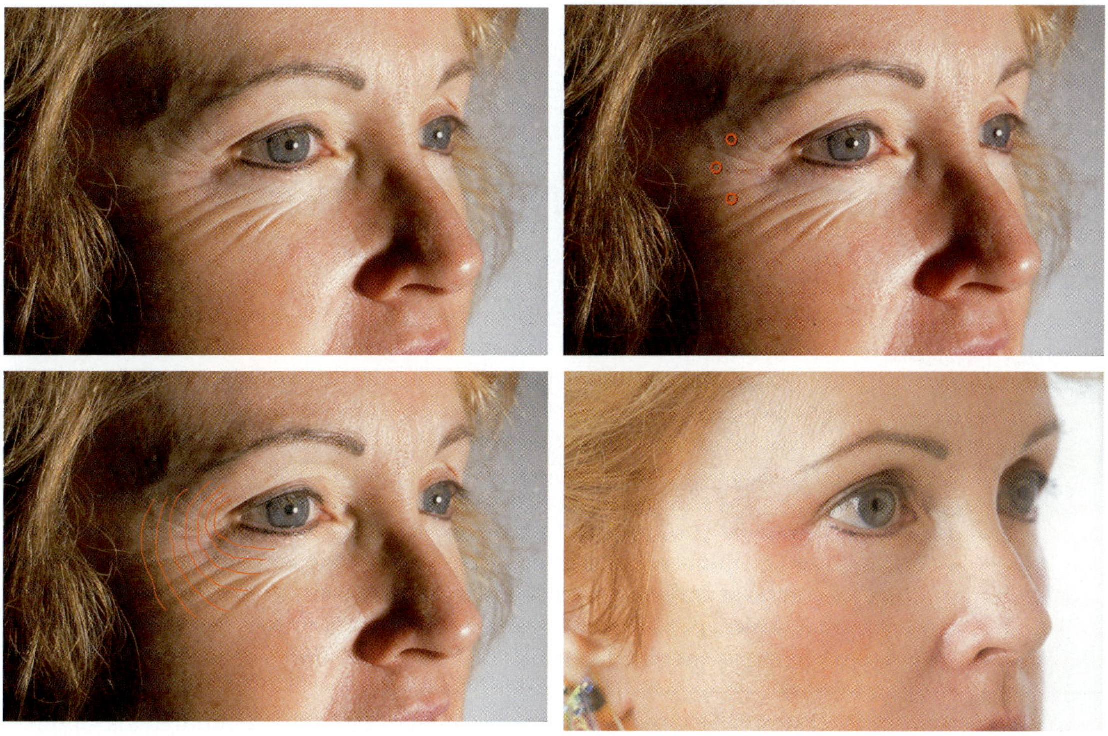

A B C D

Fig 106.1. (A) Crow's-feet rhytids. (B) Typical injection sites for radiating crow's-feet rhytids. (C) Location of underlying concentric orbicularis oculi muscle fibers. (D) Improvement in rhytids following Botox injection. (Images courtesy of Joan Kaestner, MD.)

107

Orbicularis Oculi Treatment with Botox

Samuel M. Lam

Ecchymosis occurs most readily around the eyes and should be minimized to the best of a physician's ability. Avoidance of any anticoagulant is crucial as well as close scrutiny of the skin surface for any major vessels after makeup has been thoroughly removed. Other techniques to avoid ecchymosis involve liberal use of icing and only superficial injection of Botox.

The physician should study the patient's surrounding anatomy. A malar protuberance could represent a malar bag or an orbicularis festoon. A malar bag is a descended and visible malar fat pad; a festoon is a weakened and prolapsed orbicularis-oculi muscle. If the prominence is partially or completely effaced with smiling, an orbicularis festoon is present and the physician should not inject the area as the orbicularis might prolapse further. Preexisting lower eyelid laxity may be exacerbated with Botox, and snap and lid distraction tests are informative. Patients who have wrinkles that extend all the way down the face when smiling are not great candidates for Botox therapy. Chasing these wrinkles down the face may paralyze the zygomaticus musculature and cause unwanted facial droop and loss of normal facial animation. In order to establish realistic expectations for what Botox can achieve in this area, the physician can lift the cheek up manually to evaluate what component of wrinkling is attributed to cheek movement (which cannot be safely addressed with Botox) versus what is caused by orbicularis activity by then having the patient smile. This is shown to the patient in a mirror.

The presence of brow asymmetry may also be partially or entirely corrected with Botox into the upper tail of the eyebrow on the ptotic side. The orbicularis on the contralateral side should not be injected this far supero-laterally for fear that the brow will also elevate on that side, eliminating the symmetrizing benefit. The unopposed frontalis must adequately elevate the brow, which becomes less likely with ongoing age. Botox should not be aggressively injected into the lateral outer frontalis on the descended side so that the frontalis can still act to elevate the brow after injection of the orbicularis depressor.

Compared with other upper facial areas, treatment of the orbicularis oculi tends to last a bit shorter (less than 3 months) compared with 3–4 months on average for other anatomic zones. If the Botox is lasting 2 months or less, higher dosages are warranted. Using less than 10 units of BTX per side typically is insufficient, and I have used as much as 15 units per side to achieve the desired aesthetic result.

The application of ice is very important to shrink periocular vessels as well as limit discomfort. Injection is very superficial to raise a dermal wheal, as the vascular orbicularis muscle resides immediately below the skin surface. The objective is not to inject the muscle but the subcutaneous plane, which will in turn diffuse directly into the muscle. I usually inject about four sites (with 2.5 units per site) around the eyes that correlate with where wrinkles are distributed as observed during animation (Figure 107.1). With any evidence of bleeding from the injection site, the physician applies immediate pressure with gauze for 3 minutes without removing the gauze to observe the area. Unfortunately, even if a small trickle of bleeding is observed from any injection point, there will most likely be at least some ecchymosis there. Unlike in the glabellar region, where pressure application is unsafe, it is mandatory in the orbicularis-oculi region when any bleeding is noted.

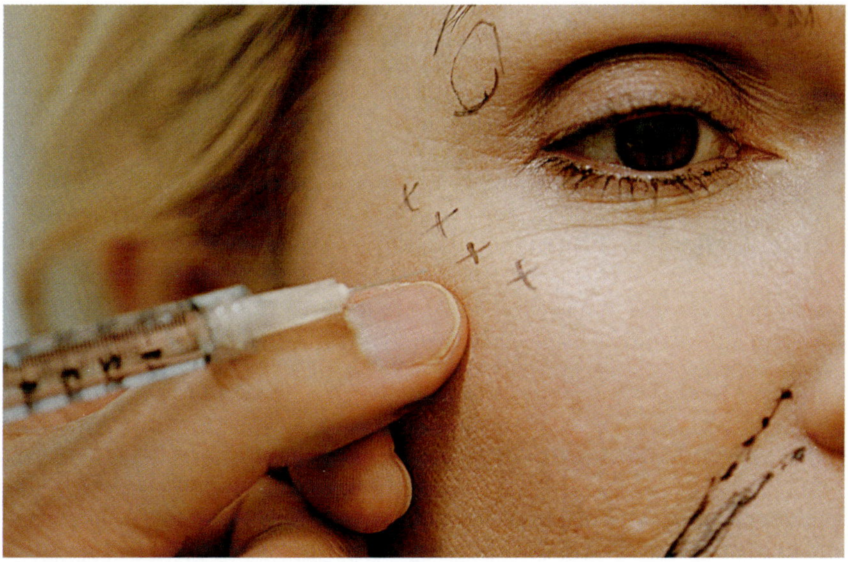

Figure 107.1. The Xs mark the areas for Botox therapy of the orbicularis oculi. Each X is treated with 2.5 units.

108

Perioral Botox Injections

Jemshed A. Khan

The perioral area responds less predictably than other treatment areas because the dynamic muscle actions associated with eating, drinking, speaking, and smiling may be impaired. A cautious approach to this area is warranted.

Only 50% of patients are satisfied with perioral Botox because of lack of perceived benefit or side effects of drooling, difficulty in puckering and whistling, impaired enunciation, or drooling.

Perioral Botox therapy may focus on the orbicularis oris muscle to relax perioral rhytids, the depressor anguli oris muscle to produce an upturn in the lateral oral commissure, or the mentalis muscle to relax a peau d'orange chin.

Orbicularis Oris Therapy

The orbicularis oris muscle must be treated cautiously with very small doses on Botox. Singers and woodwind instrumentalists must be avoided (Figure 108.1).

Depressor Anguli Therapy

The depressor anguli oris is treated cautiously to give a subtle, but pleasing, upturn to the lateral oral commissure (Figure 108.2). Caution must be exercised to avoid injecting too medially and weakening the depressor labii inferioris, which will produce a stroke-like appearance.

Originally published in: Chen WPD, Khan JA, McCord, Jr. CD. Color Atlas of Cosmetic Oculofacial Sugery. Philadelphia: Butterworth Heinemann/Elsevier. 2004.

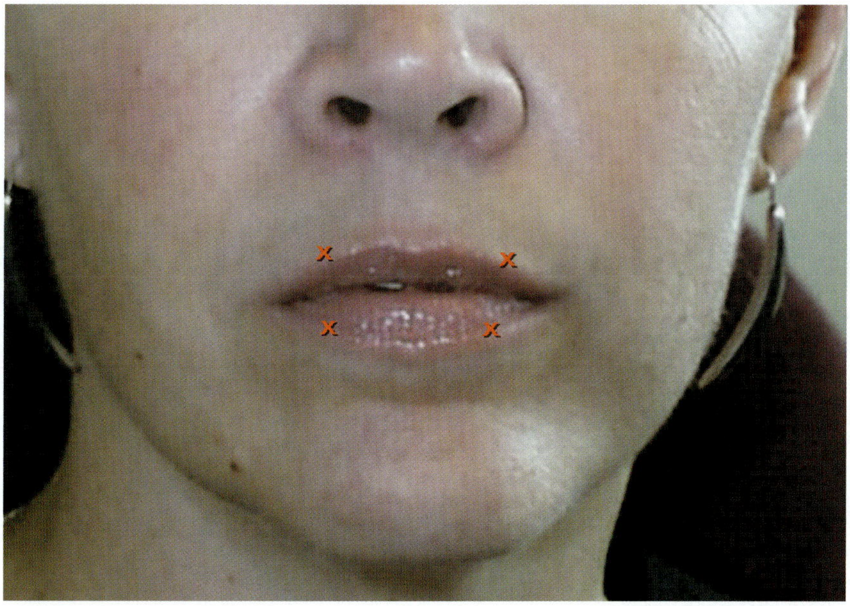

Figure 108.1. Typical treatment sites for vertical lip lines. Minute doses, i.e., 1–1.5 units per site, are delivered. Dose and number of injection sites may be gradually increased if the response is inadequate.

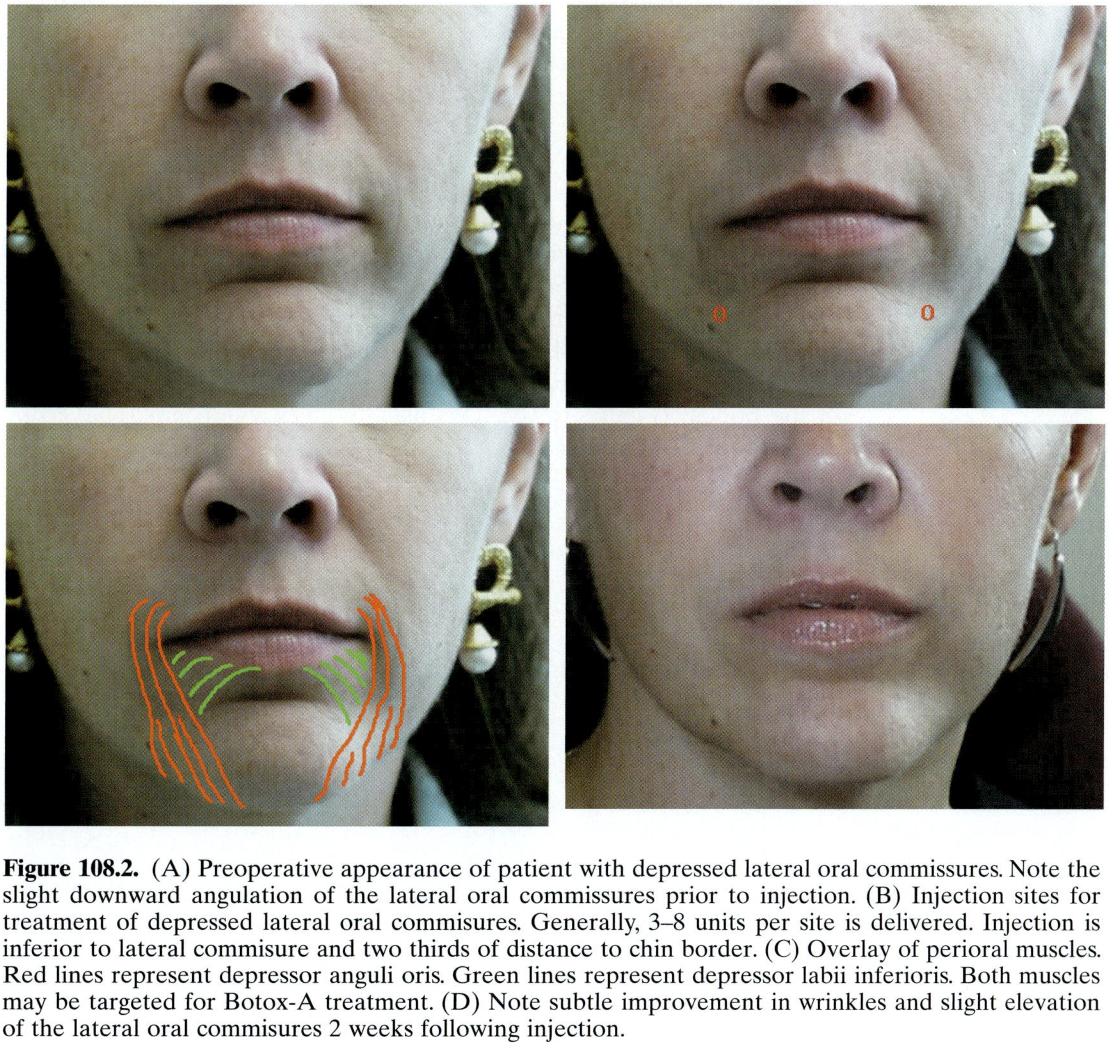

A B C D

Figure 108.2. (A) Preoperative appearance of patient with depressed lateral oral commissures. Note the slight downward angulation of the lateral oral commissures prior to injection. (B) Injection sites for treatment of depressed lateral oral commisures. Generally, 3–8 units per site is delivered. Injection is inferior to lateral commisure and two thirds of distance to chin border. (C) Overlay of perioral muscles. Red lines represent depressor anguli oris. Green lines represent depressor labii inferioris. Both muscles may be targeted for Botox-A treatment. (D) Note subtle improvement in wrinkles and slight elevation of the lateral oral commisures 2 weeks following injection.

109

Botox Injection to the Lacrimal Gland for the Treatment of Epiphora

R. Jeffrey Hofmann

Botox injection to the lacrimal gland can be useful to control epiphora in patients with no drainage system. I have had a number of patients that lost their lacrimal sac following extirpation of a tumor. Some of them refused Jones tube surgery, while others were simply poor surgical candidates. Botox injection to the lacrimal gland is very effective at controlling their symptoms of epiphora, as it is with "crocodile tears" after a Bell's palsy.

Using a 1/2″ 30-gauge needle on a tuberculin syringe, I advance the needle through the skin near the superotemporal orbital rim (Figure 109.1). I aim the needle directly posteriorly for the first 2 mm and then direct the needle superotemporally so that I am in the lacrimal gland fossa. In order to be as far away as possible from the rectus muscles or levator muscle (and avoid diplopia or ptosis), I actually touch bone with the needle tip within the lacrimal gland fossa (Figure 109.2). I then inject 0.1 cc (3.3 units) as I withdraw the needle just a millimeter (so that I am off the bones) (Figure 109.3). This usually gives significant relief from epiphora for 6–8 months.

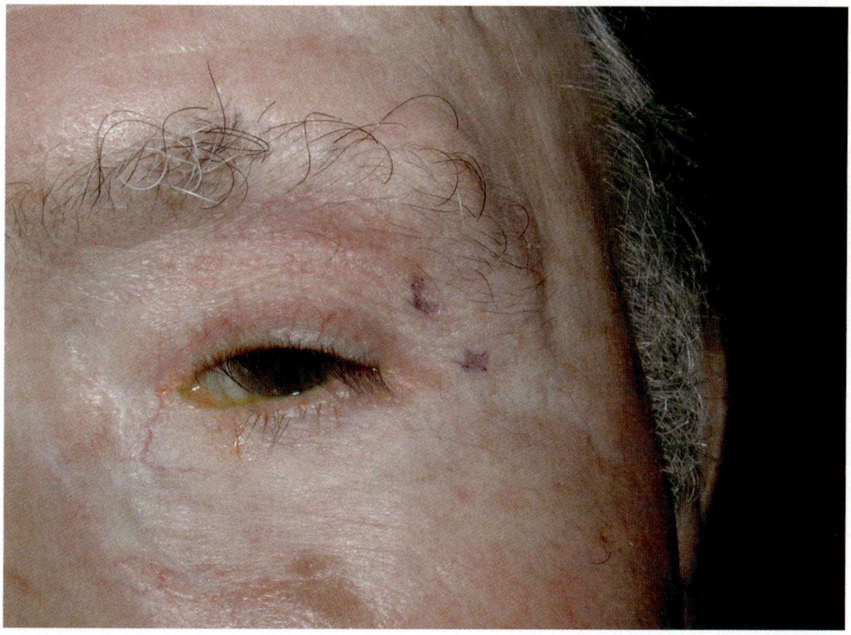

Figure 109.1. The blue "L" marks the point of injection for the lacrimal gland.

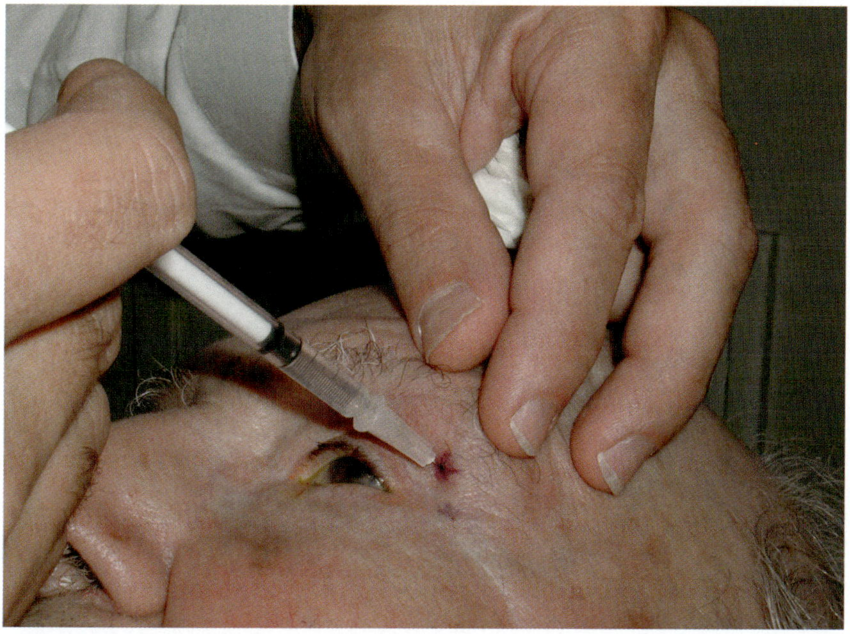

Figure 109.2. After entering the skin, the nedle is advanced posteriorly and superotemporally within the lacrimal gland fossa.

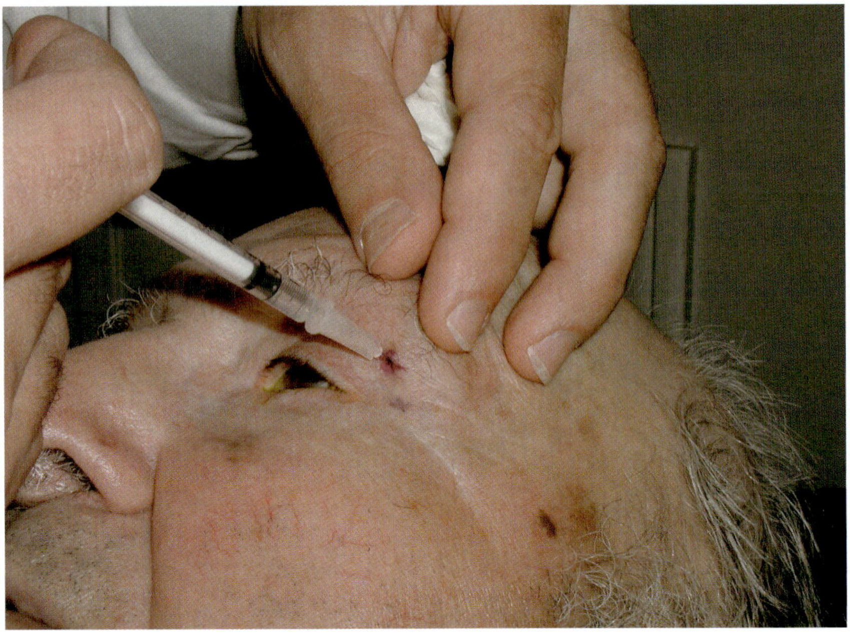

Figure 109.3. A total of 0.1 cc is injected as the needle is withdrawn 1 to 2 mm away from the bones.

110

Botox Therapy for Hyperhydrosis: How I Do It

Charles B. Slonim

Hyperhidrosis is the poor man's detection method for determining where to inject botox:

1. Paint the area (e.g., axilla) with betadine solution (a betadine wipe will do)
2. Allow the betadine to dry
3. Apply a thin layer of cornstarch or fine talc powder over the betadine
4. Shine a handheld spotlight with a 100 W bulb directly on the area
5. The areas of hyperhidrosis will be stimulated and the moisture will cause the betadine to "bleed" through the white powder or cornstarch
6. Photograph the area for documentation
7. Apply a layer of a topical anesthetic (e.g., betacaine, EMLA, etc.)
8. Inject Botox into the dermis in a grid pattern in the targeted area with approximately 1 cm between injections
9. Use 2.5 units in 0.05 cc per injection site

111

Other Uses of Botox

John R. Burroughs and Richard L. Anderson

We have had good results for hyperlacrimation by subconjunctivally injecting 1–3 units into the palpebral lobe of the lacrimal gland. This has been very helpful for patients suffering gustatory crocodile tearing from aberrant regeneration.

Severe lid retraction in active inflammatory dysthroid ophthalmopathy can be treated with a 2–10 units of Botox® given subconjunctivally, supratarsally to the upper eyelid elevator complex.

Low dose and precisely placed, Botox injections have also been helpful for the temporary management of mild to moderate blepharoptosis, with aesthetic augmentation of the vertical palpebral aperture and eyelid fissure asymmetries.

Patients with lagophthalmos and eyelid retraction, with exposure keratopathy from facial palsy, may benefit from improved ocular surface coverage by inducing a blepharoptosis (Botox tarsorraphy). When conservative treatment has been inadequate or if the patient is a poor or unwilling surgical candidate, then a Botox-induced blepharoptosis can be achieved by injecting 5–10 units in the central upper eyelid.

Spastic entropion may respond to a few units given to the lower eyelid pretarsal orbicularis.

Botox can be a "miracle" treatment for migraine headache patients refractory to routine treatments and may require large doses in corrugators, temporalis, occipitalis, and frontalis muscles, so we generally dilute the Botox with 2.5 ml (4 units/0.1 ml) of preserved saline. Careful patient questioning and examination to precisely identify trigger areas is critical. Common trigger areas are the glabella, forehead, temples, and occipital musculature.

Newer oculofacial applications include treatment of oral incontinence in facial paralysis patients. Facial and lip droop can make it difficult to drink and retain fluids and food in the oral cavity during consumption. Small doses to the unaffected side can lessen the angle and asymmetry between the two sides of the oral commissure, which can lessen the incidence or severity of oral incontinence. Injections to the unaffected forehead and face in facial paralysis patients helps provide symmetry and may help stimulate reinnervation on the affected side. Postoperative frontalis overaction following uppr blepharoplasty can also benefit from strategic placement of Botox until motor releasing has occurred.

In summary, the approved uses and off-label applications for Botox continue to expand and find high patient acceptance. Proper understanding of oculofacial anatomy is paramount for safe and effective utilization in functional and cosmetic uses.

112

Botox for Axillary Hyperhydrosis

R. Jeffrey Hofmann

I have treated a number of patients with axillary hyperhydrosis. I have tried the various methods and doses and have found that 100 units (50 units per side) is very effective for about 8 months. This is consistent with what I found with facial hyperhydrosis in Frey's syndrome.

I use 4 cc of saline to reconstitute the Botox (2.5 units per 0.1 cc). I create a grid pattern in each armpit in the hair-bearing area. Each grid is approximately 4 cm × 5 cm (or sometimes 3 cm × 7 cm, depending on the hair distribution pattern). This results in 20–21 different 1 cm × 1 cm injection sites in each armpit. Each injection is 2.5 units (0.1 cc) and is injected intradermally. Inject intradermally rather than subdermally because the target (the sweat gland) is within the dermis. It is nice to see a blanched wheal at each of the injection sites. I find it easier to inect intradermally if I hold and "pinch up" the skin with my left thumb and finger while injecting with my right hand.

Part VIII

Fillers

113

Optimizing Outcome from Facial Cosmetic Injections and Promoting Realistic Expectations

Leslie Baumann

Although the various injectable materials used to minimize the signs of aging facial skin are safe, adverse reactions can occur. Among them, bruising is by far the most common. Practitioners and patients alike can take several steps to reduce the risk of inducing such a response. While there are subtle but distinct differences in the techniques involved in injecting Botox and similar products such as Reloxin (also known as Dysport) and Myobloc as well as the various soft tissue augmentation fillers (including the collagen products Zyderm, Zyplast, Cosmoderm, and Cosmoplast and the hyaluronic acid [HA] products Restylane, Hylaform, Hylaform Plus, Captique, and Juvéderm), the approach to avoid bruising as a sequela of such procedures is the same. I have found that discussions of ways to avoid and treat bruising are part and parcel of promoting realistic expectations.

Preparations

1. Instruct patients to avoid, 10 days prior to the scheduled procedure, medications, herbal formulations, and other agents that confer a blood-thinning effect and, therefore, can facilitate bruising (Table 113.1). Tylenol, which does not affect platelet function, can be taken.
2. Applying ice to the area to be treated prior to injection and after injections may decrease bruising.
3. Note that bruising is more likely to occur in very light skinned individuals and red heads.

Posttreatment

1. Recommend that patients obtain a product containing arnica or vitamin K, and/or retinol, to apply after the procedure as a further preventive measure against bruising and/or to treat any bruises that develop.

2. Advise patients to avoid hot showers, saunas, or other exposure to heat for 6 hours after injection to reduce the risk of bruising. Also, suggest avoiding sun exposure and alcohol for 24 hours, since both have been associated with erythema.

Expectations

Tell Botox/Reloxin patients the following:

1. Treatment involves injections via a tiny needle smaller than the size of a pinhead.
2. Frown lines usually require three injections: crow's feet receive three injections per side, and lines in the forehead usually get five to eight injections.
3. Following treatment, the skin will have a few raised bumps in the area of injection that look like insect bites. These typically last about 30 minutes.
4. Having already taken precautions against bruising, patients should be reminded which products to use at the first sign of bruising.
5. All skin care and makeup use can be resumed after treatment.
6. It takes about 10 days for the full treatment effects to be seen.
7. Treatment effects last 4–6 months (Myobloc injections last about 6 weeks).

Tell soft tissue augmentation patients the following:

1. Each wrinkle will require about three to five injections to treat.

2. HA fillers are more painful than collagen injections because the collagen-containing fillers contain the anesthetic lidocaine.

3. Collagen fillers are associated with less swelling and bruising than HA fillers. Injecting first with collagen and then HA will often reduce swelling and decrease the bruising risk as well as provide the benefits of both types of fillers.

4. Collagen fillers tend to last 4–6 months.

5. Most HA products last 4–6 months. Juvéderm may last up to 1 year.

6. Sculptra, a dermal stimulator rather than filler (it stimulates the production of collagen), may last as long as 2 years. Unlike the fillers, it does not provide instant results—it is injected every month for 3–5 months until the desired result is achieved. Epinephrine can be added to the product to decrease bruising.

7. Dermal stimulators can be combined with dermal fillers or Botox/Reloxin (like dermal fillers) to achieve both immediate short-term correction and delayed long-term correction.

8. A good skin care routine, including a retinoid such as Tazorac, Differin, or Retin-A to prevent future wrinkles, is recommended. Sunscreen should be used DAILY as well as an antioxidant supplement.

It is essential to be candid with patients regarding the results and potential side effects of cosmetic facial surgery. Specific expectations should be provided by the practitioner, who should underestimate or underpromise in terms of the finished result. These are not permanent procedures. Finally, good consent should be obtained so that patients are fully informed about potential complications.

Table 113.1. Drugs and Herbal Agents to Avoid for at Least 10 Days Prior to Scheduled Injections

→ Alcohol
→ Coumadin
→ Fish oil
→ Garlic
→ Ginger
→ Ginkgo
→ Ginseng
→ Green tea
→ Nonsteroidal antiinflammatory drugs (NSAIDs)
■ Aspirin
■ Advil
■ Motrin
■ Ibuprofen
→ St. John's wort
→ Vitamin E
→ Warfarin

114

Filler Pearls: General Considerations

John R. Burroughs and Richard L. Anderson

Fillers are an outstanding adjunct to Botox and, in some situations, are superior to surgery. In our practice, we prefer the nonanimal-based synthetic fillers (Restylane, Juvederm, Perlane, and Radiess). This is because skin and allergy testing is not required and there is no risk of animal-based disease transmission. In our practice, we have found that patients have a higher acceptance for the synthetic than for animal-based products. Patient acceptance is quite high, and both the physician and patient can immediately enjoy the rejuvenative effect just following injection. We recommend patients avoid any blood-thinning agents for approximately 2 weeks prior to injections.

Hyaluronic acid fillers can be reversed by injecting a small amount of hyaluronidase.[1] The injection of 25–150 units of hyaluronidase will remove hyaluronate fillers in the event of asymmetry or overtreatment. Nitropaste can also be kept on hand to apply to the skin in case of vascular compromise.

Reference

1. Soparkar, CN, Patrinely JR, Tschen J. Erasing restylane. Opthal Plast Reconstr Surg 2004;20:317–318.

115

List of Fillers

Bradley T. Kovach

Table 115.1. List of fillers

Category	Trade name (company)	Composition	Year of FDA approval	FDA–approved indications (year of approval)	Additional clinical uses	Duration of effect
Superficial dermal fillers						
	Cosmoderm I (Allergan)	Human collagen 35 mg/ml in 0.3% lidocaine	2003	Injection into the superficial papillary dermis for correction of soft tissue contour deficiencies such as wrinkles and acne scars	Overlay of deeper fillers	2–4 months
	Cosmoderm II (Allergan)	Human collagen 65 mg/ml in 0.3% lidocaine	2005	Same as Cosmoderm I	Same as Cosmoderm I	2–4 months
	Zyderm I (Allergan)	Bovine collagen 35 mg/ml in 0.3% lidocaine	1981	Same as Cosmoderm I	Same as Cosmoderm I	2–4 months
	Zyderm II (Allergan)	Bovine collagen 65 mg/ml in 0.3% lidocaine	1983	Same as Cosmoderm I	Same as Cosmoderm I	2–4 months
Mid- and deep dermal fillers						
	Cosmoplast (Allergan)	Human collagen 35 mg/ml crosslinked with glutaraldehye in 0.3% lidocaine	2003	Injection in the mid- to deep dermis for correction of soft tissue contour deficiencies such as wrinkles and acne scars	Lip augmentation, folds (such as nasolabial folds and marionette lines), angles of the mouth	3–5 months
	Captique (Allergan)	Hyaluronic acid 5.5 mg/ml	2004	Injection in the mid- and deep dermis for correction of moderate to severe facial wrinkles and folds (such as the nasolabial folds)	Lip augmentation, marionette lines, tear troughs, angles of the mouth, prejowl sulcus, atrophic scars, others	3–5 months

continued

Table 115.1. Continued

Category	Trade name (company)	Composition	Year of FDA approval	FDA–approved indications (year of approval)	Additional clinical uses	Duration of effect
	Elevess (Galderma Phama. S.a., and Anika Therapeutics) Augmentation Product (Anika Therapeutics, Inc.)	Hyaluronic acid 28 mg/ml with 0.3% lidocaine	2006	Same as Captique	Not commercially available	Approximately 6 months
	Fascian (Fascia Biosystems, LLC)	Freeze-dried cadaveric fascia lata reconstituted with saline or lidocaine	FDA approval not required	FDA approval not required	Lip augmentation, rhytids and folds, atrophic scars	Not well known (at least 3–4 months)
	Hylaform (Allergan)	Hyaluronic acid 5.5 mg/ml	2004	Same as Captique	Same as Captique	3–5 months
	Juvederm Ultra (Allergan)	Hyaluronic acid 24 mg/ml	2006	Same as Captique	Same as Captique	6–12 months
	Restylane (Medicis)	Hyaluronic acid 20 mg/ml	2003	Same as Captique	Same as Captique	5–7 months
	Zyplast (Allergan)	Bovine collagen 35 mg/ml crosslinked with glutaraldehye in 0.3% lidocaine	1985	Same as Cosmoplast	Same as Cosmoplast	3–5 months
Deep dermal fillers						
	Hylaform Plus (Allergan)	Hyaluronic acid 5.5 mg/ml	2004	Same as Captique	Marionette lines, angles of the mouth atrophic scars, prejowl sulcus	3–5 months

	Juvederm Ultra Plus (Allergan)	Hyaluronic acid 24 mg/ml	2006	Same as Captique	Same as Hylaform Plus	6–12 months
	Radiesse (Bioform Medical, Inc.)	Calcium hydroxyapatite microspheres	2006 (for cosmetic use)	Subdermal implantation for correction of moderate to severe facial wrinkles and folds, such as the nasolabial folds; subdermal implantation for correction of HIV-associated lipoatrophy; oral/maxillofacial defects; vocal cord insufficiency; radiographic tissue marking	Cutaneous lip augmentation (not vermillion lip), age-related lipoatrophy, facial contouring, atrophic scars	9–18 months
Subcutaneous fillers						
	AdatoSil-5000 (Bausch and Lomb)	Liquid injectable silicone	1994	Prolonged retinal tamponade in complicated retinal detachments	Moderate to severe rhytids and folds, atrophic scars	Permanent
	Artefill (Artes Medical, Inc)	Polymethylmethacrylate microspheres in vehicle of 3.5% bovine collagen with 0.3% lidocaine	2006	Correction of the nasolabial folds	Moderate to severe rhytids and folds, atrophic scars	Permanent
	Autologous fat	Autologous fat	FDA approval not required	FDA approval not required	Lip augmentation, facial folds, facial contouring, lipoatrophy, dorsal hand augmentation, correction of liposuction contour defects	1 year–permanent

continued

Table 115.1. Continued

Category	Trade name (company)	Composition	Year of FDA approval	FDA–approved indications (year of approval)	Additional clinical uses	Duration of effect
	Cymetra (Life Cell Corporation)	Human cadaveric proteins, primarily collagen, elastin, and glycosaminoglycans	FDA approval not required (classified as banked human tissue)	FDA approval not required (classified as banked human tissue)	Lip augmentation, deep rhytids and folds, atrophic scars	3–6 months
	Sculptra (Dermik Laboratories)	Poly-L-lactic acid particles 2–50 μm in diameter reconstituted with 2–10 ml saline or lidocaine	2004	HIV-associated facial lipoatrophy	Age-related lipoatrophy, facial contouring	Up to 2 years
	Silikon-1000 (Alcon)	Liquid injectable silicone	1997	Same as AdatoSil-5000	Moderate to severe rhytids and folds, atrophic scars	Permanent
Subdermal implants						
	Advanta (Oceanbreeze Surgical Supply)	Expanded polytetrafluoroethylene	2000	Facial plastic and reconstructive surgery	Lip augmentation, deep rhytids and folds	Permanent
	Alloderm (Life Cell Corporation)	Human cadaveric proteins, primarily collagen, elastin, and glycosaminoglycans	FDA approval not required (classified as banked human tissue)	FDA approval not required (classified as banked human tissue)	Same as Advanta	6–12 months

Softform (Tissue Technologies, Inc.)	Expanded polytetrafluoroethylene	1998	Plastic and reconstructive surgery	Same as Advanta	Permanent
Ultrasoft (Tissue Technologies, Inc.)	Expanded polytetrafluoroethylene	2001	Plastic and reconstructive surgery	Same as Advanta	Permanent

116

Dermal Filler Pearls: the Hyaluronic Acids

John R. Burroughs and Richard L. Anderson

Our preferred hyaluronic acid dermal fillers are Restylane, Perlane, and Juvederm. Each of these has a very high safety profile and are easier to inject than Radiesse. They are outstanding for lip enhancement, including the vermillion border, perioral rhytids, and for less severe glabellar and nasolabial folds or as a superficial fine tuning to deeper filling with Radiesse. The newer, higher viscosity hyaluronic acids, however, are excellent for deep lip augmentation, nasolabial folds, and deep rhytid filling. We have found excellent success treating nasojugal ("tear trough") deformities with hyaluronic acids, which offers a nonsurgical option to cosmetic lower eyelid blepharoplasty (Figure 116.1). Patients require variable amounts depending on the desired outcome and severity of the folds. Injections deep (periosteally) or just below the orbicularis tend to cause less swelling and bruising below the eyes. The effects are potentiated by the concomitant application of Botox. We generally use the provided needle and find that direct injection with withdrawal of the needle as well as the described "feathering" technique both work well. We routinely perform the infraorbital and mental nerve blocks as previously prescribed, as lip injections are quite painful. Premark the perioral rhytids prior to the nerve blocks to ensure optimal filling.

We have found that the hyaluronic acids last longer when Botox is also injected. We recommend that patients not aggressively massage any perceived irregularities, as this can worsen bruising and swelling and the patient may inadvertently overmassage the filler out of position. We advise patients to ice the areas a few hours following injections to reduce swelling. Injection to areas of high dynamicity (the perioral rhytids) will last less time that relatively adynamic areas, such as horizontal forehead rhytids or lower eyelid tear trough defects. Perlane and Juvederm Ultra Plus contain higher concentrations and reportedly last longer than the other hyaluronic formulations. Deep rhytids may further benefit by first performing subcision with a needle (e.g., 27-gauge) followed by placement of hyaluronic filler.

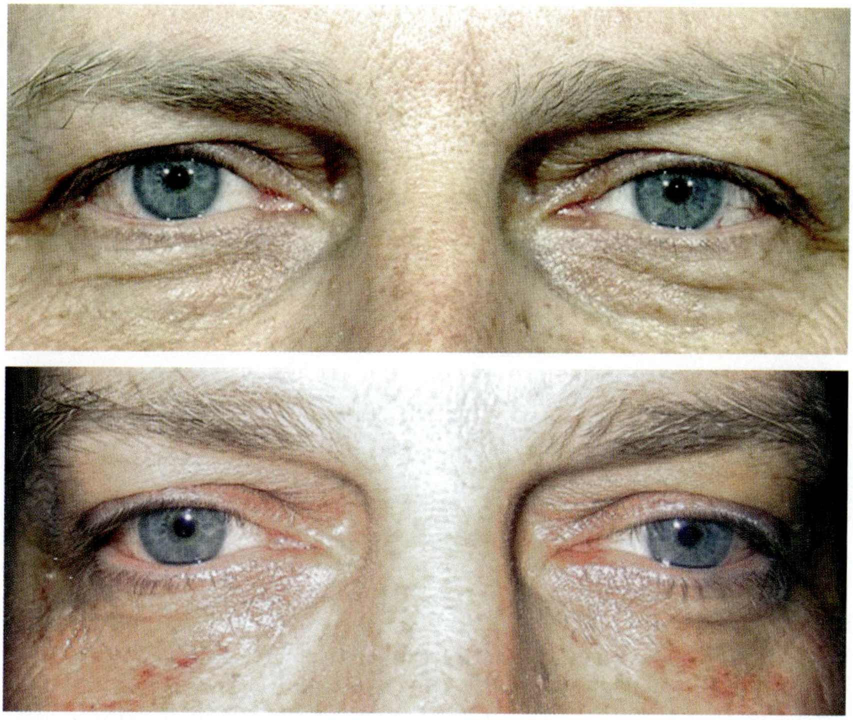

A

B

Figure 116.1. (A) Preinjection of Restylane in a patient with pronounced lower eyelid hollowness "tear trough deformities." (B) Immediately following the injections, showing the marked improvement.

117

Radiesse Pearls

John R. Burroughs and Richard L. Anderson

For deep glabellar and nasolabial folds, our preferred filler is Radiesse®. Radiesse is calcium hydroxyapatite gel. Radiesse is an excellent dermal filler for severe folds, wrinkles that require large volumes and respond well to deep placement, which is critical with Radiesse. It is recommended to inject Radiesse below the dermis to avoid visibly noticeable lumps and irregularities. For the nasolabial folds, inject slightly medial to each nasolabial fold as the natural muscular action of the facial muscles will tend to lateralize the effect and can worsen the appearance of the folds if not placed medially (Figure 117.1).

We inject with a 1.25-inch 27-gauge needle as the material is quite thick. A linear threading or fanning technique can be used to achieve linear filling or volumization. Mark the nasolabial folds prior to injection of a nerve block, which is preferred by most patients for nasolabial and lip augmentation. The nerve block is performed by injecting the upper and lower gingival sulcus with a 1.25-inch 27-gauge needle in line with the patient's pupils, which will anesthetize the infraorbital and mental nerves. Use 1–2% lidocaine with epinephrine with 1–2 ml at each injection site. It is critical to premark the nasolabial folds prior to local anesthetic injection due to distortion of the tissues and to ensure slight medialization of the filler placement. A single syringe (1.3 cc) of Radiesse is adequate for most nasolabial folds. Some patients desire or require a second syringe at a later time to achieve an optimal result. In the glabellar areas a quarter to half a syringe is all that is required. Patients should be cautioned, and placement must be precise in the glabellar region as necrosis and or visual loss has been reported with intravascular injection of fillers. In general, glabellar fold injections are not uncomfortable, and we do not inject local anesthetic, which distorts the target area. However, a small amoung (0.5 cc) of local may be injected for supratrochlear and suproorbital nerve blocks.Radiesse is not optimal for lip augmentation, as the patients often complain of lumps and irregularities. Caution must be exercised to avoid injecting Radiesse too superficially, which can cause skin necrosis. We have found Radiesse to give improvement for the reported 2 years in most of our patients.

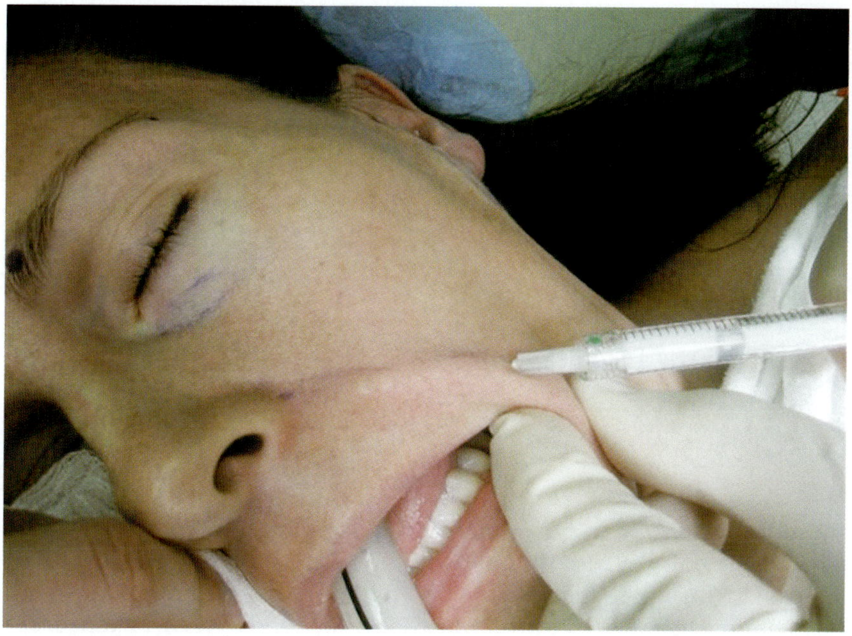

Figure 117.1. Injection of Radiesse into the left nasolabial fold. Note the slight medial placement to the premarked nasolabial fold.

118

Juvederm Pearls: Fine and Superficial Lines

John R. Burroughs and Richard L. Anderson

Juvederm is a newer nonanimal-based hyaluronic acid that has the advantage of lower viscosity allowing for easier injection. Juvederm is technically for filling minimal rhytids, particularly for perioral lines and for defining the vermillion border. It works very well to enhance the vermillion border as an adjunct to deeper lip augmentation with Restylane, Perlane, and Juvederm Ultra Plus. Superficial, fine lines may also be treated by first performingsubcision with an injection needle (e. g., 27-gauge), followed by an injection of hyaluronic acid through a 32-guage needle. The 32-gauge needle seems to thin the filler viscosity, enabling fine, superficial rhytid filling while avoiding lumps. Caution is needed with superficial filling to avoid skin color discoloration, and it is imperative to ensure that the needle is securely fastened to the luer-lock syringe to avoid accidental needle expulsion and potential ocular injury.[1]

Reference

1. Lin DJ, Sami MS, Burroughs JR, Soparkar CN, Patrinely JR. Ocular injury from local anesthetic injections: needle expulsion—the luer-lock allure. Arch Facial Plast Surg 2006;8:436.

119

Achieving Beautiful Lip Augmentation

Kimberly J. Butterwick

Consultation

Achieving successful and beautiful lip augmentation is a balance of the physician's aesthetic eye, the patient's natural anatomy, and the patient's desired look. A key to a satisfied patient is to understand the patient's concerns and goals. This is established during the consultation, in which the patient's goals for her lips are discussed. Does a patient want her lips larger or simply to have better definition when applying lip liner? Patients have unique preferences, such as whether he or she wants the upper lip larger or smaller than the lower lip or how large the lip should be. Some want central fullness, while others desire a full lip across the entire length. Theses goals are discussed in the context of the examination period. Some patients have very thin lips, which may not be amenable to the goals that they have in mind. Some have a very long distance from the nose to the vermillion border and augmentation would make a heavy protruding upper lip. Many patients are afraid to have the lip overdone and need reassurance that enhancement can be very natural and undetectable. Patients with a history of herpes simplex virus may need to be treated prior to the procedure. Allergies and filler choices are discussed as well. The discussion will therefore outline a reasonable outcome, duration, expense, risks, and benefits.

Anesthesia

The lips are by far the most sensitive area for injecting fillers of the face. I have found that ice and topical anesthetics are adequate only for the injection of collagen products that contain local anesthetic and are less viscous, flowing through tissue without resistance. For the use of any other filler, such as hyaluronic acid or fat, nerve blocks or sulcus blocks[1] are utilized with 1% lidocaine, with or without epinephrine. If the patient has numerous vertical rhytids, a sulcus block is not utilized, as the edema from the anesthetic may obliterate some of these lines. However, patients may prefer the sulcus block, because the anesthetic wears off quickly—within an hour. One should try to use the least amount of local anesthetic to achieve anesthesia so as not alter the natural anatomy of the lip. A recently described means of applying topical anesthetic to mucosal membranes has been described, but has not been reproducible in the initial attempts at our office.[2]

Choice of Filler

My filler of choice for the lips is nonanimal-based hyaluronic acid (Restylane and Juvederm). This filler has excellent longevity in the vermillion border (6–10 months), minimal morbidity, and very few side effects. Collagen products, both bovine and bioengineered, have excellent flow characteristics, but their longevity is roughly half that of hyaluronic acids. Other hyaluronic acid products (Hylaform, Perlane, Captique) are also available, and the reader may prefer some of these for ease of low versus firmness desired in the lip. Permanent or semipermanent fillers, such as Radiesse, Artefill, and Sculptra, are generally contraindicated for the vermillion of the lip due to risk of nodularity. After utilizing hyaluronic products, a seasoned patient may elect other offerings, such as silicone, new softer Gortex implants, or fat injections. Silicone is used by some practitioners, but fear of long-term side effects limits its use. Autologous fat seems to have a relatively low level of "take" in the lips compared to other sites, but does have potential for permanence without nodularity.

Anatomic Guidelines

The lip is subdivided into red and white segments at a well-defined and arched vermillion border. The philtrum is the vertical depression at the center of the upper lip, bordered on either side by philtral columns. The upper lip is generally M-shaped, with a cupid's bow representing two anatomic mounds at the highest point of the bow, with a midline tubercle. The lower lip is slightly W-shaped, with two lateral lobes and a midline groove. The upper lip is more arched, wider, and longer than the lower lip. The upper lip vermillion is generally less than the lower lip height, although this varies from individual to individual. The upper lip projects approximately 2 mm more than the lower lip.

Elements to consider when injecting the lip include:

- Upper lip shape
- Lower lip shape
- Philtral columns
- Balance of the upper and lower lip
- Texture of the lip
- Definition
- Natural movement

Technique

The patient is seated upright with the head resting on the chair. Divide the lip into quadrants and inject the right upper, the left upper, the left lower, and the right lower, in that order; switching sides of the table. First inject the vermillion border space, starting at the lateral-most aspect of the right upper lip and inject toward the center. The skin is stretched between the thumb and index finger of the nondominant hand while the needle is inserted at the vermillion border. The filler will travel along the vermillion border space to variable degrees. Hyaluronic products rarely flow along the entire border. Inject until the filler seems to stop and continue on from that point along the vermillion border. At times the vermillion space will extend above the actual vermillion into a well-defined white roll. Injecting this more superior space may result in an artificial white accentuation of this natural anatomy. I therefore try to inject on the red edge of the vermillion border space (Figure 119.1). Inject to the peak of the cupid's bow. Observe how much filler is required, then cross the table and inject the same quantity in a similar fashion. It is important to note the quantities injected, because patients will feel if one side is heavier and injected with more material than the other. Asymmetries should be considered, however. One side may require more than the other. Depending on the anatomy of the cupid's bow, inject along the cupid's bow bilaterally from the center of the bow. If the center portion of the cupid's bow is too wide, it is helpful not to inject this area as one can narrow the cupid's bow when the filler on either side pushes against it.

Then inject the left lower lip along the vermillion space starting at the lateral most aspect and injecting centrally. Usually two to three separate entry sites are required due to the material ceasing to flow along the border. It is best not to force the filler if resistance is felt to avoid lumpiness or inadvertent focal filling. The right lower lip is then injected in a similar fashion. If the patient has lost some of the natural anatomy along the philtral columns, these are injected at this time. The goal is to create a natural-appearing lip. If further volume enhancement is desired, the actual vermillion is next injected. This is often confined to the four central mounds of the vermillion itself. One or two linear threads of filler are placed along these four areas of greatest lip height. Sometimes enhancement is needed along the lateral vermillion as well if the lip is puckering or wrinkling laterally. This will widen the upper lip. To address downturning of the lower lip, the filler is also injected in and around the modiolis. As described by Klein,[3] the lateral lower lip often requires buttressing in the marionette area to prevent down turning and to fill the marionette area. It is important to treat surrounding volume loss in the lip, particularly in the marionette area, to support the extra weight that one is adding to the lip with filler.

I generally treat patients conservatively the first time with 1 ml of filler material in order for the patient to become used to the new appearance. Sudden dramatic enlargement of the lip can be rather startling to the patient or his or her family. It is preferable that the patient asks for more volume with subsequent treatment rather than feel upset with overcorrection after the first session. After filling the lips, excessive perioral muscle movement of the obicularis oris or depressor anguli oris can be addressed with small quantities of Botox.[4]

Summary

Augmentation of the lips is a very artistic and satisfying endeavor for both the patient and the cosmetic surgeon. The goals are natural enhancement, emphasizing the vermillion border, and optimizing anatomical landmarks (Figure 119.2). Atrophic volume changes in the lip and surrounding areas are addressed as well. Attention to detail involves addressing the shape of the cupid's bow, the need for enhancement along the philtral columns, and discussing with the patient his or her preferred lip shape. Small quantities of Botox to perioral muscles can enhance results and extend the longevity of the filler. Long-term goals should be considered so that if the patient wants a trendy, exciting look, the filler should be temporary. As patients become more comfortable with enhancement, more volume is added in subsequent sessions.

Inject along the vermilion side of border

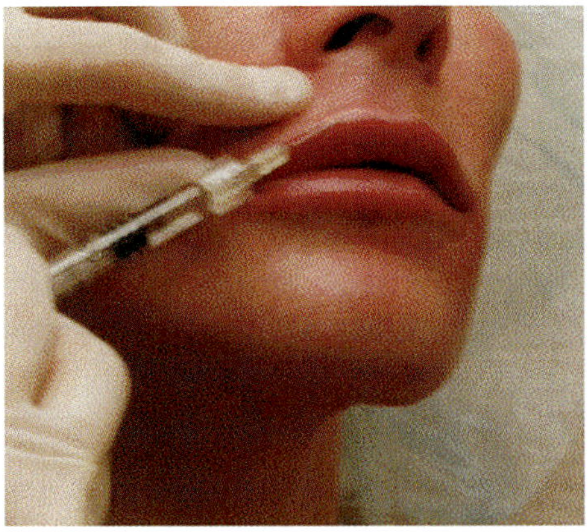

Figure 119.1. Injection along the red edge of the vermillion border rather than the white edge prevents artifical white line above the lip.

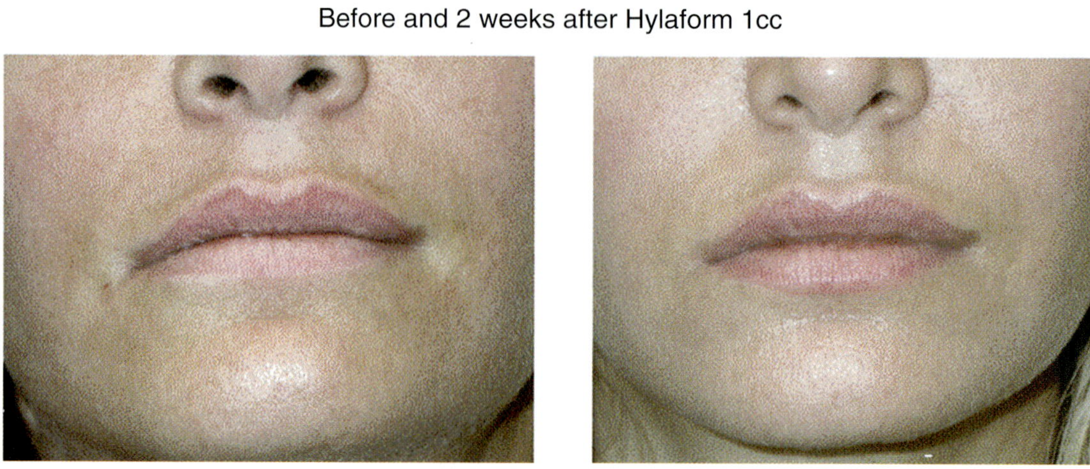

Figure 119.2. Injection of 1 ml of hyaluronate filler along the vermillion border and red upper lip. Avoiding injection of the cupid's blow narrowed its width.

References

1. Niamtu J. Simple technique for lip and nasolabial fold anesthesia for injectable fillers. Dermatol Surg 2005;31(10):1330–1332.
2. Smith KC, Melnychuk M. Five percent lidocaine cream applied simultaneously to the skin and mucosa of the lips dreates excellent anesthesia for filler lnjections. Dermatol Surg 2005;31(11):1635–1637.
3. Klein AW. In search of the perfect lip. Dermatol Surg 2005;31(11): 1599–1603.
4. Carruthers J, Carruthers A. Aesthetic botulinum A toxin in the mid and lower face and neck. Dermatol Surg 2003;29(05):468–476.

120

Restylane Injection for the Lower Eyelid Tear Trough

R. Jeffrey Hofmann

Injecting Restylane into the lower eyelid (to correct a tear trough or orbitomalar groove) is fraught with potential complications, such as bruising, lumpiness, and contour irregularities. Nonetheless, it can be done and good results can be achieved.

Adjust patients' expectations and tell them that they will most likely have some bruising, even though they do not have bruising in the lower face with Restylane.

I only use a topical anesthetic—usually ELA-Max cream. I always inject very deep along the inferior orbital rim. Inject very small aliquots (0.02 ml). While injecting, keep one finger pressed inside the inferior orbital rim to prevent the Restylane from traveling superior to the orbital rim. After each injection, apply pressure to the area to tamponade bleeding and prevent bruising. I inject greater volumes into the cheek (inferior to the orbitomalar groove or tear trough) because expanding the cheek will "push" fat superiorly toward the lid area. This treatment is much more time-consuming than Restylane injections in the nasolabial folds or marionette lines.

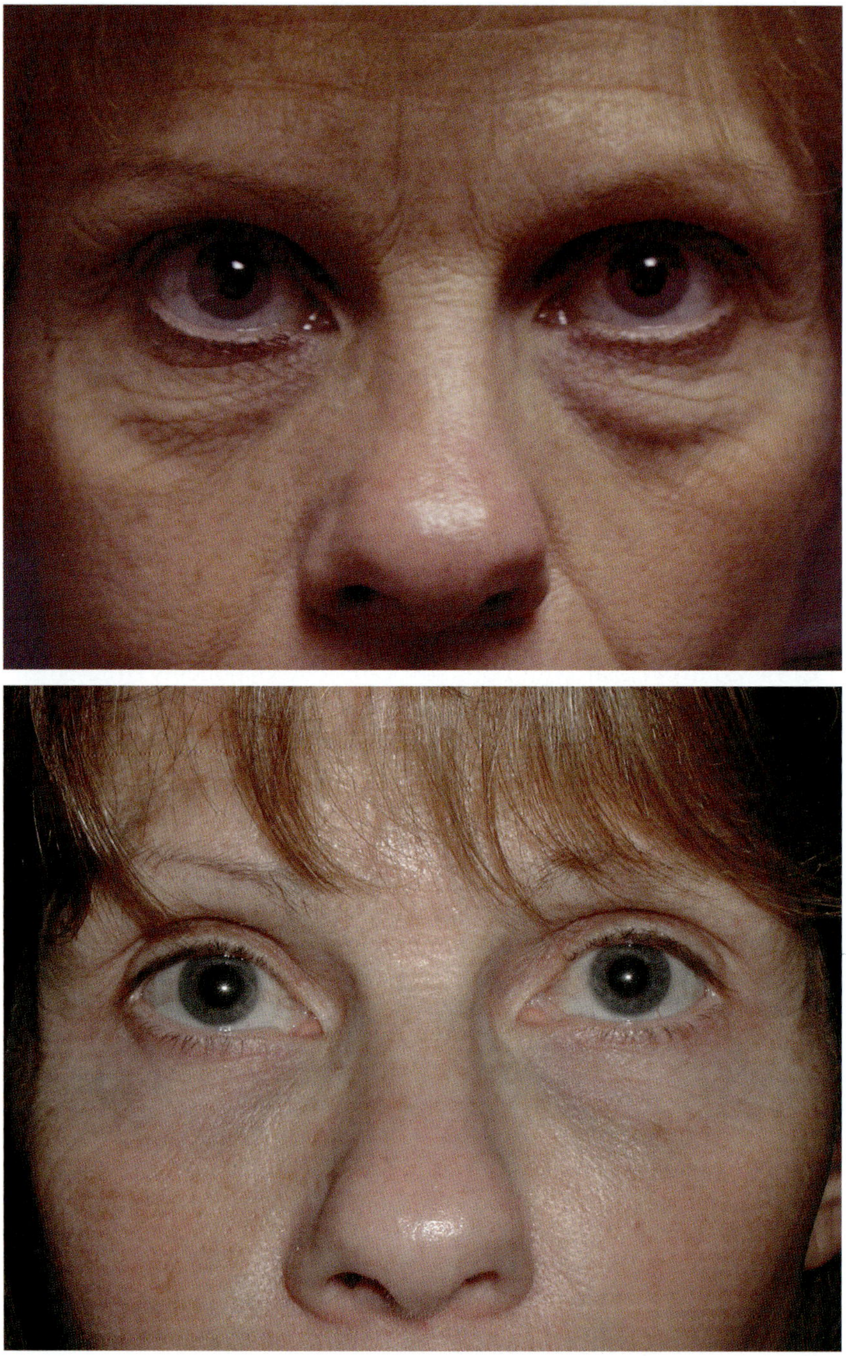

A

B

Figure 120.1. (A) Patient post lower blepharoplasty with fat repositioning. The patient declined midfacial liposculpture. Note significant midface volume loss and prominent residual tear trough. (B) Following three sessions of midfacial fillers and tear trough treatment spread over months (most recently with 4 vials of Restylane), the patient achieves appropriate facial volumization and correction of the tear trough.

121

Liquid Injectable Silicone for the Upper Third of the Face

Derek H. Jones

Liquid injectable silicone (LIS) is the most permanent of all injectable fillers employed within the United States. For certain soft tissue defects, pure liquid silicone may be superior to other currently available filling agents in properly selected patients.

LIS is controversial, with both advocates and opponents citing anecdotal data to support their position.[1–6] Advocates of LIS rely on a wealth of anecdotal data to assert that it is safe and effective if the following three rules are strictly followed:

Rule 1: Inject only pure medical grade, highly purified LIS that is intended for injection into the human body and specifically FDA approved for that purpose. To date, two LIS products are FDA approved: Silikon 1000 (Alcon Labs, Fort Worth, TX) and Adatosil 5000 (Bausch and Lomb, Rochester, NY). Both were FDA approved in the mid-1990s for intraocular injection to treat retinal detachment. Under new guidelines enacted under the 1997 FDA Modernization Act, these medical devices may be legally injected off-label for any indication deemed appropriate within a unique physician–patient relationship. Of the two FDA-approved silicone oils, Silikon 1000 is a less viscous substance and is more appropriate for injection through smaller-gauge needles, making it the more appropriate substance for tissue augmentation. It should be noted that prior to 1990, there was no FDA-approved LIS. Most LIS prior to 1990 was obtained from clandestine sources. Studies have proven that most of those products contained impurities that adversely affected biocompatibility.[7] Injection of such products prior to 1990 was extremely common, with publicity surrounding associated adverse events leading to a negative public image.[5]

Rule 2: Adhere to strict microdroplet, serial puncture technique. This is defined as injection of 0.01 cc strictly into the subdermal plane at 2- to 5-mm intervals, through a 27-gauge metal hub needle or smaller, with no double pass over a given area at any one visit. Intradermal injection should be avoided, as dermal nodules may result. Over time (1–3 months), a limited foreign body response produces a collagenous

capsule around each microdroplet, anchoring it in place and further enhancing tissue augmentation.

Rule 3: Inject small volumes at monthly intervals. Optimal correction occurs slowly over time. LIS is an oil and injected in large bolus may track along tissue planes, which gives silicone a reputation for migration. However, potential for drift is eliminated as long as small volumes are injected at monthly intervals utilizing microdroplet, serial puncture technique.

Histologic analysis of purified liquid silicone present in vivo for long periods (up to 38 years) displays impressive biocompatibility.[4] Despite rigid adherence to these rules, adverse events may rarely occur, even years after injection.[5] The most worrisome complication is granuloma formation, which clinically may appear as a firm or even rock-hard nodule in the skin. The overlying skin may reflect edema and purple, red, or brown discoloration. Such adverse events may be treated with injection of intralesional steroids and the oral antibiotic minocycline. Inflammatory adverse events have been noted to arise in conjunction with an adjacent infection, such as a sinus infection or a dental abscess. Surgical correction may be required.

For the upper third of the face, LIS may be employed for the following indications:

1. Acne scarring[3]
2. Deep glabellar furrow.
3. Temporal lipoatrophy associated with HIV[2]

The specific technique for each of these indications iswell described in the references. The reader should be cautioned that LIS, although extraordinarily useful as a permanent injectable filler, is the least forgiving of all filling agents. Physicians wishing to perform this procedure should receive appropriate training. Furthermore, different liability carriers have varied regulation regarding off-label use of LIS. In the author's opinion, until longer term studies are available with the currently available FDA-approved silicone oils, LIS should be reserved for severe atrophic acne scarring and severe HIV facial lipoatrophy, where other fillers may not work as well or be cost-effective.

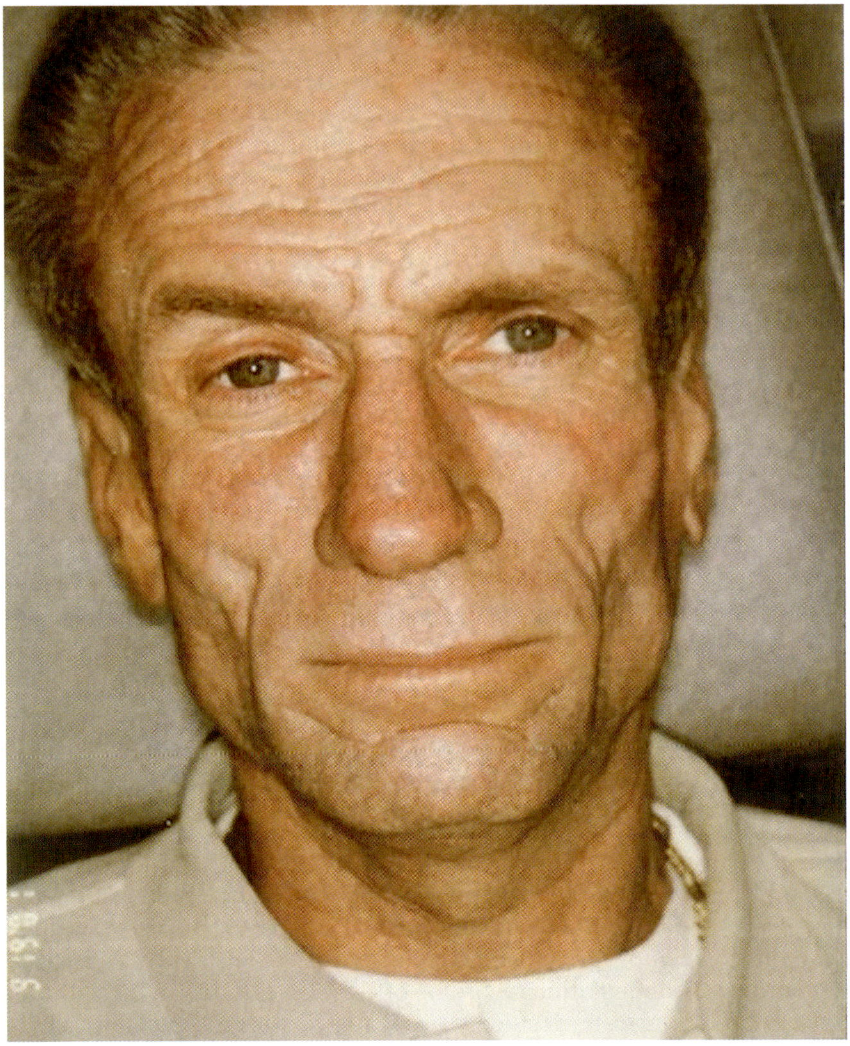

A

Figure 121.1. (A) HIV lipoatrophy pretreatment. (B) HIV facial lipoatrophy after a series of liquid injectable silicone to the cheeks, temples, and glabella. The glabella has also been treated with Botox.

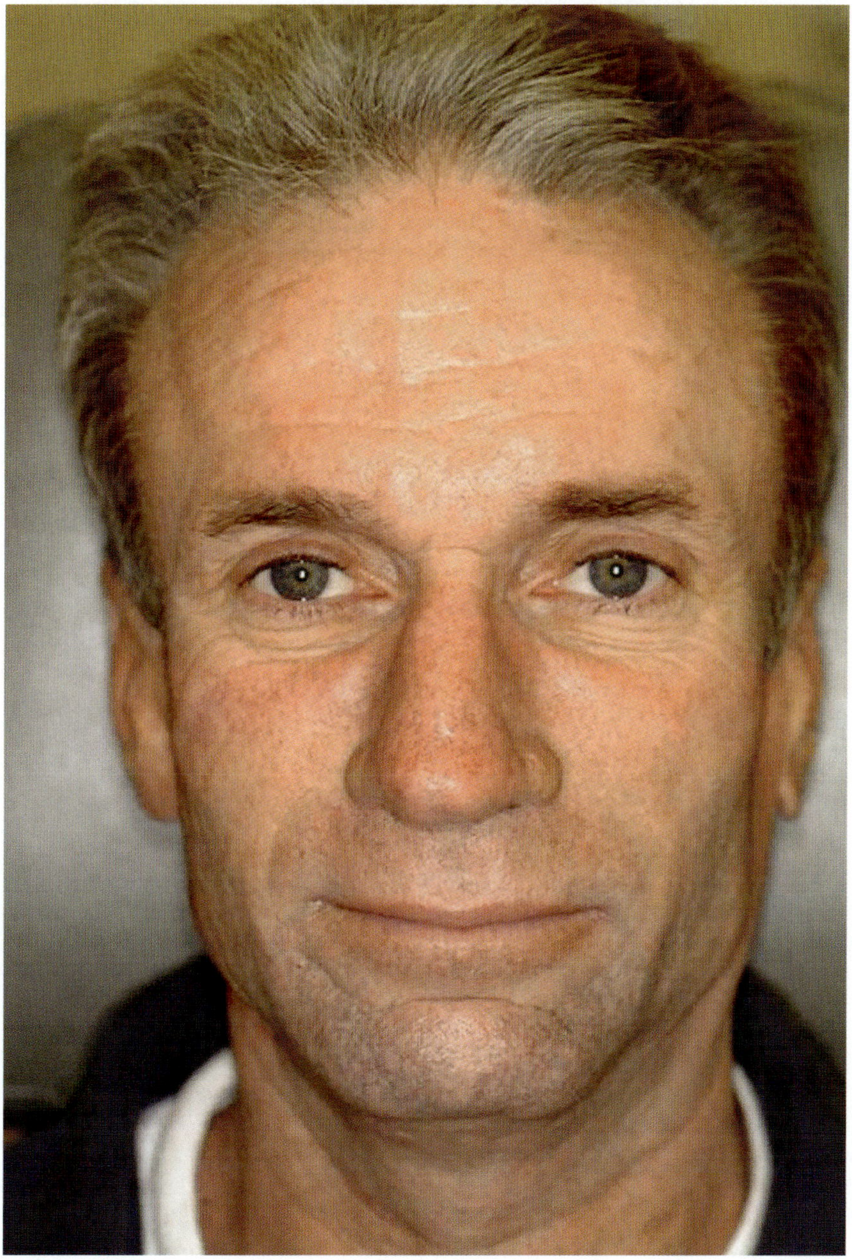

B

Figure 121.1. (*Continued*)

References

1. Orentreich DS, Jones DH. Liquid injectable silicone. In: Carruthers J, Carruthers A (ed.). Soft Tissue Augmentation. New York: Elsevier, 2005: 77–91.
2. Jones DH, Carruthers A, Orentreich D, et al. Highly purified 1000-cSt silicone oil for treatment of human immunodeficiency virus-associated facial lipoatrophy: an open pilot trial. Dermatol Surg 2004;30:1279–1286.

3. Barnett JG, Barnett CR. Treatment of acne scars with liquid silicone injections: 30 year perspective. Dermatol Surg 2005;31:1542–1549.
4. Balkin SW. Injectable silicone and the foot: a 41-year clinical and histologic history. Dermatol Surg 2005;31:1555–1560.
5. Duffy DM. Liquid silicone for soft tissue augmentation. Dermatol Surg 2005; 31:1530–1541.
6. Rapaport MR. Silicone injections revisited. Dermatol Surg 2002;28:594–595.
7. Parel JM. Silicone oils: physiochemical properties. In: Glaser BM, Michels RG (eds.), Retina, Vol 3. St. Louis: Mosby, 1989:261–277.

122

Periocular Injectables with Hyaluronic Acid and Calcium Hydroxyapatite

Robert A. Glasgold and Samuel M. Lam

Periocular rejuvenation with injectable soft tissue fillers is increasingly more popular over the past few years. The availability of new fillers provides physicians and surgeons greater flexibility in rejuvenating the periocular region while appealing to the minimal downtime, nonsurgical mindset of many patients. Volumetric enhancement around the eyes is a major new aesthetic perspective that has contributed to the implementation of injectable fillers. Periocular fat grafting in which volume is added, as opposed to conventional blepharoplasty in which volume is generally subtracted, has provided the principal impetus toward the revolution in understanding the importance of volume in periocular rejuvenation. The charm of periocular injectable fillers must be tempered with appropriate clinical judgment and technical skill to avoid potentially devastating complications. This chapter focuses on two recent injectable soft tissue fillers—hyaluronic acid (HA) and calcium hydroxyapatite (CH)—that are successfully used in the periocular region. The pearls and pitfalls of each filler are enumerated.

General Principles

The concerns in periocular enhancement with soft tissue fillers involve various complications that range from prolonged ecchymosis to blindness. Although there is no guarantee that a complication can be entirely avoided, adhering to certain principles minimizes the likelihood of these complications. Any use of nonsteroidal antiinflammatory medications, herbal medications (*Ginkgo biloba*, St. John's wort, fish oil caps, melatonin, etc.), and alcohol consumption during the week prior to treatment predispose toward ecchymosis. In the richly vascular periorbital region, use of these products is strictly prohibited or the procedure is abandoned until the patient is compliant. Liberal application of ice immediately prior to injection can also reduce the extent of periorbital ecchymosis.

Catastrophic complications that can occur with periocular injections are soft tissue/skin necrosis due to vascular obstruction and blindness from central retinal artery occlusion. Using ice immediately prior to injection minimizes the risk of intra-arterial injection. In addition, injection is performed only during needle withdrawal, watching for bleed flashback into the syringe. Any duskiness or skin color change that suggests vascular compromise is treated with topical nitropaste. Always have a supply of nitropaste at hand in the event of this unlikely complication.

Contour irregularities can arise due to technical error with injection method. Deeper placement (suborbicularis), steady injection, and vigorous massage are the principal methods to avoid a contour problem.

Hyaluronic Acid (HA)

HA has become one of the most popular choices as a soft tissue filler for facial enhancement. HA can be used effectively in the entire periocular region, including the glabellar rhytids, superior orbital rim depression, inferior orbital rim hollow, and the nasojugal trough (Figure 122.1).

To avoid contour problems, HA should be injected smoothly with a linear threading or crosshatch technique while minimizing serial punctures. The slow and deliberate injection into the suborbicularis oculi plane achieves a more uniform contour. Digital massage and manipulation smoothes out remaining contour problems and is routinely performed in the periocular region. Massage is less critical in the perioral region, but it is beneficial in the unforgiving thin skin of the periocular region.

The best candidates for periocular filling are those with limited deficiencies that can be corrected with one or two 1-ml syringes of HA. Greater contour deficiencies are better managed with autologous fat transfer. Larger volumes of HA risk contour irregularities and are cost prohibitive. Trying to camouflage a pronounced prolapse of fat in the lower eyelid using HA (or any other filler for that matter) along the bony rim can contribute to an unsightly bulge and compound the problem. The best candidates are those who exhibit mild to moderate isolated deficiencies of the nasojugal trough with or without some extension of hollowing in the remaining inferior orbital rim (Figure 122.1).

The patient should be seen 1 week after treatment when it is still relatively easy to massage out contour problems. After the second week, manipulation of the material becomes ineffective. In these cases, use of hyaluronidase can be instrumental to dissolve the HA in a matter of a few hours. This potential reversibility is a compelling reason to use HA for periocular purposes.

Calcium Hydroxyapatite

CH can provide superb enhancement in the periocular region (Figure 122.2). In several cases that we have observed, CH elicits a persistent cutaneous erythema in the nasojugal trough recalcitrant to treatment but that dissipates after many months. We have restricteded the use of CH in the nasojugal trough despite early successes. The superior orbital rim may also be a difficult area to contour.

The remaining inferior orbital rim can be enhanced but should be approached in the immediate supraperiosteal plane, i.e., deeper than just below the orbicularis oculi where HA is injected. Doing so limits contour problems with CH due to its higher viscosity. As a general rule, CH works exceptionally well in the adjacent malar depression since it provides a more potent volumetric enhancement per ml than HA and also because it comes packaged in a larger syringe (1.3 ml vs. just 1 ml with HA). When filling a complex contour deficit, it is always wiser to approach that area with a crosshatch method that facilitates a seamless result where the borders of augmented soft tissue are not seen.

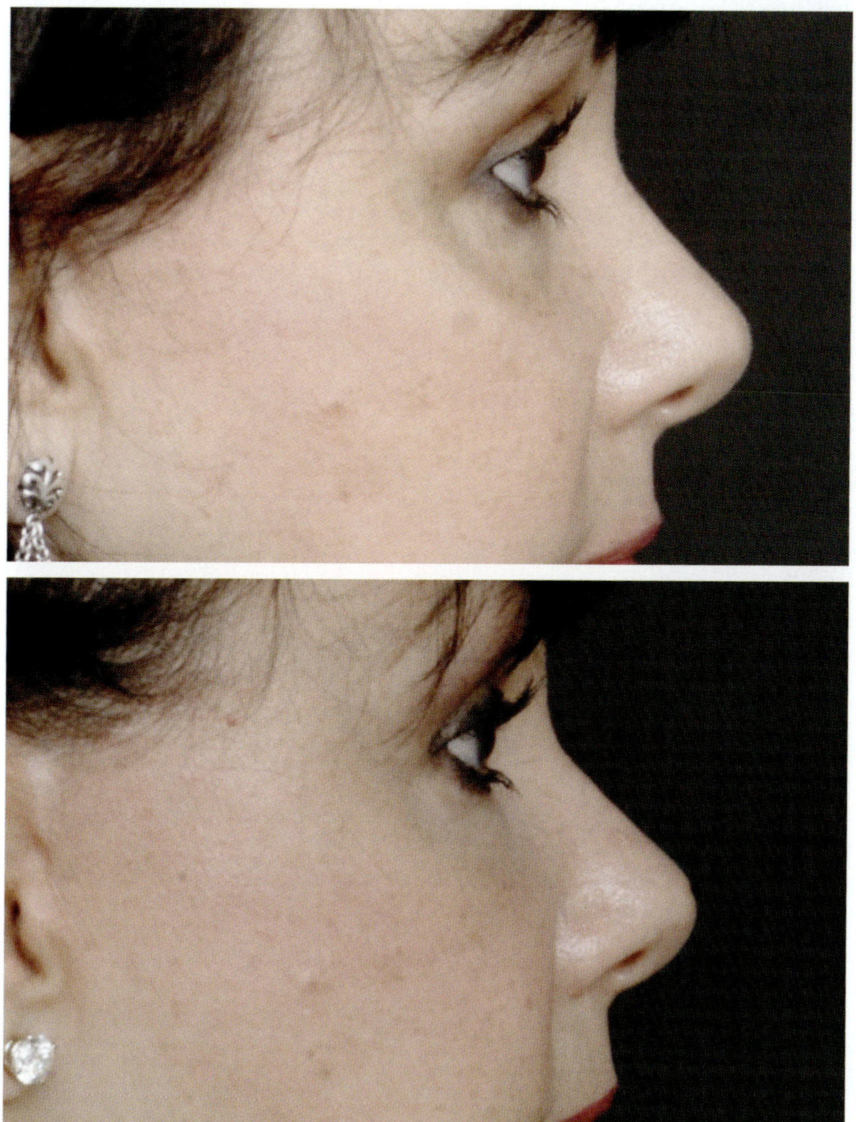

A

B

Figure 122.1. Pre- (A) and posttreatment (B) photos following Restylane injections to the nasojugal groove and inferior orbital rim depression.

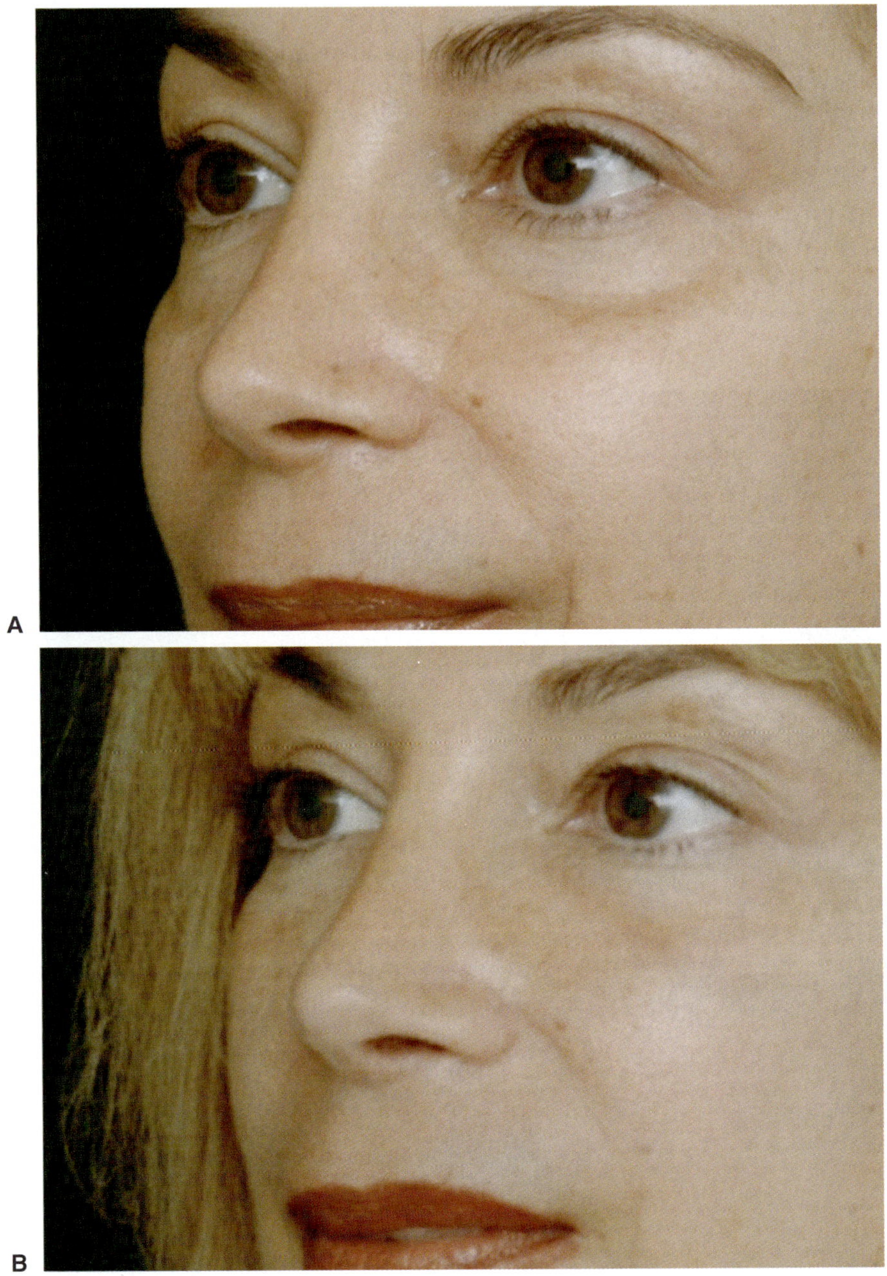

Figure 122.2. Pre- (A) and posttreatment (B) photos following Radiesse injections to the nasojugal groove and inferior orbital rim depression.

123

Pearls and Pitfalls of Botox and Filler Substances in the Upper Third of the Face

Seth L. Matarasso

The three aesthetic units that comprise the upper third of the face are the midline glabellar complex, the forehead, and the peri-ocular areas. Unlike rhytids in the lower half of the face, which are static and primarily due to cumulative photodamage and gravitational changes, wrinkles above the zygomatic arch are dynamic and are in large part a result of hypertrophy of the underlying musculature. The deep vertical lines in between the eyebrows are from chronic movement of the brow depressor muscles: the procerus, the bilateral corrugator supercilii, and the medial fibers of the orbicularis oculi (depressor supercilii). The horizontal creases of the forehead are the result of the brow elevator, the frontalis muscle, and the arciform perioribital lines (the crow's feet) are due to the lateral fibers of the orbicularis oculi muscle. There are many treatment options available to improve these lines, including surgery as well as the ever-expanding list of new filler agents and lasers. However, as with any intervention, the treatment should be aimed at the underlying pathology, and as such the treatment of choice for rhytids in the upper third of the face is chemodenervation with botulinum toxin. A small amount of botulinum toxin injected precisely into facial muscles renders them immobile and releases the superimposed cutaneous defect and rhytid (Table 123.1) Currently the sole FDA-approved neurotoxin is Botox (Allergan Inc., Irvine, CA) and the only cosmetic indication is "for the temporary improvement in appearance of moderate to severe glabellar lines associated with corrugator and/or procerus muscle activity in adult patients 65 years of age or younger." All other uses are considered off-label.[1,2]

Botox for the wrinkles and lines in the upper third of the face is safe and effective and has gained remarkable patient acceptance and is presently the most popular cosmetic treatment for both men and women. Despite the remarkable global endorsement, patients must be made aware of potential complications. The most common functional adverse events are eyelid and eyebrow ptosis. However, an additional concern that is often omitted and should be discussed with patients is their goals and the degree of the expected cosmetic improvement. It should be stressed that the mimetic lines will be reduced for approximately 3–4 months and that with each subsequent treatment the results may last longer and the lines may not be as deep, but deeply etched-in lines often require additional therapy. For complete rhytid effacement, if cost permits, patients may often require additional adjunctive therapy. An ideal combination is the administration of Botox to relax the muscles of facial expression and maximally reduce the dynamic lines and the subsequent use of a filling agent to further reduce the remaining static lines. Not only does this optimize the ultimate aesthetic result, the decreased muscle activity increases the durability of the filling substance.[3]

1. Patients who elect to undergo a procedure for facial enhancement often do not have the same expectations as those who present for medical indications. While bruising and edema are acceptable sequelae for many therapeutic procedures, they are often ill tolerated with cosmetic procedures. Patients must be made aware of these normal consequences and the associated morbidity (downtime). To reduce the incidence of bruising, medications that can interfere with the clotting mechanism (aspirin, nonsteroidal anti-inflammatory drugs) should, if medically appropriate, be discontinued for 10–14 days prior to treatment. There may also be an increased incidence of eccyhmosis as most facial injectables require a 30-gauge needle-and aspiration prior to injection to ensure appropriate cutaneous (as opposed to intravascular injection) placement is not tenable.
2. The results of Botox can be dramatic and muscle immobilization can be objectively appreciated—conversely the results of a filler can be more subtle and subjective. Standardized preoperative photographs assume an important role with soft tissue augmentation. For the physician they are a valuable learning tool as they reinforce proper technique and placement. For the patient they are more important—it is not atypical to forget the pretreatment appearance of a wrinkle, and baseline photography is unequivocal documentation.
3. Ideally, Botox should be administered initially and allow 3–4 days for the maximal effect to take place. The remaining soft tissue defect will require a smaller quantity of filler and hence lowers the total cost of the combined procedures. However, for patient convenience Botox and fillers can be done simultaneously. There is no scientific documentation of which should be injected first. Theoretically as they are placed at different levels—Botox is intramuscular and fillers are intradermal—it should not be clinically relevant. Some physicians do prefer to inject the filler before the toxin. This sequence may theoretically prevent the spread of toxin with subsequent percutanous injections and unwanted diffusion into adjacent areas with unintentional muscle weakness.
4. The selection of the filler depends upon the depth and location of the remaining rhytid and the quantity needed. The thinner, superficial fillers, those that are noncrosslinked, such as Zyderm I and II and CosmoDerm 1 and 2, are preferable. These agents contain a high saline content that is rapidly reabsorbed and therefore upon injection into the

superficial papillary dermis require overcorrection with visible blanching of the skin. As small amounts of filler are required to complement the Botox, the collagen that is commercially available in the smallest volume (0.5 cc) is recommended. Collagens notoriously have a brief longevity; using the longer-lasting hylauronans (Restylane or Juvederm) is acceptable. The tradeoff is that they do not contain local anesthesia and are more painful to inject, are associated with more edema and bruising, and are thicker and so must be placed deeper in the papillary dermis.

5. There are two primary injection techniques for dermal fillers: serial puncture and linear threading. With the former, small aliquots of a filler are sequentially deposited immediately anterior to the previous injection. This is often the preferred method, although it requires multiple entries into the skin, is more precise, and is not blinded, and therefore, unlike linear threading, there is less chance of intravascular embarrassment.

6. Patients should be placed in an upright/dependent position to accentuate rather than blunt the rhytid. Overhead lighting and magnification assist not only in appreciating the depth of the defect, but also in locating vessels that should be avoided upon injection.[4]

7. Injections into glabrous skin can be painful. To reduce the discomfort and make it a nonthreatening experience for the patient, the use of a topical anesthesia for 15–30 minutes is beneficial. Despite adequate anesthesia with cream preparations, repeated injections can dull the 30-gauge $^1/_2$ needle and increase the pain. Not only can changing the needle as needed diminish the pain, but also injecting the material slowly is helpful.

8. After successful treatment with Botox into the orbicularis oculi muscle (crow's feet), there may be residual lines laterally and in the infraocular sulcus. The lines that radiate laterally are superficial and therefore well suited to very fine fillers such as Zyderm I or CosmoDerm 1. When using bovine products it is the standard of care to have two negative skin tests documented to reduce the risk of hypersensitivity reactions.[5] The infraocular sulcus is the result of loss of subcutaneous tissue and therefore will not be responsive to Botox or a superficial filler. Soft tissue augmentation in this area restores the convexity of youth. The collagen products tend to "bead" in this area and do not provide a sustainable augmentation. More viscous products such as the hyalutonic acids (Restylane and Juvederm) are recommended in this area. This area can be approached laterally from the canthal region or inferiorly just above the bony zygomatic arch. The skin in this area is thin and very prone to eccyhmosis and contour irregularities. Placing these products deep in the submuscular plane seems to produce longer-lasting augmentation and reduce contour irregularities. The anterior threading ("push along") method acts like blunt dissection and creates a submuscular space. To reduce the potential risk of intravascular placement it may be warranted to inject in a lateral direction, away from the eye, as opposed to towards the peri-orbita. (Figure 123.1)

9. Perhaps the sine-qua-non stigma of treatment with Botox in the frontailis muscle is the intact inferior muscle fibers located immediately above the lateral eyebrow. They can on occasion be treated

conservatively with very small amounts of Botox (1.0–2.0 units). However, completely inactivating the sole brow elevator muscle may cause ptosis with lateral hooding. To avoid this it is advisable not to treat the most inferior horizontal rhytids with Botox (approximately 1.5–2.0 cm above the superior orbital rim). This does predictably result in what has been commonly known as the "Mr. Spock" or quizzical brow. A reliable remedy of these infero-lateral furrows is the use of a filler. Selection of the filler is predicated upon the depth of the wrinkle, and most dermal fillers would be acceptable in this suprabrow location.

10. Most fillers approved by the FDA are for the temporary "improvement of soft tissue contour folds and wrinkles, such as the nasolabial fold." When used above the zygomatic arch, they are considered off-label. The most significant absolute contraindication for the use of fillers lies in the glabellar region. There is a high risk of intravascular injection with fillers with consequent tissue necrosis, slough, and cicatrix formation. To avoid this complication, fillers that are robust (crosslinked with gluteraldehyde-Zyplast and CosmoPlast) should be strictly prohibited in this area. Thin agents (Zyderm I and Cosmoderm 1)are indicated for any dermal lines in this area. Even with slow deliberate superficial placement of a filler vascular occlusion can occur. This will be manifested by unexpected blanching and pain. If this occurs it can be responsive to topical vasodilator nitroglycerin paste. It may be prudent to keep this cream readily available in treatment rooms.

11. As the uses of injectables evolve, an era of facial shaping is becoming a standard practice. This is especially apparent in the brow area. Treating the glabellar complex with Botox relaxes the brow depressor muscles and by definition will produce lateral "chemical brow lift" of 2.0–3.0 mm by unopposed action of the frontalis muscle. To further accentuate elevation of the brow, a filler can be placed along the lateral tail of the eyebrow. A hylauronan can be injected in a threading manner along the superior orbital rim. Very small amounts, 0.2 cc per side, can be placed one third to one fourth of the length of the eyebrow. It may be slightly uncomfortable, but patients report an immediate lift of the brow.

12. Postinjection massage is not a universal practice, but it does locate any skip areas that have not been adequately addressed with a filler as well as reduce postinjection edema. Similarly, brief application of cool compresses or ice can be helpful in minimizing patient discomfort and erythema.

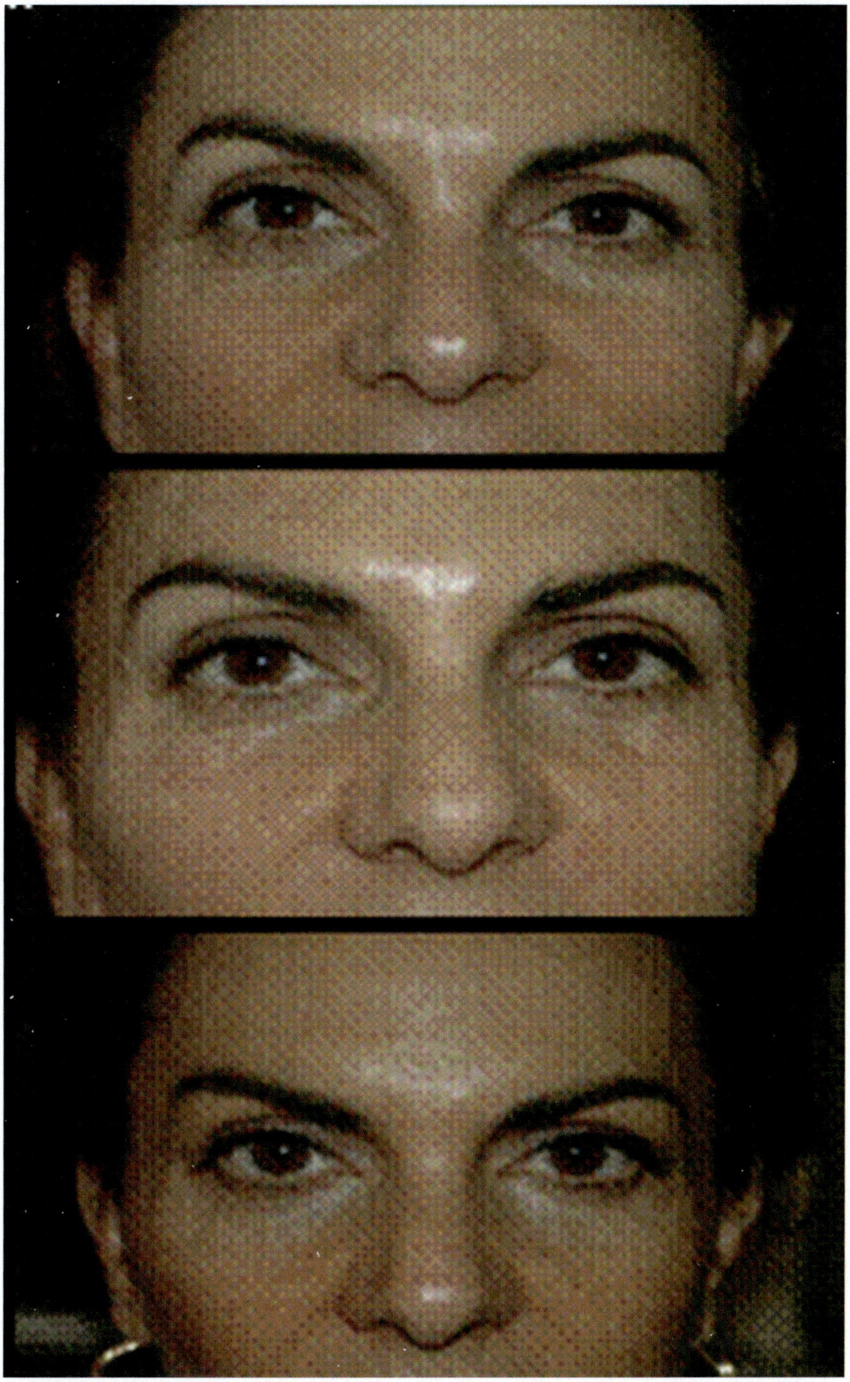

Figure 123.1. (Top) Prior to treatment of the peri-ocular rhytids. (Middle) Immediately following treatment. (Bottom) Following treatment with 15 units of Botox (per side) into the lateral fibers of the orbicularis oculi, 0.25 cc Zyderm I (per side) into the static lateral lines, and 0.15 cc Restylanc (per side) into the inferior ocular sulcus.

Table 123.1. General Dosing Guidelines for the Treatment of the Upper Third of the Face with Botox

Indication	Muscles	Units/Area
Glabella (scowl)	Procerus Corrugator supercilii Medial fibers orbicularis oculi (depressor supercilii)	25–35
Nose (bunny lines)	Nasalis	3.0–5.0
Lateral orbital lines (crow's feet)	Lateral fibers Orbicularis oculi	10–20 per side
Forehead (horizontal creases)	Frontalis	20–30

References

1. Carruthers J, Fagien S, Matarasso SL, and the Botox Consensus Group. Consensus recommendations on the use of botulinum toxin type A in facial aesthetics. Plast Reconst Surg Suppl 2004;114(6):1S.
2. Matarasso SL, Matarasso A. Treatment guidelines for botulinum toxin type A for the periocular region and a report on partial upper lip ptosis following injections to the lateral canthal rhytides. Plast Reconst Surg 2001; 108:208–214.
3. Carruthers J, Carruthers A. A prospective, randomized, parallel group study analyzing the effect of BTX-A (Botox) and nonanimal sourced hyaluronic acid (NASHA, Restylane) in combination compared with NASHA (Restylane) alone in severe glabellar /rhytides in adult female subjects: Treatment of severe glabellar rhytides with a hyaluronic acid derivative compared with the derivative and BTX-A. Dermatol Surg 2003;29:802.
4. Matarasso SL, Sadick NS Soft tissue augmentation. In: Bolognia J, Jorrizzo JL, Rapini RV, Horn T (eds.). Dermatology. London: Mosby/Harcourt Health Sciences, 2003:2439–2449.
5. Elson ML The role of skin testing in the use of collagen-injectable materials. J Dermatol Surg Oncol 1989;15:301–303.

124

Periorbital-Facial Volume Rejuvenation for Focal Deficits

John R. Burroughs and Richard L. Anderson

Management of focal volume deficits of the face has traditionally been a difficult problem, especially following trauma. We have found good success with the use of various materials. We have found fat and orbicularis tissue removed at the time of blepharoplasty or myectomy surgeries to be useful for filling volume deficits of the nasolabial folds, lips, glabellar folds, and for the lateral hollowing in myectomy patients following aggressive removal of the lateral orbicularis fibers of the upper and lower eyelids. Radiesse is an outstanding volumizer in HIV—or age-related fat atrophy. Four to 5 vials of Radiesse may be needed. It can also be used in the correction of enophthalmos.[1]

Lip enhancement is most commonly done by filler agents. We prefer the synthetic hyaluronic acid fillers for the lips as they do not carry the risk of infectious disease transmission (HIV, hepatitis, etc.) and are well tolerated and accepted by most patients. Our preferred fillers are Restylane for volume enhancement and Juvederm for fine perioral wrinkles and enhancement of the vermillion border.

In the glabellar folds, we prefer Radiesse, as it can most often be placed deep to the dermis and provides a long-lasting effect. We have used fat and orbicularis for the glabellar folds, but fixation to keep it in place is more problematic than in the lips. For more superficial glabellar folds, Restylane or the other hyaluronic acids may be injected closer to the surface.

In patients with posttraumatic bony defects, we have found good success with the use of Enduragen® acellular dermis material. This material comes in both 0.5-mm and 1-mm thickness, and it can be trimmed, shaped, stacked, and sutured to itself for deeper volume deficit restoration. Radiesse may also be injected deep into these areas or into bony deficits to raise large areas of overlying tissue for volume restoration.

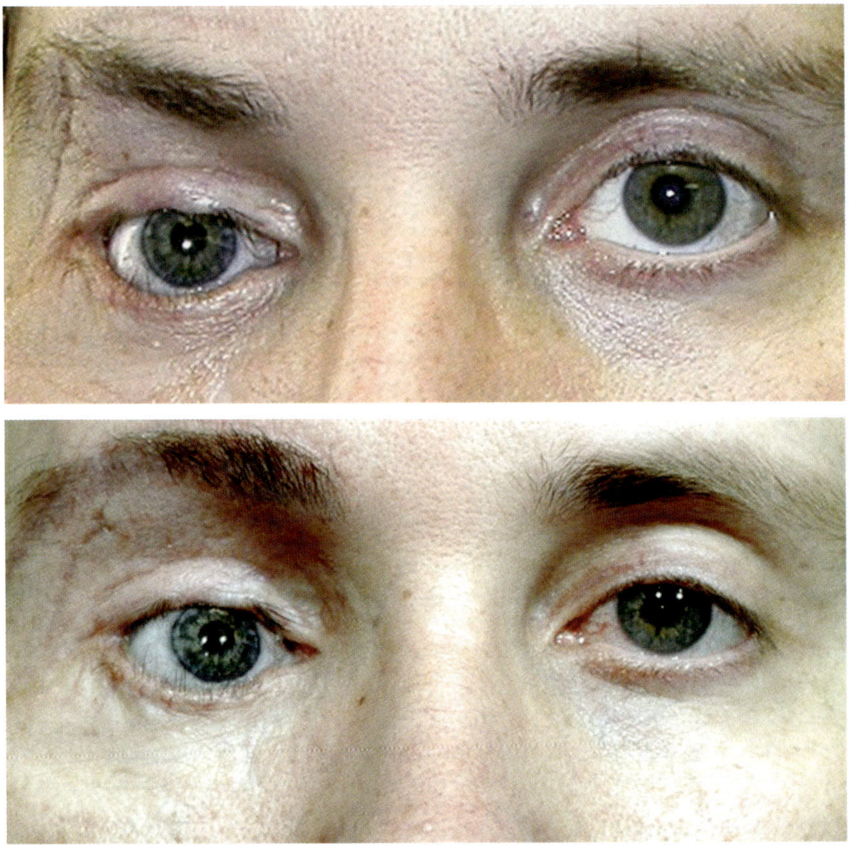

A

B

Figure 124.1. (Top) A patient who suffered severe right-sided craniofacial trauma leaving right superolateral brow bony deficiency and hollowness. (Bottom) Markedly improved brow appearance following the placement of an Eduragen graft into the right superolateral bony defect.

Reference

1. Vagefi MR, McMullan TF, Burrough JR, White GL Jr., McCann JD, Anderson RL. Injectable calcium hydroxyapatite for orbital volume augmentation. Arch Facial Plast Surg 2007;9:439–442.

125

Pearls for Periorbital Fat Transfer

Lisa M. Donofrio

Aging in the periorbital area leads to demarcation of the bony landmark of the orbital rim, unmasking of the orbital fat pads, flattening of the frontal projection of the subcutaneous soft tissue with resultant downward displacement of skin.

Two suborbital aging patterns can be appreciated. The "atrophic" pattern leads to a sunken, hollow orbit. Blepharoplasty in these patients can further accentuate the suborbital shadowing. Most patients with suborbital hollowing complain of dark circles due to the shadow cast by the globe onto the skin of the orbital bowl and relative translucency of the skin itself to the underlying vasculature. The second pattern is a "hypertrophic" change where the orbital fat appears to protrude past the margin of the orbital rim. This is always seen in conjunction with an atrophic upper cheek (except in the case where it was present in youth). As the superior portion of the malar fat pad involutes with aging, the relationship of the upper cheek to the suborbital area changes. Restoring cheek volume in these patients resets the orbital fat posteriorly in relation to the cheek.

The upper lid and brow complex undergoes similar changes with hollowing and flattening of this area and the temple, causing an inferior displacement of skin into the lid crease with concomitant lateral brow ptosis. The goal of rejuvenation of the periorbital area with fat should be to restore normal (youthful) contour. This in and of itself will often result in adequate skin redraping (Figure 125.1)

Pearls of periorbital fat transfer are as follows:

1. Use only blunt cannulas to place fat in the periorbital area. 18-gauge or smaller cannulas are suggested for smooth results with less tissue trauma.
2. Use only 1 cc syringes to inject.
3. Avoid entry at the lateral orbital rim. Avoid horizontal placement with parallel linear "threading" of fat in both the suborbital and brow areas.
4. Enter the suborbital area either through the mid-cheek (Figure 125.2), the base of the nasolabial fold, or from a tangential site on the

upper lateral cheek (Figure 125.3). Place fat in "droplets" along and perpendicular to the orbital rim. Pull the "tail" of the droplet through the tissue to blend. Enter the brow from either the hairline or the eyebrow (Figure 125.4). Avoid treatment of the eyelid skin.

5. Enter the temple from the temporal fusion line and dive deep to the temporalis muscle.

6. Stay posterior to the orbicularis occuli muscle.

7. Fat droplets should be no more than 0.05 cc total in volume per pass.

8. Place no more than 2 cc in the suborbital or brow area in one sitting.

9. Treat the neighboring areas to blend transitions and improve overall results.

10. Treat the cheek as the same "cosmetic unit" as the suborbit. Recreate the cheek–eye continuum.

11. Undercorrect. Build up the tissue in the periorbital area slowly with staged injection sessions.

A,B 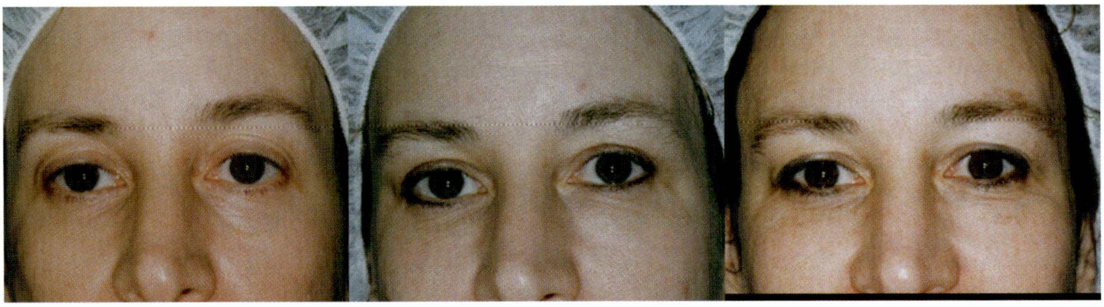 C

Figure 125.1. (A) 47-year-old female with typical age-related atrophic changes. (B) After lipoaugmentation to the suborbital, brow, temple, and cheek. (C) 2-year follow-up.

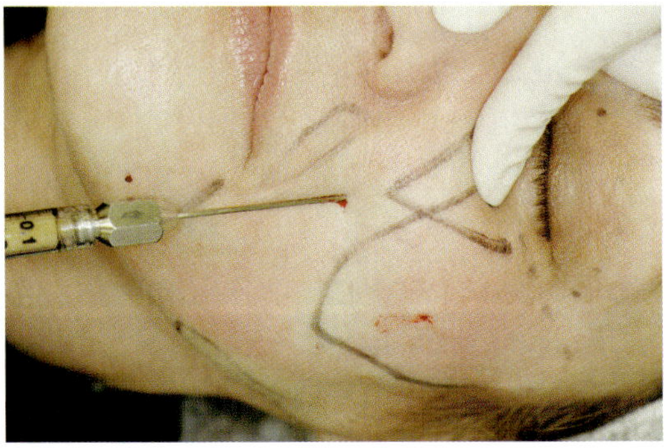

Figure 125.2. Suborbital augmentation from an inferior approach.

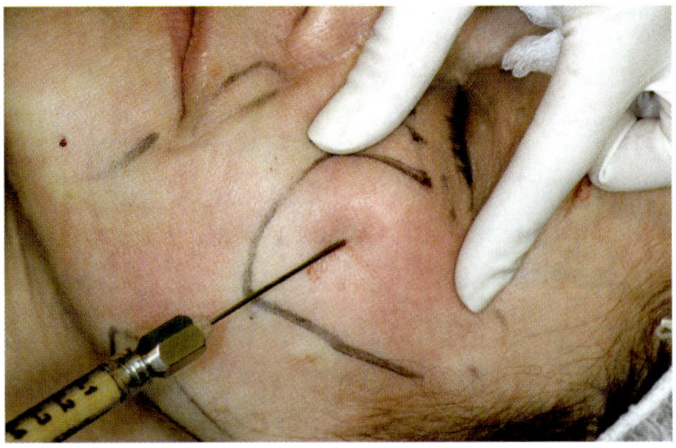

Figure 125.3. Suborbital filling from a tangential approach.

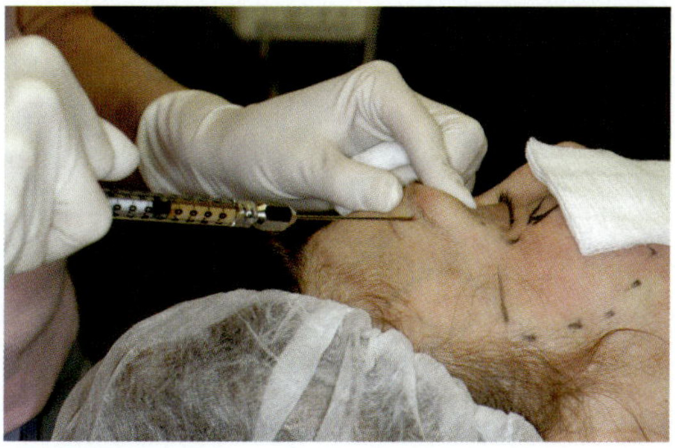

Figure 125.4. Augmentation of the brow.

126

Complementary Fat Grafting in the Periorbital Region

Samuel M. Lam, Mark J. Glasgold, and Robert A. Glasgold

Traditional blepharoplasty entails tissue excision: removing a combination of skin, muscle, and/or fat. Often tissue removal only makes an already hollow eye even more so, which accentuates the appearance of aging rather than achievihng the desired rejuvenation.

Autologous fat transfer is an integral part of our strategy toward periocular rejuvenation. We contend that volumetric depletion is a prime mechanism of the aging process. We call our approach "complementary fat grafting" to emphasize the role that blepharoplasty plays when combined with fat grafting to achieve the optimal aesthetic result.

The technique described in this chapter relies on blunt manual harvesting of fat with minimal negative pressure on the syringe and blunt cannulas to infiltrate. Blunt cannulas for fat infiltration permit unparalleled safety and minimize tissue trauma. The majority of local anesthetic is infiltrated into the recipient sites with the same blunt infiltrating cannula used for fat grafting. The fat is processed with centrifugation for 3 minutes at 3000 rpm and decanted. Atraumatic, purified fat that is bluntly injected in micro-droplets across multiple tissue planes helps optimize fat cell viability and thereby potential longevity of the result.

The primary goal in fat grafting is to frame the eye. Although fat grafting truly provides wonderful rejuvenation across the lower half of the face, especially in the prejowl region, the anatomic territory that achieves the most remarkable aesthetic impact with fat grafting is the periorbital region, which includes the cheek. With the aging process, the luster and beauty of the eye is detracted by the loss of volume that surrounds and supports the eye. Use of fat grafting facilitates rejuvenation by restoring the lost frame around the eye. Cheek enhancement with fat grafting is an extended frame for the eye. A youthful face exhibits a confluence between the lower eyelid and the cheek in which the two areas are united; one of the objectives of fat grafting is to restore this union between the lower eyelid and cheek.

To truly efface a prominent eyebag, or steatoblepharon, a higher volume of fat may be required. When approaching the orbital rim, the use of a conservative amount of fat reduces periocular complications. In fact, almost all complications that arise from autologous fat transfer in the face arise in the unforgiving periocular region. Approximately 2 ml of fat transplanted to the inferior orbital rim is a safe starting point. A higher volume risks the development of overcorrection that is difficult to correct. We find that a conservative transconjunctival blepharoplasty works well in reduction of excessive prolapsed fat. The surrounding tissue bed is undisturbed so that concurrent fat grafting can be easily undertaken. With only mild steatoblepharon, autologous fat transfer or a transconjunctival blepharoplasty alone may suffice to attain the desired rejuvenation. A conservative skin-only upper blepharoplasty combined with fat grafting along the hollowed superior orbital rim can create the best outcome with minimal morbidity.

Very small amounts of fat should be infiltrated per pass with the standard 1 cc Luer-Lock cannula, approximately .02–.03 of an ml per pass. The plane of injection is relatively deep in the immediate supraperiosteal plane. Superficial injection with larger boluses of fat per pass is associated with visible contour irregularities. The injection of fat along the inferior orbital rim is best carried out from an inferior mid-cheek location rather than from a laterally oriented site. The nondominant hand is used to palpate the orbital rim to ensure that the cannula tip passes gently across the rim and protect the globe from injury.

A systematic approach to periocular injection with symmetric volumes allows ideal rejuvenation and minimal problems. We begin by dividing the inferior orbital rim into medial and lateral halves, injecting each half with 1 ml of fat, as described. An additional 0.5 ml is added per half of the rim for more visibly sunken orbital rims. The nasojugal trough can is then filled with an additional 1 ml of fat. It is more aggressively augmented with 1/10 ml per pass along the planes of least resistance.

The lateral canthus and lateral superior orbital rim are augmented from a lateral port 2–3 cm lateral to the lateral canthus. At times it is difficult to pass the cannula tip through fibrous adhesions near the lateral canthus. Gentle pressure overcomes these ligamentous restrictions without avulsing vessels. 0.5 ml of fat is sufficient to fill the depression near the lateral canthus. The lateral superior orbital rim can be enhanced easily by following a plane of least resistance. With 1 ml of fat, the appearance of a cigar roll along the borders of the injected superior orbital rim should not cause alarm, as it is temporary.

A sunken upper eyelid sulcus may be a product of prior overzealous blepharoplasty, aging, or the patient's anatomy. The surgeon should approach this deficiency with great caution. Correction of this deficiency is associated with a relatively long recovery time, on the order of several weeks to months. Also, it can alter a patient's look so that the patient feels that his or her identity is changed.

Fat grafting and volume restoration have assumed a greater role in periorbital rejuvenation. Viewed in a complementary fashion, fat grafting is effectively combined with standard blepharoplasty and tailored to individual anatomy, aesthetic deficits, and concerns.

127

Autogenous Orbicularis and Fat as a Filler

John R. Burroughs, Michael T. Yen, and Richard L. Anderson

In patients who would like a longer-lasting effect and are undergoing a blepharoplasty surgery, we have used the removed fat and orbicularis as an autogenous graft to the nasolabial folds, lips, and glabellar folds.

We routinely place orbicularis grafts into the superolateral portion of the tissue removal in our myectomy patients. And we elevate and suspend the SOOF pads in the lower portion of the tissue removal. This not only helps with incision closure, but helps avoid postoperative hollowing routinely seen in the lateral eyelids of postmyectomy patients. Overcorrection can occur, so the orbicularis grafts need to be thinned and trimmed to just the area requiring volume augmentation. Over time, the orbicularis grafts shrink to approximately 50% of the original size as partial resorption and fibrosis occurs.[1]

In the lips, the orbicularis needs to be finely chopped by placing it in a specimen container and using a 15 blade or scissors to finely chop it into small particles. It can then be injected into the lips from the lateral oral commisure with a large-bore needle along the length of the lips or into the nasolabial folds. Great care must be taken in the glabellar region to avoid injecting into large vessels, which may cause necrosis of tissue or even potential vision loss. Many patients already undergoing eyelid surgery prefer the use of their own readily available autologous tissues over synthetic or animal-based products for filling these types of defects.

Reference

1. Yen MT, Anderson RL. Orbicularis oculi muscle graft augmentation after protractor myectomy in blepharospasm. Ophthal Plast Reconstr Surg 2003;19(4):287–296.

Part IX

Skin Rejuvenation

Section One

Skin Care

128

Skin Care 101: The Basics

Diane S. Berson

Patients undergoing rejuvenation procedures should be counseled regarding fundamental skin care to enhance the cosmetic outcome. Basic cleansing, moisturizing, and sun protection can be combined with prescription and cosmeceutical agents that address discoloration, wrinkling, and irregular tone and texture. Appropriate postsurgical wound care will also ensure faster healing and a better cosmetic result.

Basic Skin Care

Cleansing is an essential component of skin care that removes dirt, oil, environmental pollutants, and bacteria from the skin. Mild products such as liquid cleansers, foaming washes, and syndet bars containing mild synthetic surfactants (Neutrogena, Cetaphil, Dove, Olay) are recommended. Abrasive cleansers should be avoided so that the skin remains intact for surgery. Patients should gently rub with their fingers or a soft washcloth and avoid vigorous scrubbing. They should gently pat dry, rather than rub, and then apply a moisturizer to seal in the dampness. Moisturizers hydrate the skin and restore the epidermal barrier, thereby decreasing transepidermal water loss (TEWL). This is essential for keeping skin smooth and supple and will ensure optimal healing by protecting from dryness, irritation, and infection. Patients with dry skin should use moisturizers with emollients such as glycerin and hyaluronic acid (humectants that bind water) and petrolatum (occlusives which trap water). Those with sensitive skin should avoid products containing fragrances and additives, and those with oily or acne-prone skin might prefer light noncomedogenic moisturizers containing silicone oils. Daily sun protection is imperative; it prevents premature aging of the skin and the development of skin cancer and postoperatively will decrease post-inflammatory hyperpigmentation. An SPF of 30 with broad-spectrum protection against both UVA and UVB should be worn on a daily basis.

Preoperative Skin Care

Topical agents can be used as an adjunct to cosmetic procedures. Prescription retinoids (tretinoin, tazarotene, adapalene) improve the appearance of photodamaged skin. They help smooth tone and texture, reduce pigmentation, and improve the appearance of fine lines and wrinkles. Regular use of topical retinoids before resurfacing procedures, such as chemical peeling and lasers, aids in reepithelialization. Retinoids are usually applied to the skin at bedtime. Cosmeceuticals can be used along with sun protection to prevent sun-induced inflammation and to further improve the appearance of photodamaged skin. Antioxidants protect the skin against the effects of free radicals formed by ultraviolet light radiation. These include vitamins C, E, and B, vitamin A (retinol), green tea, co-enzyme Q_{10}, idebenone, and soy. Products containing collagen-stimulating pentapeptides are another option. The combination of cosmeceuticals in the morning with prescription retinoids at bedtime helps to protect and repair the skin and is continued after healing for maintenance.

Patients who may be at risk for developing postinflammatory hyperpigmentation after surgery are prescribed topical bleaching agents, such as hydroquinone, for a few weeks preoperatively. This includes patients with darker skin tones and those with photodamage undergoing ablative procedures. The ideal preoperative regimen for these patients would include a bleaching agent and SPF in the morning, along with a prescription retinoid at bedtime.

Skin Care After Rejuvenation Procedures

Intensive wound care is essential after ablative procedures such as chemical peels and laser resurfacing. Recovery can take up to 2 weeks. Soaking the affected areas with water, saline, or 0.25% acetic acid every few hours will help loosen crusting and remove debris. Occlusive bland emollients containing petrolatumis used for the first few days. This enhances barrier function, retards water loss, and aids in reepithelialization, thus facilitating repair and recovery. It also ensures an optimal outcome and minimize undesirable effects such as discomfort, redness, swelling, and crusting. Areas that are itchy, inflamed, or irritated can be soothed with milk, cold water, and ice compresses. Gentle cleansing is resumed after 1–2 days, and as healing progresses emollient ointments are switched to lighter moisturizers.

During the postoperative period patients should be instructed to minimize facial manipulation; traumatizing wounded areas will increase the incidence of infection, postinflammatory hyperpigmentation, and scarring. Daily sun protection prevents persistent erythema and hyperpigmentation. After the skin has healed, camouflage makeup is used to help conceal redness, discoloration, and scars.

Posttreatment skin care and a maintenance regimen with mild cleansing and moisturizing, combined with sun protection and appropriate topical cosmeceuticals, bleaching agents, and prescription retinoids enhance the cosmetic outcome of surgery.

129

Retinoids for the Cosmetic Patient

Kenneth R. Beer

Background

Cosmetic procedures to restore lost volume and relax muscles allows cosmetic surgeons to reverse several cardinal signs of the aging face. However, reversal of these symptoms does nothing to restore the epidermis to a more youthful appearance. Fortunately, there are treatments ranging from laser resurfacing to chemical peels to cosmeceuticals to topical retinoids to accomplish this goal.

Topical retinoids have been used in dermatology for decades, and the first report of their use for cosmetic indications by Kligman. Originally approved for the treatment of acne, retinoids were subsequently noted to reverse fine lines and wrinkles. Microscopically, these drugs demonstrate a remarkable ability to restore the dermis and epidermis to a more organized, thickened appearance. Clinical trials performed with tretinoin applied for several months were notable for significant reductions of lentigines and other stigmata of aging. Additional benefit stems from improvement of keratinocyte organization.

Derived from retinol (a vitamin A derivative), these compounds vary in the degree of oxidation as well as the chemical structures added to the parent compound. Retinol is converted to all-*trans*-retinoic acid (tretinoin) by the body, and the latter compound is 20-fold less effective than tretinoin. A second retinoid used for cosmetic indications is tazoratene. Tazoratene has been shown to be at least as effective as tretinoin for remodeling of the epidermis and dermis. At the present time, this molecule has been marketed as a treatment for acne and psoriasis as well as photorejuvenation. One drawback to its use is the high rate of irritancy. Adapalene, another of the topical retinoids, has gained acceptance as a topical treatment for mild to moderate acne. To date it has not been formulated in a vehicle that is optimal for cosmetic indications.

Tretinoin originally had a concentration of 0.025%. Later generations increased this to 0.05 and 0.1%. In addition, emollient vehicles and "microsponge" technology have been employed to enhance tolerability of the product and increase patient compliance. One compound popular for its antiaging effects is the 0.05% tretinoin emollient cream Renova. When used for several months, this product produces skin that appears more youthful histologically as well as clinically. The role of the retinoids for cosmetic indications is expanding rapidly. Clinicians now routinely incorporate these products into their topical treatment regimens. They may be used with nonprescription cosmeceuticals such as glycolic acids, green tea, growth factors, vitamin C, and a host of other products. The optimal skin care regimen incorporating retinoids with these products has yet to be defined and most likely requires some trial and error based on the skin type of the individual being treated.

Retinoids also have a place as adjunctive therapy to "prime" the skin. Treatments using chemical peels, lasers, intense pulsed light, and perhaps even poly-l-lactic acid may be affected by the degree to which the epidermis and dermis have been pretreated with retinoids. Retinaldehyde 0.05% has been shown to improve outcomes of nonablative laser treatments. More studies of this type need to be performed to discover whether treatment with retinoids improves surgical outcome with various cosmetic procedures.

Quite simply, almost all cosmetic patients should be using retinoids. Patients who are irritated by the use of these products should use low concentrations of them or apply them twice per week until they are able to tolerate stronger or more frequent applications.

In my practice, the retinoid that I use the most is tretinoin. Typically, I begin my patients on the 0.025% cream. Whenever possible, I use the Retin A brand of tretinoin because I am comfortable with the vehicles used for the family of products and I am confident in the consistency of the product. Generic products may not always be from the same manufacturer, and this may result in varying concentrations and vehicles, which can affect patient compliance.

For patients who are Fitzpatrick type I or II, I instruct them to apply the cream every other night. They are instructed to apply the cream to dry skin, as applying it to moist or wet skin may increase the risk of irritation. After approximately 6–8 weeks, they are instructed to try to increase the application to nightly. If the skin becomes irritated, they are told to continue every other night usage for another 6–8 weeks before trying to increase the frequency again. Some patients simply will not tolerate daily usage of retinoids, and for these individuals, I use another product such as a green tea, vitamin C, or growth factor–containing product on their "off" nights. This enables me to be certain that the patient is using something nightly (which I believe increases compliance) as well as to provide the patient with the benefits derived from using another cosmeceutical. I will vary the cosmeceutical used based on the patient's goals, skin type, budget, and experience in the past. Many patients use green tea products with retinoids, and there appears to be a synergistic effect.

Patients who tolerate the 0.025% cream for 3 months may progress to the 0.05 cream. As patients tolerate this, increase the concentration that they use. For most patients, the 0.05% cream is as high as they can tolerate, although some patients, particularly those with type III or IV skin, can go to the 0.1%. Several of my cosmetic patients who have used retinoids for decades have graduated to the 0.1%. Interestingly, they report very little irritation and minimal photosensitization.

Microsponge technology and an emollient base are variants of the basic tretinoin formula. Adding the emollient makes the product slightly less irritating, and it has a role for a select few patients. The microsponge technology delivers the active ingredient more efficiently. In practice, it is easier and less expensive to maximize the concentration of the traditional formula before migrating to the more expensive microsponge.

Tazoratene is packaged for cosmetic usage as Avage®. This product will restore the epidermis and dermis to a more youthful appearance clinically and histologically. It does not seem to have the patient acceptance of Retin A and may be slightly more irritating. I use this product intermittently and prescribe it much the same way as I do Retin A, beginning with the lower concentration and graduating to a stronger product after several months. One potential benefit of using Avage is that there is no generic substitute, so that if you prescribe this drug the patient will get it.

As previously mentioned, I believe that many cosmetic patients will benefit from pretreatment with retinoids. Patients undergoing nonablative laser, intense pulsed light, and perhaps injections of poly-l-lactic acid should benefit from treatment with retinoids. For patients undergoing nonablative laser or intense pulsed light, treatment with the 0.025% concentration should be utilized for at least 6 or 8 weeks to maximize outcomes. In theory, the inhibition of metalloproteinases caused by treatment with tretinoin should increase the collagen formation with injection of poly-l-lactic acid. To date, there are no studies to demonstrate that this is the case, but from a theoretical perspective, treatment with tretinoin for 6–8 weeks prior to injections as well as throughout the course of the treatment makes sense.

In conclusion, most cosmetic patients can benefit from the use of retinoids. They are great adjuncts for rejuvenation and potentially may increase the utility of various cosmetic procedures performed. Retin A has the longest record of safety and efficacy in this category, but other products are available, and more are on the horizon.

Suggested Reading

Gilchrest BA. Treatment of photodamage with topical tretinoin: an overview. JAAD 1997;36:S27–S36.

Griffiths CEM, Russman AN, Majmudar G, Singer RS, Hamilton TA, Voorhees JJ. Restoration of collagen formation in photodamaged human skin by tretinoin (retinoic acid). N Engl J Med 1993;329:530–535.

Kang S, Leyden JJ, Lowe NJ. Tazarotene cream for the treatment of facial photodamage. Arch Dermatol 2001;137:1597–1604

Kligman AM, Grove GL, Hirose R, Leyden JJ. Topical Tretinoin for photodamaged skin. J Am Acad Dermatol 1986;15:836–839.

Kligman Am, Leyden JJ. Treatment of photoaged skin with topical tretinoin. Skin Pharmacol 1993;61(suppl):78–82. (Review).

Mordon S, Lagarde JM, Vienne MP, Nocera T, Verriere F, Dahan S. Ultrasound imaging demonstration of the improvement of nonablative laser remodeling by concomitant daily application of 0.05% retinaldehyde. J Cosmet Laser Ther 2004;6:5–9.

Rokhsar C, Lee S and Fitzpatrick R.Review of photorejuvenation: devices, cosmeceuticals or both? Dermatol Surg 2005;31:1166–1178.

130

Evaluation of Skin Lesions in the Cosmetic Patient Made Simple: Actinic Keratosis

Brent R. Moody

Actinic keratoses (AKs) are the earliest form of malignant transformation in the skin. The primary initiator of this malignant transformation is exposure to ultraviolet radiation, which explains their clinical predilection for the head and neck, dorsal hands, and extremities. Many times, patients with AKs will present chiefly with what they perceive to be a cosmetic complaint, such a dry or rough skin. In the context of an aesthetic practice, recognition of AKs has important medical implications for the patient. Left untreated, AKs can progress into invasive squamous cell carcinoma.

The clinical presentation of AKs is variable, but certain features are commonplace. Typically AKs are found in light-skinned Caucasians. AKs tend to be palpable, and early lesions can be felt more easily than seen, hence the complaint of dry or rough skin. More advanced lesions exhibit greater degrees of hyperkeratosis and are readily visualized. Figure 130.1 illustrates a field effect of actinic damage with discrete lesions. A common misperception is that AKs are only found in the elderly. These lesions can be identified in patients in their twenties. Particular attention should be paid in those patients with risk factors for the development of AKs: light skin, excess sun exposure, or artificial UV source use, such as a tanning beds.

There are multiple modalities available for the management of AKs. Factors in the selection of treatment are patient goals, compliance with treatment regimens, and physician experience. Table 130.1 highlights the most commonly utilized treatments for AKs. Prevention strategies are simple, but patient compliance can be low. Patients should be advised to practice sun avoidance, wear sun-protective clothing and hats, and utilize broad-spectrum sunscreens.

Table 130.1. Treatments for Actinic Keratosis

Modality	Advantages	Disadvantages	Comments
Cryosurgery	1. Effective, especially for thicker lesions 2. Physician administered	1. Treats individual lesions only 2. Risk of hypopigmentation 3. Physician experience and skill important	1. Longstanding traditional therapy 2. No issues with patient compliance 3. Hypopigmentation may be unacceptable in some patients
Topical 5-fluorouricil	1. Can treat broad areas and address subclinical lesions 2. Long history of safety and efficacy	1. Requires patient to apply 2. Prolonged erythema and potential crusting	1. Commonly utilized topical treatment 2. Requires good patient education regarding treatment course
Topical Imiquimod	1. Can treat broad areas and address subclinical lesions	1. Requires patient to apply 2. Erythema and crusting. Frequency and duration of adjustment	1. Newer topical agent 2. Some evidence to suggest that can induce long term clearance
Photodynamic therapy (PDT)	1. Can treat broad areas and address subclinical lesions 2. Physician administered	1. Photosensivity after treatment for 24–36 hours 2. Erythema and sunburn like reaction 3. Requires physician to be familiar with treatment protocols	Evidence suggests that PDT has a photorejuvenation effect that decreases erythema and rosacea, which may be desirable in the cosmetically sensitive patient
Chemical peels/Laser ablation	1. Can treat broad areas and address subclinical lesions 2. Physician administered	1. Requires physician to be familiar with treatment protocols 2. May have prolonged healing and erythema	Has well known cosmetic benefits

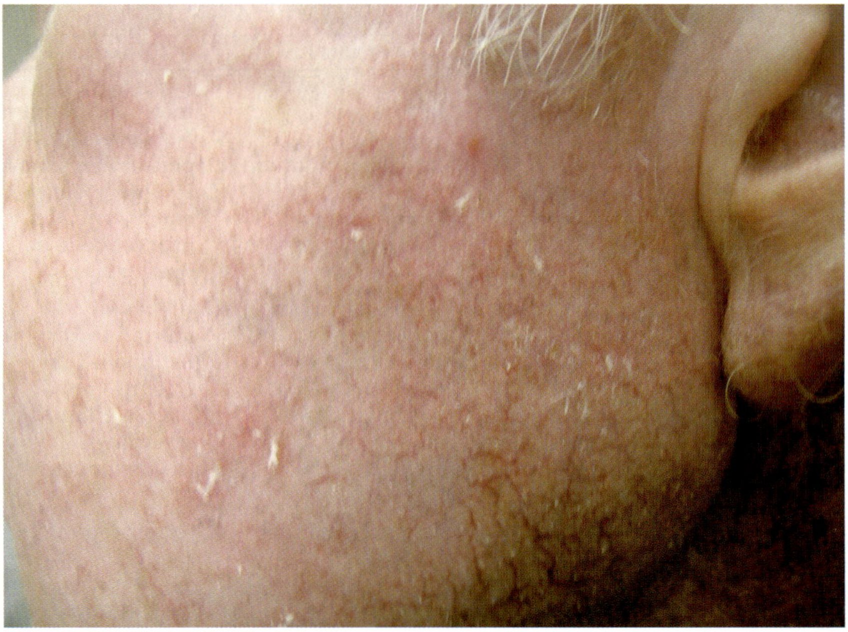

Figure 130.1. typical actinic keratoses manifest as rough scaly papules.

Section Two

Nonablative Therapy

131

Chemical Peels for Facial Rejuvenation

Andrew J. Kaufman

Chemical peeling is an underutilized but powerful procedure for improving the surface texture and color of photoaged skin. Benefits include a long-standing safety and efficacy profile and relative ease to learn and perform. The procedure is tailored to the problem, and chemical peels are inexpensive in relation to the technological gadgetry popular in cosmetic surgery. A key component to successful peeling is proper patient and indication selection. Chemical peeling works best for treatment of fine lines, dyschromia, rough texture or actinic keratoses, and superficial acne scarring. Patients with fair complexions and light-colored hair and eyes are generally easier to peel with less risk of pigmentary change. Patients with dark complexion and brown hair and eyes have a greater risk of postoperative hyperpigmentation.

One of the greatest uses of chemical peels is in combination with other procedures such as Botox or laser resurfacing. While Botox inhibits movement of specific muscles and softens rhytides, a chemical peel helps to further improve the remaining fine lines or wrinkles. With laser resurfacing I prefer to use an Erbium:YAG laser to resurface deeper lines in the periorbital and perioral areas preceded by a medium-depth chemical peel over the rest of the face (peel *before* laser resurfacing, not after). I use the precision of the laser to reach the depths of specific deeper wrinkles, while improving milder photoaged changes over the entire face. A combined approach avoids demarcation between laser and nonlaser areas.

Some of the pearls that I have found useful in chemical peels:

1. Preoperative treatment with tretinoin. A more even and deeper peel is accomplished, healing is quickened, milia are minimized, and the effects of bleaching agents are augmented. All patients use sunscreen before and after peels, and patients with a higher risk of postoperative hyperpigmentation use bleaching agents (e.g., hydroquinone). Place all patients on valcyclovir or acyclovir prior to a medium-depth chemical peel to decrease the risk of herpes simplex infection.
2. Avoid patients at higher risk of delayed wound healing or scarring, including patients who received Accutane in the last 12 months. Other higher risk patients are on corticosteroids, are immunosuppressed,

smoke, or have unrealistic expectations. Avoid a medium-depth peel over surgically undermined areas (e.g., rhytidectomy) for 6 months.

3. Purchase chemical peel supplies from medical supply organizations rather than your local pharmacy to avoid any problems or discrepancy in the concentration of the acids used. (Concentrations are weight-to-volume.)

4. Medium-depth chemical peels are usually accomplished using a combination of Jessner's solution or glycolic acid followed by 35% trichloroacetic acid (TCA). Concentrations of TCA greater than 40% have an unpredictable risk of delayed wound healing or scarring. Cleanse and degrease the skin with acetone before applying a single coat of Jessner's solution with gauze pads. After the Jessner's solution is dried, 35% TCA is applied with cotton-tip applicators or gauze pads to give an even, light frost. When using glycolic acid, apply 50–70% glycolic acid and leave it on for 2 minutes. If the patient complains of significant burning, shorten the application time and neutralize the glycolic acid with tap water. After neutralization for 2 minutes or less the area is toweled dry and 35% TCA is applied for an even frost. For deeper rhytides or areas with greater sun damage, apply additional TCA to get a deeper, whiter frost. Cool, wet compresses and a hand-held fan are used to comfort the patient after the TCA has dried and frost appeared.

5. Many patients tolerate the procedure without any anesthesia, but most patients receive Vicodin and Valium 30 minutes preoperatively.

6. Edema of the treated area is common for the first 48 hours and is minimized by head elevation and nonsteroidals. Wound care consists of skin hydration via liberal application of water to the treated areas. Acetic acid compresses (one tablespoon to one pint luke-warm water) twice daily decreases the risk of infection. Once peeling begins, a bland ointment, such as Aquaphor, is applied several times daily to keep the area moist and speed reepithelialization. Once healed, the patient starts a noncomedogenic sunscreen and sun-protective measures and may restart tretinoin and hydroquinone.

7. Patients are seen frequently in the postoperative period and are instructed to return for any symptoms suggestive of an infection, delayed wound healing, scarring, or pigmentary problem. An early sign of herpes simplex infection is increasing pain beginning a few days after a peel. One of the earliest signs of a scar is persistent erythema and pruritus. It is much easier to treat complications of chemical peeling at an early stage.

8. I frequently use medium and superficial chemical peels. A series of superficial peels (e.g., glycolic, salicylic, Jessner's, or low-concentration TCA) is well suited for younger patients with fine lines and dyschromia. Medium-depth peels work best for older patients with more extensive actinic damage. For severe actinic damage and deep rhytides I prefer to use a laser rather than deep phenol peels. While one can cause permanent hypopigmenation with a carbon dioxide lasers, I feel that I have better control over the depth of injury using a the Erbium:YAG laser.

9. One final pearl is to start out with superficial peels and ideal patients (blond hair, blue eyes, light complexion). Develop a sense of comfort and build upon your experience before performing deeper peels or dealing with patients at greater risk of pigmentary alteration.

132

Nonablative Laser and Light Facial Rejuvenation

Jeffrey S. Dover

Nonablative laser and light treatments provide an alternative to traditional full-face laser resurfacing, an ablative modality in which carbon dioxide and/or erbium:YAG lasers are used to remove the entire epidermis and portions of the dermis. While results in expert hands are impressive, the recovery period last several weeks and the risk/benefit ratio is high. As an alternative, nonablative treatments improve skin texture and tone, some improve wrinkles or surface irregularities including scarring, and some additionally address dyspigmentation and/or erythema and telangiectasia. The epidermis is not visibly disrupted in nonablative treatment. Nonablative resurfacing is attractive to physicians and patients alike because, contrary to ablative resurfacing, there is little downtime. Fractional laser resurfacing lies somewhere between true ablative laser resurfacing and non-ablative devices. Fractional erbium:YAG and fractional CO_2 lasers used at low energies and pattern density do not ablate the epidermis, and are effective in improving sun induced brown pigmentation and fine to moderate wrinkles.

A significant number of wavelengths of both visible and infrared radiation applied to the skin have the ability to induce dermal fibroblasts to produce a zone of new collagen within the papillary dermis. It remains to be determined which of the different wavelengths is most effective at inducing this change.

Numerous laser and light devices, including the KTP laser (532 nm), pulsed dye laser (585 nm, 595 nm), intense pulsed light (IPL) devices (515–1200 nm), Nd:YAG lasers (1064 nm Q-switched, 1064 nm long-pulse, 1319 nm, 1320 nm), diode lasers (980 nm, 1450 nm), Er:Glass laser (1540 nm) and light emitting diodes have been adapted to be effective in, or specifically developed for, nonablative resurfacing. The mid-infrared devices, including 1320, 1450, and 1540 nm devices, appear most effective for wrinkle and acne scar reduction. Red color and vascular lesions are best addressed by vascular-selective devices, such as the KTP, pulsed-dye, and long pulsed Nd:YAG lasers. The Q-switched Nd:YAG laser also has efficacy for pigmentation as does, but the KTP laser and IPL devices, by virtue of their broad emission spectrum, appear the most effective for simultaneous treatment of both red and brown patches.

Differences between before and after results can be subtle and not always seen easily, even in side-by-side photographic comparisons. However, the popularity of these treatments among patients and physicians strongly suggests that differences, while not always easy to quantify, are likely real.

Patient Selection

Deciding which patients are best suited for nonablative rejuvenation depends in part on understanding what they want so that it can be determined if nonablative therapy is likely to provide these results. Good candidates for nonablative resurfacing tend to be relatively young, usually 25–65 years of age, and have minimal sagging of the face. Patients should understand that skin texture will improve and fine lines in particular will be softened, not eradicated. Cumulative aesthetic benefits from nonablative resurfacing are similar in type though less in magnitude than the results of ablative resurfacing. Additionally, since changes will occur gradually, typically after three to six or more treatments, those receiving nonablative treatments should not expect dramatic results immediately.

These treatments are variably painful. The infrared sources are the most painful of these non-ablative procedures and usually require topical anesthesia for the procedures to be tolerable. Mild erythema and edema do occur following each treatment, but these sequelae remit within minutes to a few hours or may be concealed with cosmetics. Intense treatments can elicit moderate erythema and edema, which may peak 1–2 days after treatment and tend to subside a day or two later.

Infrared vs. Pulsed Dye

In general, it is important to distinguish between the infrared nonablative devices (1320 nm, 1450 nm, 1540 nm) on the one hand, and pulsed dye lasers, IPLs, and 532 and 1064 nm Nd:YAG lasers on the other. Infrared lasers, while uncomfortable, are associated with only a few hours of redness and swelling, while side effects and longer duration tissue effects are routine with the other devices.

Dark-skinned patients or those with a tendency to develop hyperpigmentation after skin injury can often safely undergo nonablative infrared therapy. The lasers are less susceptible to pigmentary complications, and patient skin color is less important when using these. With the noninfrared devices, treating tan patients is more risky, and skin color problems after treatment, more likely. Although recent evidence indicates that, in most cases, dark-skinned and Asian patients seldom develop pigmentary abnormalities after nonablative treatment, the risk of hyperpigmentation and hypopigmentation in such patients is still greater than in lighter skinned patients.

Postoperative Care

After nonablative treatment, little if any post treatment care is usually required, except with the fractional devices where keeping the skin moist is essential to rapid comfortable healing. Unusually stringent sun protection is not necessary after nonablative therapy although patients should refrain from active sun-seeking behaviors for a few days thereafter.

Patients who prefer to continue to receive maintenance therapy for the texture and color of their facial skin will often be satisfied with nonablative resurfacing. After the standard course of three to six nonablative facial treatments separated by 3–4 week intervals, treatments can be continued indefinitely on a 3 to 4 times/year basis. Some patients may choose to receive subsequent treatment courses on different devices to obtain cumulative benefits.

Choosing a Device

Lasers and light sources should be chosen so that the features most bothersome to the patient are best addressed. Most devices are relatively specific, in that they are better for some purposes.

1. Wrinkle or acne scars do moderately well with mid-infrared lasers but better results are seen with fractional resurfacing.
2. Rcd color is bcst trcatcd with vascular-selective KTP, long pulsed Nd:YAG, and pulsed-dye lasers and IPL.
3. Brown color is best treated with pigment-selective 532 KTP, Nd: YAG, and Q-switched lasers and IPL.
4. Texture and color, including red and brown color, can be collectively modestly improved by many different devices. IPL is a particularly effective hybrid modality, but even better textural improvement is seen with fractional resurfacing, albeit with more downtime. The infrared lasers are notable in their inability to effectively treat color.

In general, the less specific the patient objective, the greater the likelihood of satisfaction with nonablative therapy. Thus, patients who want removal of a particular feature, like redness or brown spots, or a particular wrinkle, tend to be less pleased after treatment than those interested in overall facial skin rejuvenation. Specific complaints are better treated with a laser device and setting specific for that indication (e.g., a Q-switched laser for lentigines, or a pulsed-dye laser with purpura for a spider angioma).

Device-Specific Pearls

KTP or Frequency-Doubled Nd:YAG laser (532 nm)

Good for red, vessels, brown, and texture
Excellent for small-caliber focal facial telangiectasia and lentigines.

Full face treatments help diffuse redness, small vessels, dyspigmentation caused by lentigines and fine wrinkling.

Start by tracing individual vessels then using a bigger spot the entire face is "painted."

Pulsed-Dye Laser (585 nm, 595 nm)

Good for red, vessels, and texture

Excellent for facial telangiectasia, diffuse erythema and also appears to improve fine vessels.
Recommend a series of at least 3 treatments spaced 4–6 weeks apart.
Patients favor purpura free treatments using long pulse durations the 10 msec domain.

Intense-Pulsed Light Device (500–1200 nm)

Good for red, brown and texture

Ideal for diffuse facial improvement in color, tone and texture.
A series of 5 to 6 treatments performed monthly is recommended.
The addition of 5-ALA applied 30–60 minutes in advance of treatment optimizes improvement in color and texture as well as fine lines.

Long-Pulsed Nd:YAG laser (1064 nm)

Good for red and texture

Mid-Infared Lasers (1320 nm Nd:YAG, 1450 nm diode, 1540 nm Er: Glass)

Best for texture, wrinkles and texture
Do not help color

A series of 5–6 treatments recommended.
Acne scarring improves better than fine to moderate wrinkles. Most see little improvement for the first 4 treatment but with the final 2 treatments in the series seem to make the biggest noticeable difference.
Pain during treatment is common, and can be somewhat mitigated with topical anesthesia.

Fractional Resurfacing Lasers

Best for brown color, acne scars, and wrinkles

A series of 4–6 treatments recommended.
Acne scarring and fine wrinkles improve better than moderate wrinkles. Improvement is seen even after one or two treatments.
Pain during treatment is common, and must be mitigated with topical anesthesia usually with additional air cooling.

Low Intensity Sources

Light Emitting Diodes treatments are painless, brief and appear to improve texture to some extent and may also improve redness.

Laser and Light Sources for Skin Rejuvenation

Infrared Lasers
- Cool Touch 1320 nm YAG
- Smooth Beam 1450 nm Diode
- Aramis 1540 nm Er:Glass

Visible Light Lasers
- Pulsed Dye (585 nm, 595 nm)
- Pulsed 532 nm (KTP)

Broad Band Light Sources
- Intense Pulse Light (515–1200 nm)

Low Intensity Sources
- Light Emitting Diodes

133

Mesotherapy for Cosmetic Periocular Enhancement

Samuel M. Lam and Gustavo H. Leibaschoff

Mesotherapy has continued to gain popularity throughout the United States during the past several years. It has been a mainstay of therapy in Europe for 50 years,. Many different formulations exist to treat a wide range of aesthetic and nonaesthetic conditions and are classified into allopathic and homeopathic branches. We focus on allopathic therapy and separate mesotherapy from phosphatidylcholine treatments, which are also discussed.

The primary objective of mesotherapy in the periocular region is to restore the dermal-epidermal junction that breaks down during aging, which manifests as surface wrinkles and poor skin tone and texture. The allopathic medicines used in mesotherapy are designed to reconstitute the dermo-epidermal junction and to improve local circulation, thereby enhancing the youthful appearance and condition of the skin. The efficacy of mesotherapy does not relate to the quantity of medicinal product but to the selection of an appropriate site-specific formulation.

The formulation that we currently use is based on years of experience, with slight modifications to improve efficacy. One of the principal ingredients of our face-specific formula is vitamins. Vitamin A increases the flexibility of the skin by regulating the growth of epidermal cells. Vitamin E is a potent antioxidant that maintains tissue integrity by combating toxic peroxides. Vitamin C stimulates the synthesis of collagen and inhibits the synthesis of unwanted melanin. Vitamin B is indispensable for the proper biologic balance of the skin. Vitamin K plays a major role in the regulation of the microcirculation. Amino acids are also employed that form the basis of tissue architecture. A combination of minerals (sodium, potassium, calcium, and magnesium) bound as salts is also instrumental in rejuvenation of the skin. Hyaluronic acid (noncross-linked) is recognized as an important component in facial mesotherapy to replace the lost hyaluronic acid that occurs with aging. It is the principal constituent that helps to recolonize the extracellular matrix, improve skin hydration and elasticity, and diminish fine rhytids. Blufomedil and pentoxtphylline are useful to improve the local microcirculation, and tretinoin and glycolic acid are also vital for skin enhancement. These components can be compounded by a compounding pharmacist.

Delivery

We use two principal methods to deliver the medicine to the desired site: needle injection and a no-needle method of aquaporation delivery. The former method is more accurately performed with a mesogun that controls the depth and measures a standard amount of medicine delivered per pass. We use a 1/2-inch 30-gauge needle that penetrates approximately 1 mm deep near the dermal-epidermal junction. The no-needle method is a newer technology that has shown good efficacy.

Perform sessions weekly for the first month then biweekly for the second month, followed by monthly treatments. The frequency in the first 2 months is mandatory but is individualized thereafter based on age, skin type, and treatment outcomes.

Mesotherapy provides excellent panfacial rejuvenation and can lessen wrinkles that would otherwise be unsafe to treat with Botox therapy or difficult to manage with medium-depth chemical peeling. Mesotherapy treats wrinkles that appear in animation and can soften static wrinkles somewhat.

Phosphatidylcholine

Another injectable combination, phosphatidylcholine mixed with deoxycholate, is often confused with mesotherapy. Unlike mesotherapy, which targets the dermal-epidermal junction, phosphatidylcholine/deoxycholate is administered more deeply into the fat to effect local lipolysis. Phosphatidylcholine/deoxycholate is used, but is not an equivalent to liposuction. This drug combination is marketed in Europe as Lipostabil from Aventis Laboratories. It is unsafe in the postseptal periocular region, as there have been four reported cases of blindness to date when used to treat steatoblepharon. Phosphatidylcholine/deoxycholate should only be used in experienced hands in other parts of the body, as it can cause skin or muscle necrosis if injected in improper quantities and depth. It is associated with discomfort, erythema, and edema for several days after treatment, which is expected and discussed preoperatively.

Section Three

Ablative Therapy

134

Skin Rejuvenation Techniques: General Considerations

Erin L. Holloman and Sterling S. Baker

Most patients want cosmetic and rejuvenative procedures with minimal to no downtime and visible results. The services most cosmetic surgeons offer run the spectrum from topical treatments (light chemical peels, microdermabrasion), to nonablative lasers and light sources, to radiofrequency skin tightening, to injectable fillers and Botox, to more traditional ablative skin resurfacing with chemical peels, lasers, or dermabrasion. Every office may not be able to offer every device or service. The most important keys are to listen to the patient, identify goals, and decide if those goals can be achieved with the techniques available. Obtain informed consent even on the most mundane procedures, but most importantly, ensure that the patient has realistic expectations.

Patient Evaluation

This is probably the most important step in discussing skin rejuvenation techniques with prospective patients. Realistic expectations have to be discussed before the procedure or you will have unhappy patients who are willing to share their dissatisfaction. A patient wanting a surgical result needs to have surgery, or at least agree to realistic results from a nonsurgical procedure.

An excellent idea, especially for ablative skin rejuvenation, is to show patients a photo book of the daily postoperative recovery period at the initial consultation. This is the best way to properly consent the patients and prepares them for exactly what to expect.

One of the most important patient history questions to ask is about use of Accutane in acne patients wanting to undergo laser skin resurfacing. Reepitheliazation can be delayed after its use. Wait at least 6 months and preferably a year before pursuing ablative resurfacing.

Surgical Planning

The gold standard of surgical skin rejuvenation techniques is laser skin resurfacing. This is usually performed as a one-time procedure, although it can be repeated. In contrast, most nonablative services need to be planned in a series of treatments. Microdermabrasion is best done in 4- to 6-weekly sessions. Most intense pulsed light (IPL) treatments require from three to six sessions, depending on the goal.

Anesthetic Techniques

The beauty of many of the nonablative techniques is that they don't require much anesthesia. Light chemical peels, microdermabrasion, IPL, and most vascular lasers are performed without any anesthesia. Radiofrequency skin tightening occasionally requires oral pain meds or sedatives with the newest algorithms. It is no longer a good idea to do multiple nerve blocks, as patient feedback during the procedure is important. Laser resurfacing is done under either general anesthesia or conscious sedation depending on the size of the area to be treated.

Surgical Procedure

During CO_2 laser skin resurfacing, change directions of the pattern of treatment with each pass. Avoid aggressive laser treatment along the angle of the mandible as this can scar easily. Gently wipe away "char" at the end of every pass. Feather the laser pattern in between treated and untreated areas to prevent obvious demarcation lines.

Postoperative Care

Have simple handouts for postoperative care for each different type of procedure. A good precautionary habit is to have patients sign that they received the instructions at the preoperative consultation, during which the instructions for postoperative care are thoroughly discussed. Most of the nonablative treatments require very little postop care. Never forget to tell everyone to stay out of the sun. Ablative resurfacing patients have to follow rigorous guidelines for safe and effective healing. It is always a good idea to see these patients frequently postoperatively in order to monitor progress.

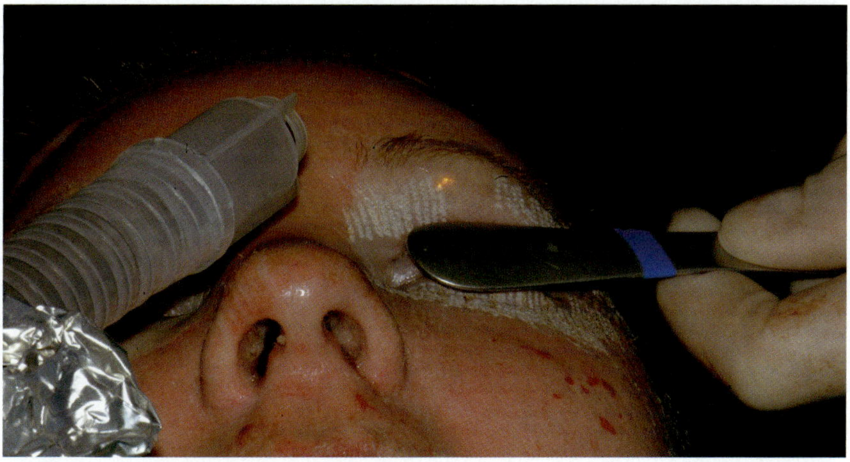

Figure 134.1. This patient is undergoing ablative laser skin resurfacing around the eyes. Notice the laser safe instrument protecting the eye and the smoke evacuator removing the plume. (Photo courtesy of Erin L. Holloman, MD.)

135

CO_2 Laser Skin Resurfacing Prophylaxis

Jemshed A. Khan

Large raw exposed facial areas following resurfacing may invite devastating bacterial cellulitis (*Staphylococcus aureus*, *Streptococcus pyogenes*, and *Pseudomonas aeruginosa*), primary herpes simplex, or reactivation of latent herpes simplex with disseminated facial scarring. To achieve therapeutic levels at the time of treatment, physicians may prescribe prophylactic antibiotic and antiviral medications prior to surgery (Table 135.1). Medications are continued for 12 days or until reepithelialization is well established. All resurfacing patients, except those undergoing very small treatment areas, receive a preoperative oral antibiotic, usually ciprofloxacin hydrochloride (Cipro®) 500 mg orally B.I.D. for 14 days, beginning 48 hours prior to surgery. Acyclovir (Zovirax®), a thymidine kinase inhibitor that is active against human herpesviruses, may be prescribed as 400 mg orally every 8 hours for 14 days, begun at least 2 days prior to surgery.

Table 135.1. Resurfacing Prophylactic Preoperative Care

Indication/Class	Generic name	Brand name	Recommended
Antibiotic	Ciprofloxacillin	Cipro	Most cases
Antiviral	Acyclovir	Zovirax	Most cases
Antifungal	Fluconazole	Diflucan	Not recommended
Bleaching agent	Hydroquinone	Various	Fitzpatrick IV,V,VI
Bleaching agent	Kojic acid	Generic	Fitzpatrick IV,V,VI
Anticomedogenic	Tretinsin	Retin A	Neutral
Steroid	Hydrocortisone	Various	Use with Retin A
Sunscreen	Various	Various	Neutral

Originally published in: Chen WPD, Khan JA, McCord, Jr. CD. Color Atlas of Cosmetic Oculofacial Sugery. Philadelphia: Butterworth Heinemann/Elsevier. 2004.

136

CO_2 Laser Resurfacing Immediate Postoperative Care Prior to Complete Epithelialization

Jemshed A. Khan

Wound care is designed to hasten the resolution of erythema and minimize postinflammatory hyperpigmentation subsequent to reepithelialization (Table 136.1). Topical application of hydrocortisone cream 1% at bedtime for up to 6 weeks after surgery will minimize both conditions. Postinflammatory hyperpigmentation is also reduced by the prophylactic use of sunscreen SPF 30 or greater for 12 weeks after surgery. Topical hydroquinone cream 4% may be applied at bedtime to speed the resolution of hyperpigmentation.

Table 136.1. Resurfacing Postoperative Care Prior to Epithehalization

Indication/Class	Generic name	Brand name	Recommended
Antibiotic	Ciprofloxacillin	Cipro	Most cases
Antiviral	Acyclovir	Zovirax	Most cases
Antifungal	Fluconazole	Diflucan	As needed
Occlusive dressing	Various	Various	Not recommended
Occlusive topical	Petroleum jelly	Vaseline	Recommended
Occlusive topical	Various	Aquaphor	Recommended
Steroid cream	2.5% Hydrocortisone	Various	Recommended
Wound care	Acetic acid	na	Recommended

Originally published in: Chen WPD, Khan JA, McCord, Jr. CD. Color Atlas of Cosmetic Oculofacial Sugery. Philadelphia: Butterworth Heinemann/Elsevier. 2004.

137

Products Used in CO_2 Laser Resurfacing Wound Care: Late Postoperative Care After Complete Epithelialization

Jemshed A. Khan

After re-epithelialization has occurred, treatment is directed toward reducing erythema and postinflammatory hyperpigmentetion (Table 137.1).

Table 137.1. Resurfacing Postoperative Care After Epithelialization

Indication/Class	Generic name	Brand name	Recommended
Steroid cream	Hydrocortisone 2.5%	Various	Recommended
Sunscreen SPF > 25	Various	Various	Recommended
Concealer	Various	Various	Recommended
Bleaching agent	Hydroquinone	Various	If pigmenting
Bleaching agent	Kojic acid	generic	If pigmenting
High-potency steroid	Clobetasol propionate	Temovate-E	If prolonged erythema—Caution: use 1 week only

Originally published in: Chen WPD, Khan JA, McCord, Jr. CD. Color Atlas of Cosmetic Oculofacial Sugery. Philadelphia: Butterworth Heinemann/Elsevier. 2004.

138

Monopolar Radiofrequency Tissue Tightening

Elizabeth F. Rostan

Background

Noninvasive tissue-tightening technologies rely on laser or radiofrequency (RF) energy to deliver heat to tissue without damaging the upper layers of skin. This heating of the tissue results in mechanical and molecular changes to produce tightening of the skin. Immediately this heating produces collagen contraction, then subsequent wound healing leads to new collagen production and wound contracture. The upper layer of skin is protected most frequently with a cooling mechanism or by utilizing low energy. There are currently multiple devices that claim noninvasive tissue tightening.

The devices utilizing radiogrequency include monopolar RF (ThermaCool device by Thermage, Hayward, CA), combined diode laser/bipolar (Polaris device by Syneron Medical, Yokeam, Isreal), and combined vacuum/bipolar RF (Aluma device by Lumenis, Santa Clara, CA). Other devices use laser or broadband light sources to heat the skin and include broadband light (Titan device by Cutera, Brisbane, CA and StarluxIR device by Palomar, Burlington, MA), and long-pulsed 1064-nm Nd:YAG lasers (multiple manufacturers). The rest of this discussion will focus on monopolar RF skin tightening.

Technology

Monopolar RF tissue tightening was first introduced in 2002 as the ThermaCool device by Thermage, Inc. (Haywood, CA). It was the first device marketed for noninvasive skin tightening. The ThermaCool device, which has FDA 510K approval for the treatment of facial rhytids and more recently for skin tightening of eyelid skin and nonfacial areas, utilizes monopolar RF energy to heat deeper dermal structures leading to collagen renewal and tightening.

The ThermaCool device utilizes a capacitively coupled treatment tip as the active electrode which is used in conjunction with a return electrode that is placed at a distant site on the patient. This treatment tip is cooled with multiple small bursts of cryogen during each treatment pulse in order to protect the upper layers of skin while the deeper structures are heated. Activation of the treatment tip against the skin creates an electric field under the tip. Tissue resistance in the skin and subcutaneous tissues generates heat from radiofrequency energy. The depth of tissue heating is related to the dimensions of the treatment tip. The first-generation treatment tips were 1.0 cm^2 and 1.5 cm^2 and produced tissue heating to a depth of about 2.5 mm. Newer 3.0-cm^2 tips penetrate more deeply, while smaller tips designed for use on eyelid skin have a much more limited depth of penetration (Figure 138.1).

Patient Selection

The best candidates for monopolar RF tissue tightening are those with mild to moderate degree of skin laxity of the face and neck. All skin types can be safely treated. Patients with thinner skin or less adipose tissue achieve greater degrees of tightening than those with heavier faces. In evaluating patients, I use gentle pressure laterally on the areas of interest to determine the degree of movement of the tissue. In the evaluation of the cheek and jowl area, if the amount of tissue that can be moved easily with one's fingertips is mild to moderate, then I feel the patient is an appropriate candidate for ThermaCool treatment. If the amount of lax tissue is very significant, such that a large amount of tissue would have to be excised during a face or neck lifting procedure, then that option is discussed with the patient. I do perform ThermaCool procedures on patients who I feel would benefit more from a surgical procedure in instances where the patient states he or she has no interest in surgery at all or if there are medical conditions that make the patient a poor candidate for surgery.

In evaluating candidates for ThermaCool procedure of the forehead, I again like to be able to detect fairly significant tissue movement when pushing up on the skin of the forehead toward the hairline. If there is minimal movement or if the tissue feels very tight, do not recommend RF treatment for browlifting. If I can't move the tissue with physical pressure, then RF treatment is not going to be able to move the tissue either. The lifting achieved with ThermaCool treatment in the forehead area is not as longlasting as other areas. Botox relaxation of the brow depressors is performed in most patients who elect to have RF treatment of the forehead area in order to remove the antagonistic effect of these muscles.

RF treatment of the eyelid skin is a new treatment with limited experience. A recently published study demonstrated that some patients, despite having as many as 700 pulses of RF energy, had no demonstrable improvement in eyelid skin laxity. For RF treatment of the eyelids, I prefer patients with mostly excess thin, loose skin to a mild to moderate degree. Patients with heavier eyelids require more significant fat pad resection in a blepharoplasty procedure.

For RF tissue tightening of the neck, the ideal candidate has mild skin laxity and no significant laxity or platysmal muscle bands (Figure 138.2).

It is recommended that treatment of the neck be combined with that of the cheek, as tightening of the cheek tissues often reduces neck laxity. If there is significant adipose tissue in the neck along with loose skin, I recommend that RF treatment be done immediately following tumescent liposculpture of the neck. This combination treatment is performed in patients who may have some skin laxity remaining after liposculpture alone. Again, monopolar RF tissue tightening will not replace a surgical procedure for those patients with significant skin laxity. I do not observe any tightening of loose platysmal bands after RF treatment. This should be clearly explained to patients prior to treatment.

For RF treatments on nonfacial skin, the most commonly treated area in my practice is the lower abdomen. I sometimes combine RF with tumescent liposuction in this area in surgical patients I judge to have excess skin that may be inadequately addressed with liposuction alone. The best candidates for RF tightening of lower abdominal skin are those with loose skin only and very minimal excess adipose tissue. This is typically seen in thin, fit women who have had children and have excess skin but otherwise tight abdominal structures. I do not commonly recommend treatment for other nonfacial areas (breasts, buttocks, thighs, arms) as I feel the results are inconsistent and often less than patient and physician expectations.

Realistic expectations are important for RF treatment of any area. The results typically are not dramatic and not well demonstrated by photographs. Sometimes the main aspect of improvement, especially in the cheeks, is how tight or firm the skin feels or that the skin resists gravity upon bending down.

Treatment

Current treatment protocols utilize multiple passes over the treatment area. Treatment grids with squares the size of the treatment tip are placed on the skin. This guides the placement of the tip during the treatment. Generally the grids are placed in the direction of desired tightening such as superior-lateral on the cheeks and vertical on the forehead. In most cases, at least one pass is applied over the entire treatment grid and then multiple passes (up to five) are performed over the areas of greatest movement or "lifting or anchor points" such as over the lateral cheek and zygoma and along the jawline to tighten the cheek and jowl area. In areas of loose skin the skin is kept taut with the nontreating hand so that the treatment tip is applied uniformly to the skin. When treating the forehead, I do not treat areas that do not move with pressure and instead focus on areas that are freely moveable.

Stretching the skin over certain anchoring points, such as pulling the lower cheek skin up to the zygoma, while applying the RF pulse can further enhance the tightening effect. Some physicians advocate pinching the skin in areas of excess adipose, such a heavy jowls or under the chin, and applying the tip to the pinched area. This is done in an attempt to cause deeper tightening and possible reshaping of fatty areas and should be used judiciously and only by experienced users. Pulse stacking is to be avoided as the heat build-up can lead to skin depressions.

Early experience with very high fluence demonstrated the risk of skin atrophy. Treatment settings are now more moderate and based more on patient tolerance and feedback. Many physicians give patients oral anxiolytics and/or oral or intramuscular narcotic pain medication prior to RF treatment. General or IV sedation is not recommended because of loss of patient feedback regarding pain of the treatment. For the same reason, nerve blocks are not recommended. Topical anesthetics are used only numb the cooling sensation and do not help with the deep heat sensation. If topical numbing cream is used, then care should be taken to completely remove it prior to treatment as any residual on the skin surface is felt to increase the risk of a skin burn.

In the treatment of skin laxity of the upper and lower eyelid, a combination of tips is used. I first treat the brow, orbital rim, and temple area with a 1.0- or 1.5-cm^2 tip. I also include treatment of the thicker upper eyelid skin just below the brow in this area. This skin is pulled above the bony orbit and the treatment tip only applied to skin overlying the bone. Then I treat the thin skin just above and directly overlying the globe and lower eyelid with the eyelid tip. A plastic eye shield must be placed prior to treatment. Metal eye shields should not be used during RF treatment.

Conclusion

Monopolar RF tissue tightening can be an effective, safe, nonablative way to achieve tighter skin in carefully selected patients. Results are modest and do not approach that achieved by surgery.

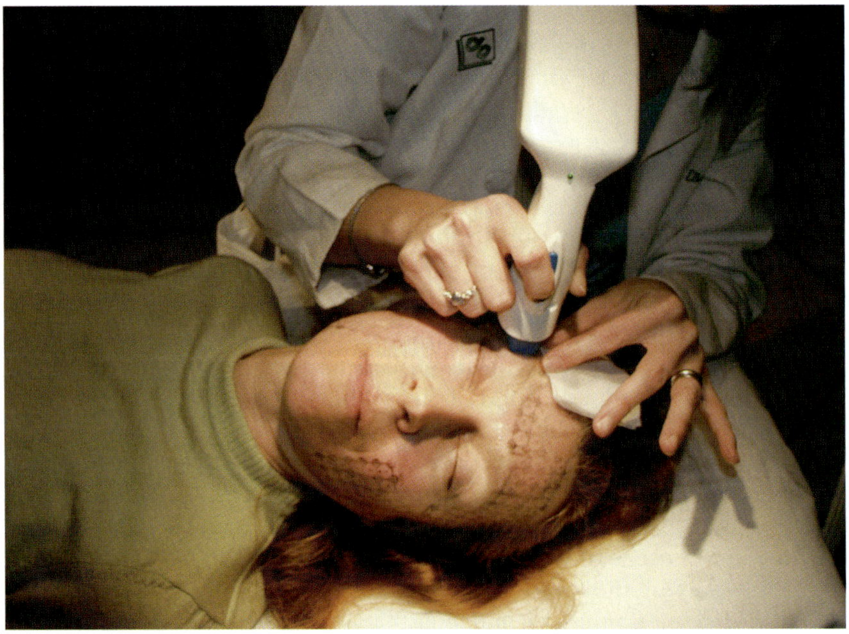

Figure 138.1. Treatment of periorbital area with a 1.5-cm^2 tip. The treatment tip is applied to thicker skin that is pulled over the bony orbit.

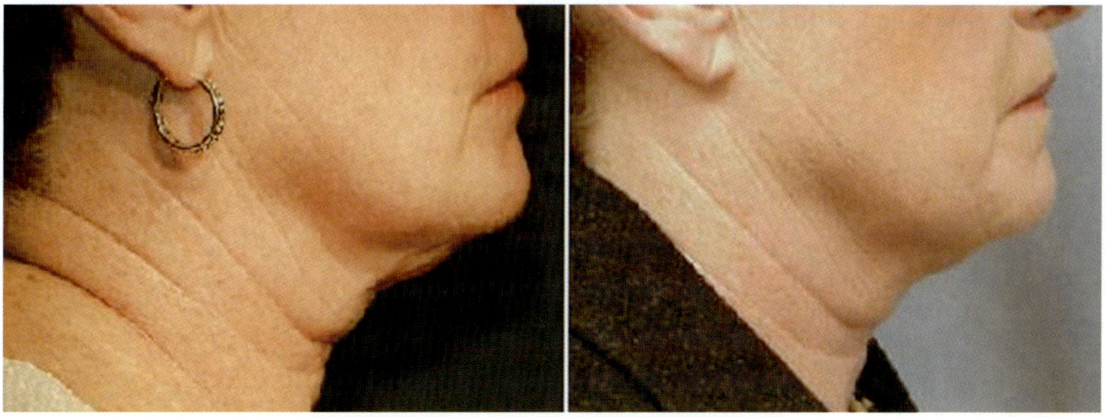

Figure 138.2. Before and after neck treatment.

139

Dual-Mode Erbium-YAG Laser Skin Resurfacing

John B. Holds*

Ablative laser skin resurfacing may give dramatic benefit in skin rejuvenation, although at the cost of significant risk, side effects, and healing time. Two lasers with significantly different physical effects but similar final surgical results are employed: short-pulse CO_2 and erbium-YAG (Er:YAG) lasers (Table 139.1). The absorption coefficient of water and tissue at the near infrared wavelength of the Er:YAG laser is 18 times that of the CO_2 laser. For this reason, the Er:YAG laser at a short pulse-width is almost purely ablative. The longer pulse duration and greater thermal damage in Table 139.1 for Er:YAG refers to lasers with a long pulse width coagulative mode. Moderate to deep chemical peels and dermabrasion can achieve results comparable to laser skin resurfacing in smoothing the skin and eradicating rhytids, with some similarities in healing.

The short-pulse CO_2 lasers were available first and are familiar to surgeons performing laser skin resurfacing. The Er:YAG lasers have been available for over 10 years, although the early lasers were underpowered and lacked both a thermal mode for deeper rhytids and a computerized pattern generator handpiece to achieve uniform application. There is a perception that Er:YAG lasers are only effective for fine wrinkles and will not treat deeper rhytids.

Multiple studies have documented CO_2 and Er:YAG treatment to be equivalent or near-equivalent in facial laser skin resurfacing. Hughes[1] noted the measurable skin contraction with Er:YAG skin resurfacing which progressed over 6 weeks of healing and persisted throughout the study. Khatri et al.[2] noted significantly less prolonged postoperative erythema after Er:YAG treatment with a much lower risk (5% vs. 43%) of hypopigmentation, and Ross et al.[3] noted equivalent results between Er:YAG and CO_2 lasers when treated to equivalent depths.

For more than 9 years I have used a Sciton Contour dual-mode Er:YAG laser that has not only a high power output (45 W) equal to the

---

*Dr. Holds has no financial interest in Sciton Corporation and receives no consultant or other fees from that company.

better CO_2 lasers, but also a variable thermal mode achieved through the use of a longer pulse width, which delivers some thermal effect. This has been an effective and versatile laser, and with this device I have been able to achieve surgical results in over 1500 cases measured in rhytid reduction and correction of dyschromia that equal the results I was able to previously achieve with the CO_2 lasers. The ultimate advantage of the dual-mode Er:YAG laser is the faster healing time and the marked decrease in risk of scarring or permanent depigmentation. Reepithelialization time and duration of erythema both appear to be significantly less with Er:YAG treatment.

Key Elements of Procedure

Patient Selection and Preparation

Patients with Fitzpatrick 1 or 2 skin type are much easier to work with. Patients should strictly avoid sun exposure for a month before and 2 months after surgery. Patients who tan readily or have significant dyschromia will benefit from preoperative treatment with bleaching creams such as 4% hydroxyquinone and/or a retinoid such as tretinoin 0.05% cream.

Preoperative counseling must focus on a frank informed consent, which dispels any misinformation the patient may bring to the visit. A discussion of expected downtime and review of procedural and postoperative photographs of similar patients will promote a realistic appraisal of the plan at hand.

In patients with no history of herpes simplex outbreak who are undergoing upper facial treatment only, such as periocular treatment, I do not generally prophylax with an antiviral medication, and I have only seen one outbreak of herpes simplex ever in such patients. Patients undergoing lower face or full-face laser are prophylaxed with valcyclovir (Valtrex) 500 mg twice daily, beginning 2 days preoperatively and continuing for 5 days postoperatively. Antibiotic prophylaxis is generally determined by other patient features.

Procedure

Up to 2–3 aesthetic units can generally be treated in an office procedure room with nerve blocks and tumescent anesthesia using a buffered 0.2% lidocaine mixture (epinephrine 1:800,000). It is possible to perform full-face treatment in office, although general anesthesia is preferred.

There are a number of treatment paradigms used by different practitioners. The parameters below are in reference to a Sciton Contour dual-mode Er:YAG laser. Micrometers of ablation are calculated at 4 $\mu m/J/cm^2$ energy fluence.

It is appropriate to use the higher coagulative settings in areas of thick skin with the most profound wrinkles, such as the perioral area. An extra coagulative pass similar to pass two is often needed in those areas. Thinner skin areas such as the eyelids generally receive energies on the lower end of those noted above, as do the cheeks.

Postoperative

Immediately postoperatively the patient is occluded with petrolatum ointment such as Vaseline or Aquaphor Natural Healing Ointment. Alternatively, a sheet dressing such as 2nd Skin (Spenco) may be applied and taped in place or held with a compressive stockinet. Dressings must be changed every day, and the ointments are generally reapplied after soaking with a dilute cool solution of white vinegar (1 ml vinegar/50 ml water) approximately every 3 hours while awake.

Patients are seen routinely at days 1, 3, 6, and 12–14. Depending on the depth of treatment, cover-up makeup can be worn 8–14 days after surgery. Erythema is variable, lasting 1–6 months, depending on the patient's skin and depth of therapy. Ultraviolet light exposure is strictly avoided for the first month postoperatively. In patients in whom postinflammatory hyperpigmentation is likely to be a problem, this is initially apparent 4–6 weeks postoperatively.

Conclusion

Dual-mode Er:YAG laser skin resurfacing is an effective treatment for photoaging skin changes. Appropriate case selection, patient counseling, and preparation will allow for optimal results with appropriate surgical technique and postoperative care. Equivalent results to CO_2 skin resurfacing can be obtained with lesser amounts of postoperative erythema and risk of hypopigmentation (Figure 139.1).

Table 139.1. Comparison of Physical Properties of Er:YAG and CO_2 Lasers

	Er:YAG	CO_2
Wavelength (nm)	2940	10,600
Thermal damage (μm per pass)	5–100	50–75
Tissue ablation (μm)	20–120	50–60
Pulse duration (μs)	100–50,000	1000

Table 139.2. Sciton Contour Typical Full-Face Settings (Low-High)

Pass	Ablation (μm)	Coagulation (μm)
1	60–90	0
2	60–90	25–100
3	60–90	0–50

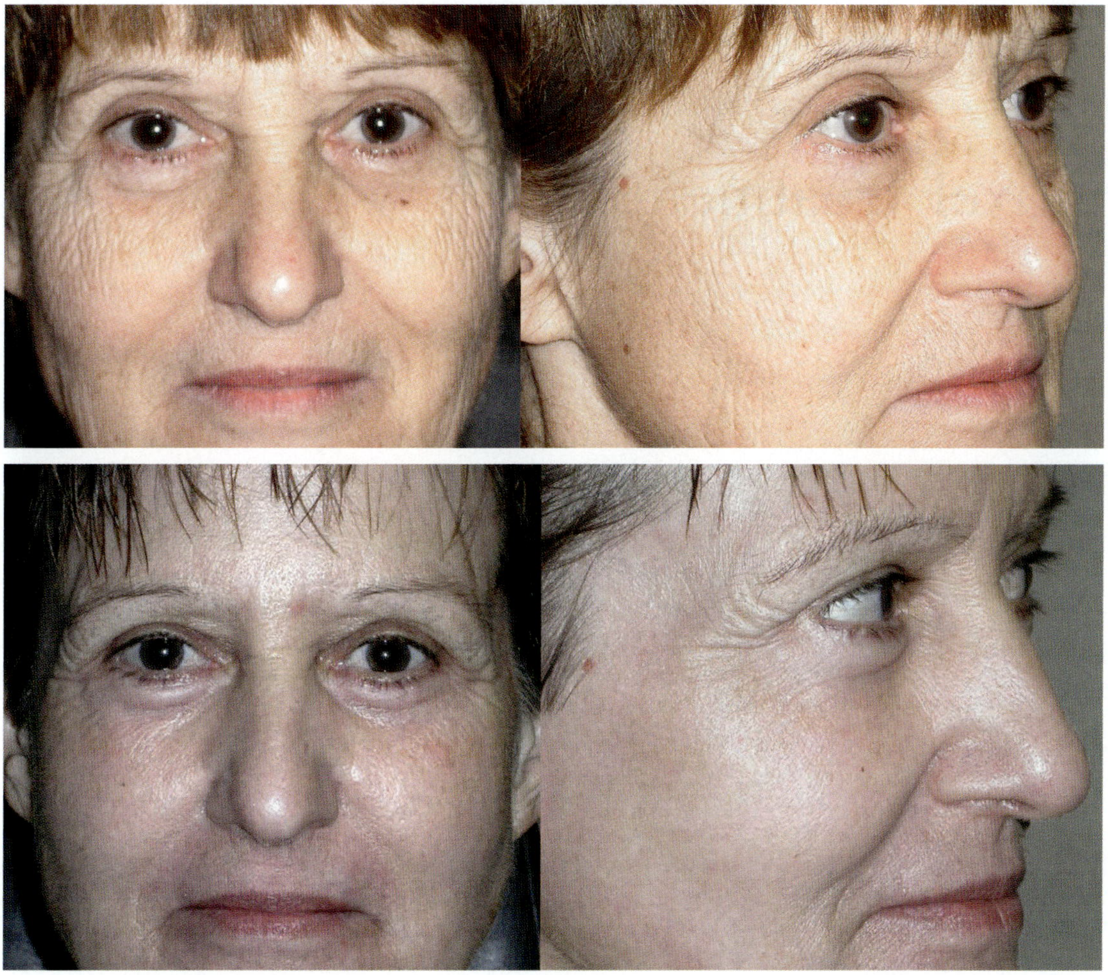

A

B

Figure 139.1. Patient shown (A) preoperatively, and (B) 6 months postoperatively.

References

1. Hughes P. Skin contraction following erbium:YAG laser resurfacing. Dermatol Surg 1998;24:109–111.
2. Khatri KA, Ross V, Grevelink JM, Magro CM, Anderson RR. Comparison of erbium:YAG and carbon dioxide lasers in resurfacing of facial rhytides. Arch Dermatol 1999;135(4):391–397.
3. Ross EV, Miller C, Meehan K, Pac, McKinlay J, Sajben P, Trafeli JP, Barnette DJ. One-pass CO2 versus multiple-pass Er:YAG laser resurfacing in the treatment of rhytides: a comparison side-by-side study of pulsed CO_2 and Er: YAG lasers. Dermatol Surg 2001;27(8):709–715.

140

Fraxel Treatment

Howard Conn

I have been using Fraxel in my practice for four years. The Fraxel effect on the skin is similar to CO_2 Ultrapulse ablation but without the wound care and downtime. The Fraxel energy is absorbed by water, as is the CO_2, but ablates microscopic spots of epidermis and dermis so that the adjacent, healthy tissue seals the wounds in a matter of hours.

If you are familiar with CO_2 Ultrapulse resurfacing, you can adapt to Fraxel very quickly. The patients can apply makeup the next day. It is useful for reducing brown spots, dyspigmentation, and mild to moderate wrinkles due to sun damage. It improves the crepe appearance and texture of the skin. Because the system applies thousands of microscopic spots, the improvement of the treated areas is uniform without skip areas that one sees with lasers utilizing stamping technology. I am treating face, neck, chest, hands, arms and legs with excellent results.

Here are a few tips to improve comfort and efficacy using the Fraxel re:store (SR1500):

1. Apply a mixture of topical 7% lidocaine and 7% tetracaine for one hour over the treated areas. A stronger concentration of lidocaine is not necessary.
2. It is essential to use the Zimmer Cryo 5 cooler for patient comfort.
3. There are two variables to consider: energy and treatment level. The energy level is roughly directly proportional to the depth of penetration of the laser. The treatment level determines the percentage of the skin treated during the session. Higher treatment levels results in greater inflammation. Therefore for superficial brown pigmentation, I use an energy setting 20–30 mJ with treatment level of 8–9. For moderate wrinkles I use 30–50 mJ with treatment level 9–11. More inflammation results in more collagen production. In treating severe wrinkles and acne scars I treat with 50–70 mJ and treatment level 9–11.
4. Screen patients for their propensity to develop postinflammatory hyperpigmentation. In these patients, I use a lower energy setting and lower treatment level and prescribe hydroquinone postoperatively.
5. The eyelids are a particularly sensitive area when treating with energy setting of 40 mJ and treatment level of 10 and above. I inject

subcutaneously small quantities of a mixture of 50 ml 1% lidocaine without epinephrine to which I add 2 ml of hyaluronidase (150 units/ml) and 6 ml of 8.4% sodium bicarbonate.

6. When a patient has a history of repeated HSV (cold sores), I prescribe Valtrex 2 gm orally every 12 hours on the day of treatment.

7. Treat only two areas at a time. This means face and neck, neck and chest, etc. This will minimize anesthetic toxicity.

In January 2008 Reliant Technologies introduced the Fraxel re:pair, a fractionated delivery system that utilizes a CO_2 laser instead of the mid-infrared laser used in the Fraxel re:store. This is a one-time ablative laser treatment that provides superior skin tightening for older patients with moderate to severe wrinkling due to sun damage. In addition to treating the face and neck, I use the re:pair device in conjunction with CO_2 laser blepharoplasty to treat periorbital wrinkles. The skin re-epithelializes in 48 hours with this system.

The advantages of the fractionated CO_2 delivery system versus Ultrapulse resurfacing are:

1. More rapid re-epithelialization, 2 days vs. 7 to 10 days
2. Less patient discomfort
3. Less wound care
4. Fewer postoperative visits and telephone calls
5. No skip areas or overlap because of scanning delivery
6. More skin tightening
7. No hypopigmentation
8. Ability to fine-tune depth of energy and density
9. Ability to treat off face

I employ the following protocol for Fraxel re:store cases:

1. Vicodin, Xanax 1 mg preoperatively.
2. Keflex and Valtrex in the perioperative period
3. Topical 23/7% xylocaine/tetracaine
4. Nerve blocks and local infiltration with 1% xylocaine, plain with hyaluronidase and sodium bicarbonate as noted above.

Part X

Thread Lift

Editors'Note: Reports on long-term outcome with the Contour Thread-Lift led Surgical Specialties Corp. to withdraw this product from the market in the summer of 2007. At this time, two FDA-approved products are being marketed for facial anesthetic surgery: The Silhouette Midface suture by FCI Ophthalmics and the Endotine ribbon by Coapt Corp. The editors have no personal experience with either device and are following developments in this field. The various thread lifting techniques have a history of initial enthusiasm followed by promotion, widespread adoption, reports of inadequate results, and abandonment. The reader is cautioned to oberve but only cautiously to adopt these techniques.

141

Pros and Cons of Contour Threads for Upper Facial Rejuvenation

Michael S. Kaminer

For decades surgeons have attempted to create a more youthful appearance of the periorbital region, including techniques to reshape and position the eyebrow complex. The downfall of some treatments is their invasive nature. To address this, surgeons have recently turned to the use of barbed sutures to elevate and reposition brows. The most noteworthy of these suture techniques is the Contour ThreadLift (Surgical Specialties, Reading, PA). Although the elevation of brows using barbed Contour threads is still considered a surgical procedure, it is much less invasive than traditional surgical procedures used to elevate the brow. However, as always with a new surgical procedure, there are issues to consider before incorporating the Contour ThreadLift into everyday practice.

Advantages

1. The procedure is performed entirely with local anesthesia. Supplemental oral sedation is not required, but can be of benefit (Valium, Ativan).
2. The incisions for placement of threads are tiny and do not require suturing or surgical closure.
3. There are no bandages required following the procedure.
4. A simple surgical tray is all that is required. Expensive equipment and setup are not needed.
5. The technique is relatively easy to learn, in particular for surgeons skilled at aesthetic surgery of the upper face.
6. The threads are quite strong and can support and handle a relatively heavy load in terms of skin weight and thickness.
7. The threads can be placed in a customized fashion for each patient, enabling the surgeon to tailor treatment to create a brow shape and location that fits the particular features of any given patient.
8. Although overcorrection at the time of surgery is recommended, the surgeon can subtly correct the amount of brow elevation. This is accomplished by simply relaxing part of the thread's pull with simple

manual pressure. Anesthesia is not required for this postoperative thread relaxation, which can be performed during a routine postoperative visit.

9. There is a high level of patient satisfaction, particularly given the limited morbidity and invasiveness of the procedure.

Disadvantages

1. The threads have only recently been approved by the FDA (May 2005). Long-term follow up studies have not been performed.

2. Past experiences with threads for other face lifting procedures have proven, in the long term, to be less than satisfactory. It remains to be seen whether the Contour threads will meet a similar long-term fate.

3. The amount of brow elevation obtained without excising skin is limited in some patients, limiting the utility of the ThreadLift procedure.

4. There is competition in the minimally invasive world of brow elevation from techniques such as Thermage and Botox. It remains to be seen whether the Contour ThreadLift will provide any long term advantages over these two less invasive options.

5. Thread extrusion remains a real problem, particularly when technique is less than optimal.

6. Threads can sometimes be seen under the skin when placed too superficially.

7. If threads are not fixated properly to the galea, migration can cause a reduction of long term efficacy as well as extrusion.

8. There is reluctance on the part of some patients to have a foreign material such as a thread placed under their skin.

Contour threads at present are a useful alternative for minimally invasive elevation and repositioning of the eyebrow region. Long-term follow-up studies are clearly needed to confirm the longevity and utility of this interesting procedure.

142

Periocular Suture Lifts: Brow and Malar Repositioning

Samuel M. Lam

The advent of various minimally invasive procedures for periorbital rejuvenation has revolutionized the practice of cosmetic surgery. Despite these advances, the prospective surgeon should always be cautioned about the efficacy, risks, and longevity of any novel approach.

Suture lifts have been introduced as a limited-downtime, in-office procedure that can provide some degree of periorbital and facial rejuvenation but should not be construed as an equivalent to a surgical lift like brow, midface, or lower facelifting. Nevertheless, in the correct patient with proper preoperative education, these new noninvasive treatments can provide satisfactory results.

Although many types of suture lifts exist, they can be most easily classified into two major categories: a closed, no-incision approach using floating, bidirectional cogged sutures and an open, tiny incision approach using superiorly anchored, unidirectional cogged sutures. This chapter is not intended to advocate the use of any particular brand of suture. Instead, a basic strategy will be outlined for each technique, and clinical efficacy based on over 100 procedures during a 2-year period will be discussed.

The closed technique (also known as the featherlift, Russian threads, or APTOS sutures) relies on floating sutures that are anchored to the surrounding tissues by virtue only of the tiny cogs that are distributed across the entire length of each suture. The cogs face toward the center of the suture in a bidirectional fashion and are used to support and hold the tissue like a hammock. The sutures are fabricated from 2-0 polypropylene like those used in the open technique (discussed below). An 18-gauge $3^1/_2$-inch spinal needle is used to pierce the subcutaneous tissue while the tissue is elevated and supported at the desired position. After the spinal needle has been properly inserted, support is removed and the tissue observed to be held in the desired elevated position by the spinal needle. The inner stylet of the spinal gauge needle is removed. The bidirectional needleless suture is then inserted through the spinal needle until equal ends of the suture are exposed at both sides. While the assistant holds one end of the exposed suture firmly in hand, the surgeon withdraws the spinal needle and the tissue is then held in place by the suture. This sequence of maneuvers is repeated until the entire face has been suspended.

The open technique (also known as Threadlift, Contour lift, endo-APTOS) relies on unidirectional cogged sutures that are distributed along a partial length of the suture with the remaining suture bare of cogs but affixed with a needle to a fixed tissue point like the galea, deep temporal fascia, preparotid fascia, or mastoid fascia. The Contour Threadlift uses clear 2-0 polypropylene suture that has a long straight Keith needle affixed to the barbed end and a curved needle attached to the bare end of the suture. Transcutaneous entry points are made at the superior limit of fixation. These incisions need only be approximately 1–2 mm long to accommodate passage of the needles through each one. A sharp-tipped iris scissors can be used to create these abbreviated incisions with a gentle spreading motion through the skin. The Keith needle is passed through one of the lower incisions and exits inferiorly through the skin and subcutaneous tissue that the surgeon wishes to elevate. The Keith needle is passed under the immediate subdermis in a sinusoidal pattern changing a slight angle every 1 cm in order to create a better tensile lift. An additional suture is then passed through the other incision down to a similar inferior exit point in the same sinusoidal pattern. The Keith needle is then cut off and discarded from both sutures. Each suture is then drawn from the inferior exit point until all of the barbs (cogs) begin to disappear under the upper entry incisions. At this point, the length of both exposed sutures from the superior incisions should be equal. The curved needle is then used to pass through the same incision up through the superior, central third incision while purchasing some deeper tissue along the way. The other paired suture is passed through to the central upper incision in the same manner, andthey are tied with the knot buried. The sutures are not tied down with excessive tension, as the skin will be redraped superiorly to the appropriate elevation in the following step. The surgeon's hand then sweeps superiorly to lift the tissues upward. Elevation of the tissue is observed and the patient questioned whether the aesthetic change is acceptable. Fine-tuning of the lift is performed. The exposed suture are cut flush with the skin.

As with any procedure, success is predicated on preoperative counseling with patients regarding the expected aesthetic benefits. No matter what changes occur, the result will not be equal to a facelift. If the patient uses his or her hand to draw the face upward to express the desired aesthetic change, the expected change may be at best half of that. Exclusion criteria include a very heavy-faced individual with thick tissues. Younger patients between 35 and 50 years of age are better candidates simply because they have lesser needs. Suture lifting can also be used as a touch-up for previous surgery that misses the mark by a small margin.

In our experience, the closed technique fails to adequately address the brow and lower face but can provide acceptable malar/mid-face elevation. The open technique that relies on a superior point of fixation has proven to be a more reliable method of achieving brow, mid-face, and lower face support. The closed technique can be used as a substitute or in conjunction with the open technique in the mid-face, especially in longer faces in which the needle is harder to pass with the open method.

Accumulated personal experience and judgment will help guide further care in each surgeon's hands. Because the tissue elevation is conservative, combined techniques can yield a more identifiable change. For example, concurrent botulinum toxin (Botox) and hyaluronic acid (Restylane) can be used in conjunction with a suture lift to increase the aesthetic impact. In these cases, 1 + 1 may equal 3 in terms of the perceived benefit.

Although the procedure is relatively short and is performed in the office setting, complications can still arise. Generally speaking, the patient exhibits swelling with either method for several days and can usually return to work in a few days, e.g., over an extended weekend. With the open technique, some skin bunching along the superior limit of fixation can persist for 3 weeks. For individuals with shorter hairstyles, camouflage may be difficult. Ecchymosis may be significant and disfiguring for a few days to weeks. Avoidance of nonsteroidal anti-inflammatory medications and herbal medications that predispose toward bleeding is imperative preoperatively. Liberal use of ice for the first 24–48 hours after the procedure lessens postoperative edema and ecchymosis. Suture migration is more commonly encountered with a nonfixed suture used in the closed method but can occur with the open method. Extrusion of the suture is managed by removal of the offending suture. For the open technique, removal of the suture from the inferior point is more easily accomplished than in a retrograde fashion from the superior end.

The future of cosmetic surgery will reveal increasingly minimally invasive techniques. However, with any method, clinical efficacy must be established in a discernible and durable fashion. The results of suture lifting must be borne out with the test of time.

143

Contour Threads Technique Pearls

Michael S. Kaminer

Several technique elements can be implemented by the surgeon to improve results and potentially improve longevity and predictability of contour thread (Surgical Specialties, Reading, PA) lifting. These include:

- Ensure consistent and accurate fixation of the threads to the galea, preferably posterior (cephalad) to the existing hair line.
- Bending of the insertion trocar can allow the surgeon to more precisely contour the trocar to the shape of the patient's brow. This enables easier placement of the thread, ensuring proper positioning.
- Make sure that the exit point for the thread is inferior to the brow at all points.
- Use enough threads to specifically contour and position the brow to where you feel it is most appropriate.
- Failure to use enough threads in elevating the brow can lead not only to long-term failure, but also an unnatural appearance of the brow.
- For many patients, three pairs of threads (a total of six threads) are used to elevate the brow. This will include one pair at the lateral brow bilaterally. In addition, a pair of threads will be placed centrally, with a single thread going to the ipsilateral medial brow from a mid line insertion point for the pair.
- In some patients, elevation of the lateral brow is all that is required to achieve the desired cosmetic result. In these patients, only two pairs of threads would be needed, each placed at the lateral brow.
- Avoid a direct vertical placement of the threads at the lateral brow, attempting more of an oblique insertion and course. This limits visibility of the threads postoperatively and improves the final aesthetic outcome.
- Introduce the threads in a zigzag fashion. This in effect lengthens the amount of thread placed subcutaneously and therefore distributes the load of the skin over a greater length of thread, in the end improving potential longevity.
- Place threads in a deep subcutaneous plane.

- Make sure when trimming the threads at the conclusion of the procedure to set the threads deep into the subcutaneous space and not allow the end of the thread to irritate the underside of the dermis.
- Overcorrect slightly at the time of surgery, anticipating a long-term relaxation of the amount of lift. The surgeon can always release some of the elevation achieved by the threads 2–4 weeks postoperatively with a simple procedure in the office.

144

Combined Modalities for the Correction of Asymmetric Brow Position

William P. Mack

The surgical correction of asymmetric brow position can prove to be a challenge for the cosmetic oculoplastic surgeon. The ideal surgical approach would result in an improvement of the asymmetric brow position through a minimal incision with an emphasis on limited recovery time for the patient.

The workup of the patient with asymmetric brow position should include any history of seventh cranial nerve paralysis, particularly if of recent origin, as further testing may be needed to determine any underlying pathology. If after complete testing, the diagnosis is Bell's palsy, then possibly delaying any surgical intervention to assess any potential improvement in the brow position should be considered. Preoperative examination should also include evaluation of any underlying unilateral ptosis on the ipsilateral side of the superiorly positioned brow. Chronic unilateral ptosis can result in an elevated brow position secondary to compensatory frontalis muscle contraction.

Many surgical approaches, including coronal, mid-forehead, direct, pretrichial, endoscopic, internal browpexy, and other transblepharoplasty techniques, can be utilized to achieve correction of brow ptosis. While many of these approaches have proven to be successful for correcting bilateral brow ptosis, results of the less invasive surgeries are not as predictable for the correction of asymmetric brow position. Recent advances in less invasive modalities with minimal incisions can now be incorporated into our surgical planning to achieve desirable results with decreased postoperative recovery time.

The described procedure is performed as an outpatient surgery under local anesthesia. Preoperatively, the patient is placed in a sitting position to assess the degree of brow asymmetry and also to document any underlying ptosis and/or dermatochalasis (Figure 144.1). The patient is then placed in the supine position and attention is directed to the inferiorly positioned brow where three small incisions are made a few millimeters posterior to the hairline. After limited undermining in the area of the incisions, two 2-0 polypropylene barbed sutures (Contour threads™) are inserted and directed in a sinusoidal pattern to exit just inferior to the brow. The two barbed sutures are then contoured to raise the brow to the desired height and contour. At that point, the two sutures are tied a few millimeters behind the hairline and two to three interrupted 6-0 plain gut sutures are used to close each skin incision.

Attention is then directed to the contralateral brow, where chemical denervation with Botox is performed to relax the frontalis muscle to lower the brow to the desired height and contour. Typically, the Botox treatment dosage to achieve this goal is in range of 4–8 units. Following correction of the brow position, attention is directed to the eyelid region, where blepharoplasty/ptosis repair is performed as necessary to achieve the desired cosmetic goals. In addition to the previously described brow technique, the patient in Figure 144.1 required bilateral upper eyelid blepharoplasty and left upper eyelid ptosis surgery to achieve maximum aesthetic results (Figure 144.2).

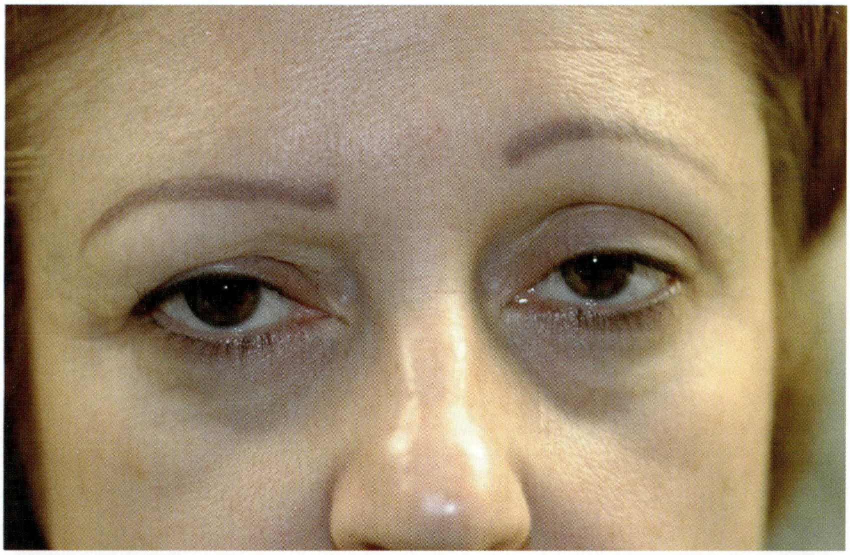

Figure 144.1. This 58-year-old patient is shown preoperative sitting position, with evidence of brow asymmetry, dermatochalasis, and ptosis.

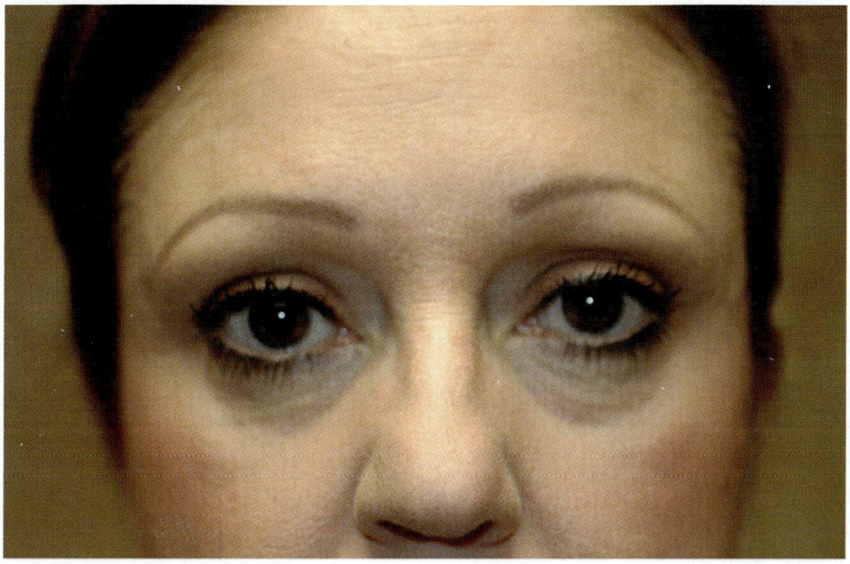

Figure 144.2. Postoperative result following right brow barbed suture lift, left brow Botox chemical denervation, bilateral blepharoplasty, and left upper eyelid ptosis repair.

Part XI

Other Cosmetic Procedures

145

Repair of the Torn Earlobe

Yoash R. Enzer

Ear piercing has been practiced since the time of ancient civilizations, not only to call attention to female beauty, but also to make statements about social status. More recently, popular cultural trends have resulted in an increased incidence of multiple ear piercing and male ear piercing. As a result, earlobe tears are an increasingly commonplace complaint among patients presenting to the cosmetic surgeon.

There are various classifications of earlobe tears. Partial tears refer to a vertical elongation of the earring hole and are sometimes referred to as "slit earlobes" (Figure 145.1). Complete tears of the earlobe are also referred to as "split earlobes," or "cleft earlobes" (Figure 145.2).

The mechanism for earlobe tears can be acute trauma (i.e., earring pulled through the earlobe). However, many patients report an indolent progressive elongation of the earring hole until it eventually becomes a complete tear. Conventional wisdom has it that this is due to wearing heavy earrings. Others have described earlobe necrosis due to clip-on earrings.[1,2] More recently Raveendran showed that many of these patients had chronic dermatitis and hypothesized an allergy to gold.[3]

Repair of earlobe tears may seem simple and straightforward. In fact, it requires great precision, much like closure of an eyelid margin or the lip vermillion. If one edge is off by a millimeter, it is obvious, and you will have a dissatisfied patient. Furthermore, this is made more complex by the fact that the patient will want to wear earrings again as soon as possible after the repair; this will place a constant mechanical load on the repair again and predispose to repeat tears (Figure 145.3).

Multiple techniques have been proposed for repair of the torn earlobe. Straight line closure after excision of the epithelial tract is the simplest method of repair.[1] However, one of the main concerns is the significant risk of recurrent hole elongation or complete tears.[3] For this reason, others have proposed elaborate flaps such as L-plasty, Z-plasty, or inverted V-plasties.[4–6] Some authors have advocated preservation of the original ear piercing hole or immediate repiercing at the time of repair.[4,5] Some have suggested converting partial tears into complete clefts.[4]

Questions to Ask the Patient

1. Was there a traumatic event that led to the earlobe tear?
2. Did you wear heavy or dangling earrings?
3. What was the metal composition of your earrings?
4. Do you have any skin sensitivities to other jewelry?
5. Was there any history of chronic earlobe inflammation or discharge?
6. Have you ever had the earlobe repaired in the past?
7. Are you planning to wear pierced earrings again? Can you go without them for 3–4 months?

Basic Principles

1. **Remove the entire epithelial lining of the piercing tract and earlobe tear.** Unless the patient has a clear history of trauma or very heavy earrings to cause the tear, these individuals are predisposed to this problem, and therefore the entire tract and original hole should be closed to minimize the chance of recurrence.

2. **If more than 75% of the distance between the earlobe piercing hole and the inferior edge is slit, convert the partial tear into a complete tear.** This will optimize the final cosmetic result.

3. **Use one or more Z-plasties along the vertical axis of the complete tear.** These flaps will accomplish two important tasks: first, they will lay down a series of zigzagging scar tissue thereby lending strength to the repair; second, a Z-plasty will provide vertical elongation, which is important to prevent the appearance of an indentation at the earlobe margin afterwards (due to scar contracture).

4. **When faced with a complete tear, draw a line along the center of the earlobe margin on both sides before infiltrating with local anesthetic, and always close the earlobe margin first.** This will give the proper three dimensional alignment and make it easy to close the remainder of the tear.

5. **Close the earlobe margin with overcorrected everting sutures.** This will allow the margin to end up flat after healing is complete.

6. **Do not pierce earlobe again for at least 3 months.**

Surgical Technique for Complete Earlobe Tears

1. Draw a line along the center of the earlobe margin on both sides of the tear before infiltrating with local anesthetic.

2. Mark along the inside of the tear where the incision is to be made (inverted V).

3. Infiltrate the entire earlobe with 1% xylocaine with 1:100,000 epinephrine. I add 200 units of hyaluronidase to a 50 cc bottle of the anesthetic in order to enhance the spread of the anesthetic solution and minimize the distortion of the tissues.

4. Cleanse the entire earlobe area with Betadine solution and place sterile drapes around the field.

5. Make an incision along the center of the inverted "V" tear on both sides to split the tear into anterior and posterior flaps. Although one can use a #15 blade, I think it is easier to perform the incision with the fine tip of the Ellman radiofrequency cautery unit. *Note: Although some authors suggest using a dermal punch to remove the epithelium lining the tear, I do not find this practical or helpful.*

6. Using curved blunt Stevens scissors, spread in the plane between the two flaps to mobilize the tissues. Remove any subcutaneous fibrosis that is binding down the edges of the incisions. Alternatively, these tissue edges can also be resected. *Note: some authors advocate using a chalazion clamp or cutting on a tongue blade to get better control of the floppy earlobe. This may be helpful in some patients.*

7. Square off the margin edges with a #15 blade on both sides to insure there is no notch postoperatively. This may be a time when cutting on a sterile tongue blade is helpful.

8. Close the earlobe margin first. This is a similar concept to closure of an eyelid or vermillion laceration in order to get accurate three-dimensional alignment. Using the previously marked center of the margin as a guide, place a 5-0 absorbable suture such a chromic gut or polyglactin 910 subcutaneously with the knot superior. Then place 6-0 fast absorbing gut or polypropylene vertical mattress sutures medially, centrally, and laterally to get good wound eversion.

9. Make Z-plasty incisions if the length of the tear is adequate. These can either be full thickness, or the Z-plasty on the lateral flap can be the mirror image of the Z-plasty on the medial flap. Make the incisions over the tongue blade to stabilize the earlobe. Your assistant can stabilize the earlobe inferiorly with a skin hook, but take care not to place any traction in order to avoid wound distortion. Transpose the flaps and suture closed (lateral flap first) with 5-0 polyglactin 910 subcutaneous sutures and 5-0 fast-absorbing gut or 6-0 polypropylene sutures through the skin edges in standard fashion. *Note: The Z-plasty closure will provide vertical elongation to the earlobe so as to prevent notching at the margin after scar contracture. This will also makes the scar less obvious and decrease the likelihood of recurrent tears.*

10. Clean the area, and dress with Bacitracin ointment. Have the patient keep the incisions moist with the ointment for 5–7 days until they return for suture removal.

11. Tell the patient to return for a check of the wound in 3–4 months. If it is well healed and the incision is soft, consideration can then be given to repeat piercing at that time. If possible, place the new piercing anterior or posterior to the original hole.

Surgical Repair for Partial Torn Earlobes

1. For partial tears greater than 75% of the distance between the piercing hole and the earlobe margin, convert to a complete tear and follow instructions above.

2. For partial tears less than 60–70% of the distance between the piercing hole and the earlobe margin follow only Steps 2–6 as noted above. Because the tear is partial, the earlobe margin is intact and will provide proper three dimensional alignment for the repair. For tears in between 60 and 75%, the surgeon will have to use his or her judgment.

3. If the partial tear is small, it can be closed with a straight line in three layers: close the subcutaneous layer with buried 5-0 polyglactin 910 sutures; close the lateral flap with vertical mattress 6-0 fast-absorbing gut or polypropylene interrupted sutures; and finally, close the medial flap with interrupted sutures of the same material.

4. If the partial tear is larger, close with a broken line or W-plasty. Remove two triangles from the anterior edge, and make mirror image incisions on the posterior edge. Close with a circlage of subcutaneous 6-0 polyglactin 910 sutures through the apices of the flaps, and then interrupted 5-0 fast-absorbing gut or 6-0 polypropylene sutures through the skin edges in standard fashion. *Note: If the earlobe is thick, the W-plasty only needs to be done for the lateral flap, and the medial flap can be closed with 5-0 or 6-0 polyglactin 910 sutures subcutaneously, and 5-0 fast-absorbing gut or 6-0 polypropylene sutures through the skin.*

5. Follow Steps 10 and 11 as noted above.

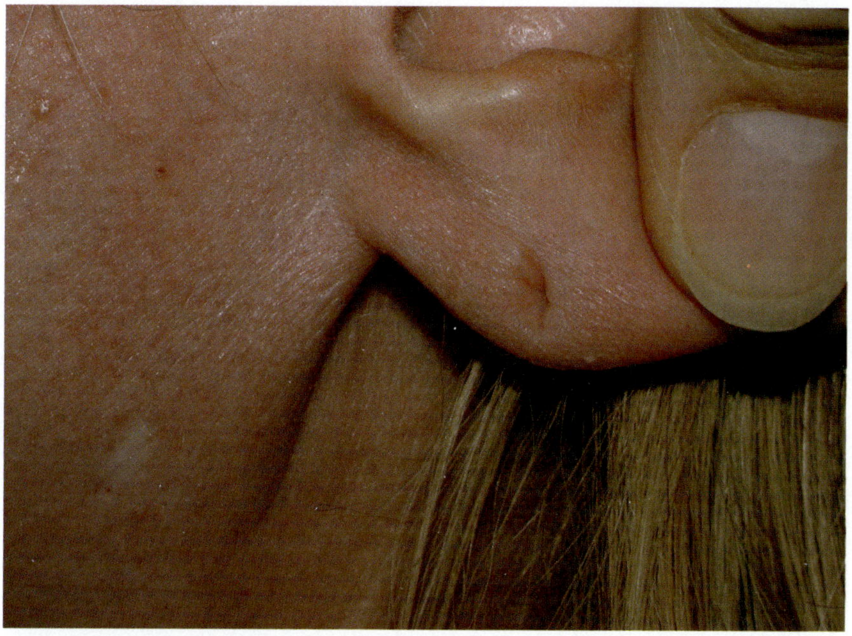

Figure 145.1. Partial earlobe tear, approximately 75% of the distance between the piercing hole and the earlobe margin.

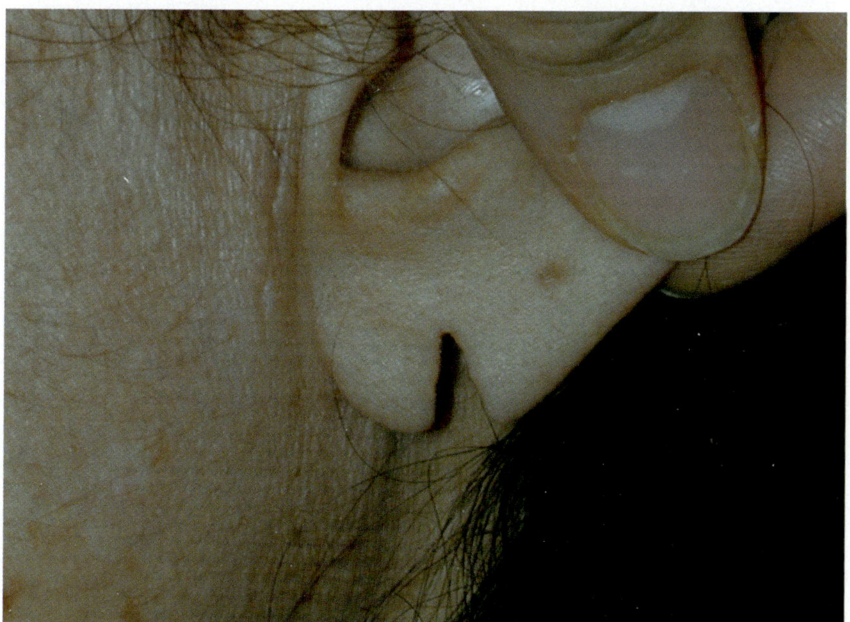

Figure 145.2. Complete earlobe tear.

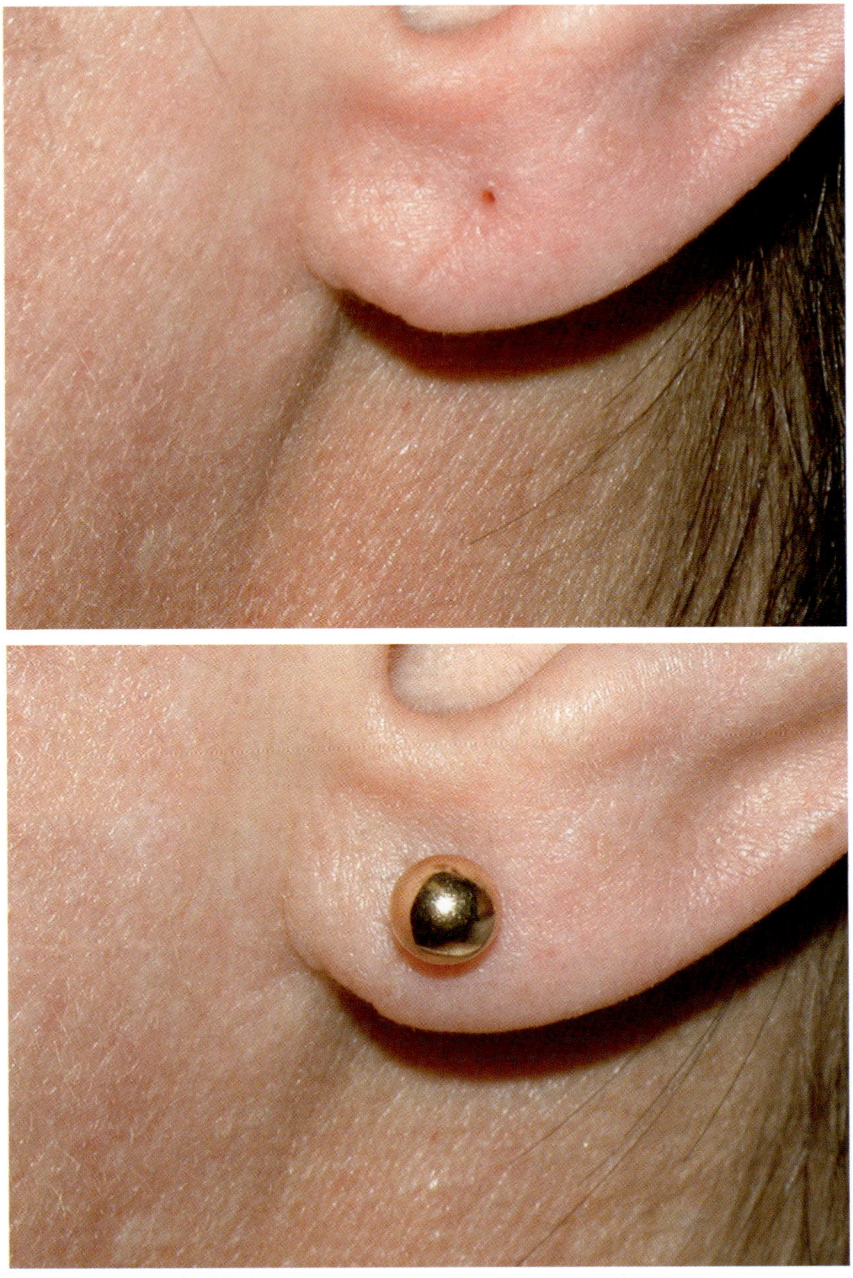

A

B

Figure 145.3. Successful repair of complete torn earlobe. Note the naturally smooth earlobe margin.

References

1. McLaren LR. Cleft ear lobes: A hazard of wearing earrings. Br J Plast Surg 1954;7:162.
2. Wallace AF, Garretts M. A case of necrosis of the ear lobes. Br J Plast Surg 1960;13:64.
3. Raveendran S, Amarasinghe L. The mystery of the split earlobe. Plast Reconstr Surg 2004;114:1903–1909.
4. Boo-Chai K. The cleft earlobe. Plast Reconstr Surg 1961;28:681–688.
5. Niamtu J. Eleven pearls for cosmetic earlobe repair. Dermatol Surg 2002; 28:180–185.

146

Upper Lip Lift as a Complementary Technique in Facial Rejuvenation

Oscar M. Ramirez and Camilo O. Reyes

Introduction

The lip lift is a relatively easy and controlled surgical procedure that has a long-term effect and may be modified to each patient's facial anatomy and aesthetic goals. The descent and enlargement of the upper lip depend on the gravitational effect, weakness of collagen bundles and elastic fibers in the skin, and diminution of bone structure. In order to achieve a better result the lift lip can be combined with others complementary procedures such as a fat injection to obtain fullness and give the vermillion eversion and rolled dermis graft under the philtrum columns for height enhancement and illusion of narrowing. This procedure may be performed under local anesthesia or as a part of full face lift.

Preoperative Markings

The preoperative markings are drawn before the injection of local anesthetic (Figure 146.1). We mark the important landmarks of the upper lip, which include the border of the lip, the philtrum columns and the midline. Based on those references, we mark the planned area of incision, which includes a curved linear incision from the implantation of the ala, close to the nasolabial fold going around the ala, continuing inside the nostril sill and the base of the columella. Symmetric marking of more or less the same length and shape is done on the contralateral side. Another symmetric marking of more or less the same length is done inferiorly into the upper lip. The lower incision marking is drawn to allow the maximal lateral elevation of the lip. This can be modified for a more central elevation depending of the patient's desires and surgeon's aesthetic goals.

Technique

The surgery is performed under local infiltration of 1% xylocaine with 1:100,000 epinephrine solution. About 5 cc of this is injected in the entire area. Using the #67 beaver blade, we proceed with excising the segment between the intervening lines down to the orbicularis oris muscle (Figure

146.2). The muscle is respected and kept intact. To avoid bunching up the tissues and allow eversion of the vermillion border, we proceed with undermining the skin off the orbicularis oris muscle for about 3 mm inferiorly. This also allows the eversion of the skin borders at the suture line. Hemostasis is done with bipolar cautery. To allow better reshaping of the cupid's bow, we proceed with undermining with a blunt micro cannula the philtrum columns on the right and on the left. This produces an elevating effect of these structures. Fragments of dermis/fat graft are obtained from the undersurface of resected skin and introduced in the tunnels beneath the philtrum columns. We then proceed with closing the incision upon the advancement of the upper lip in two layers with 7-0 interrupted Prolene sutures for the deep subdermal layer and 6-0 Prolene sutures for the skin. We strongly recommend closing the opening of tunnels in order to keep in place the dermal grafts. The suture line is dressed with mastisol and micropore sterile tapes.

As a complementary procedure, if vermillion eversion and fullness is needed, micro fat injection can be done at the same time using "cell friendly" Ramirez micro cannula (Tulip Biomedical Company, San Diego CA).* An average of 4 cc of fat is injected into the upper lip. For aesthetic balancing fat can also be injected into the lower lip (6 cc as an average).

Discussion

We aim to have at least 3 mm of tooth show at rest. The exact amount resected will depend upon the vertical height of the maxilla and the length of the lip. Those that have a longer upper lip in youth and those that lose more maxillary vertical height with aging will need a larger amount of resection.

We have received requests using dermal graft taken from the same skin resected to increase the height of philtrum columns. It is important during the undermining of the tunnels to keep in mind always to do it in a conservative way, because the sockets must be fit to avoid the displacement of the dermal grafts. These tunnels must be closed in an independent way with a nonabsorbable suture, such as 6-0 or 7-0 prolene.

For augmentation of the lip volume, we prefer autologous tissue as opposed to alloplastic materials. Small amounts of fat are injected in the inner side of vermillion through puncture wounds in the corners of the mouth using the described micro cannula. If the fat graft is partially reabsorbed in the next few months, more fat can be reinjected later.

Conclusion

The lip lift provides an effective tool for correcting a natural tendency of the upper lip to cover the upper teeth during aging (Figures 146.3–146.6). There is a dramatic improvement in the patient's facial aesthetic appearance during the smiling and at rest. We strongly recommend this technique as a part of surgical armamentarium to achieve a youthful face.

---

* Dr. Ramirez is an Unpaid member of the Medical Advisory Board of Tulip Biomedical. He does not receive any royalties for these canulas.

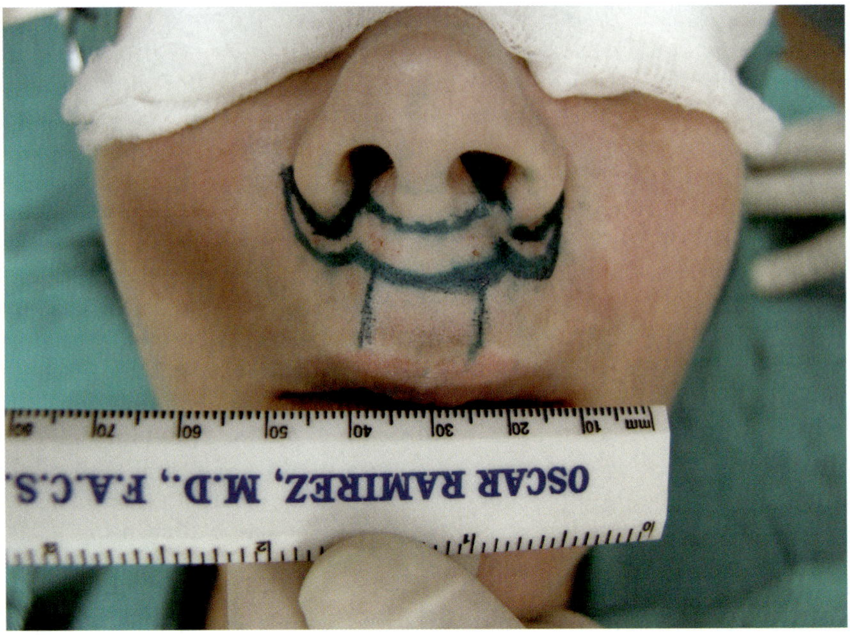

Figure 146.1. The shape of the resected skin resembles the horns of a bull. The width of the strip is about 5 mm as its narrowest and about 8 mm at its widest.

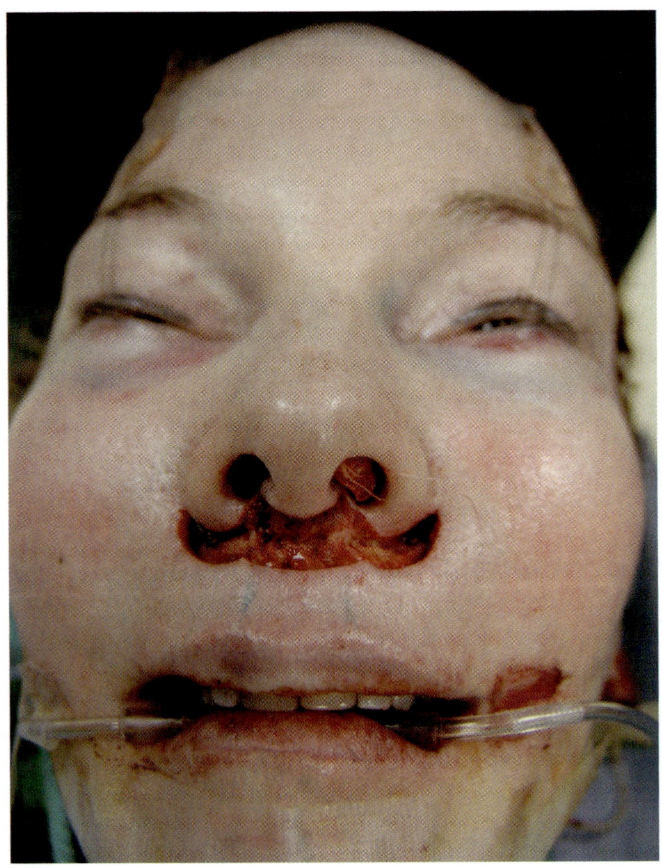

Figure 146.2. Front view in the same patient. Notice the strip of skin resected Observe that excision extents into the nostrils.

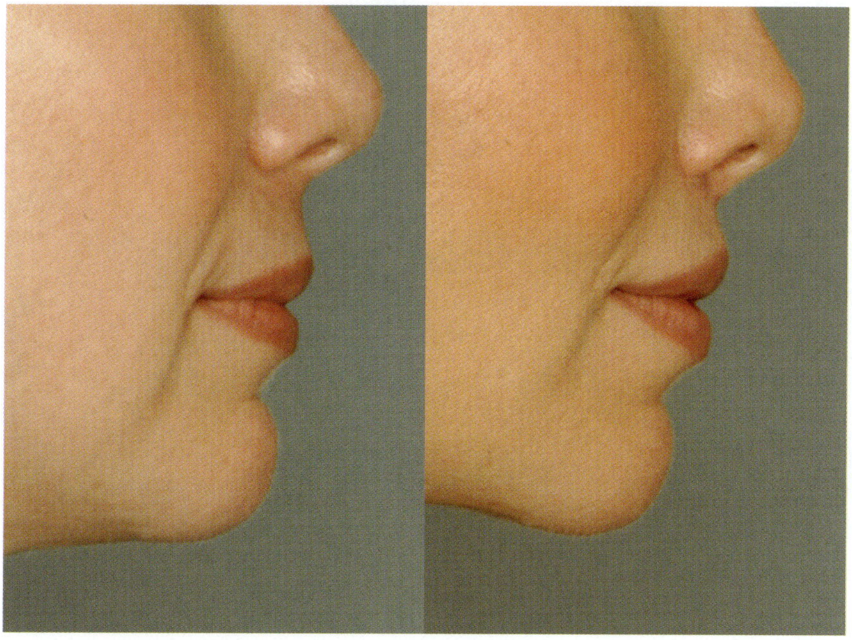

Figure 146.3. Lateral view of the same patient. Notice the fullness and eversion of the vermillion. She has a more youthful appearance.

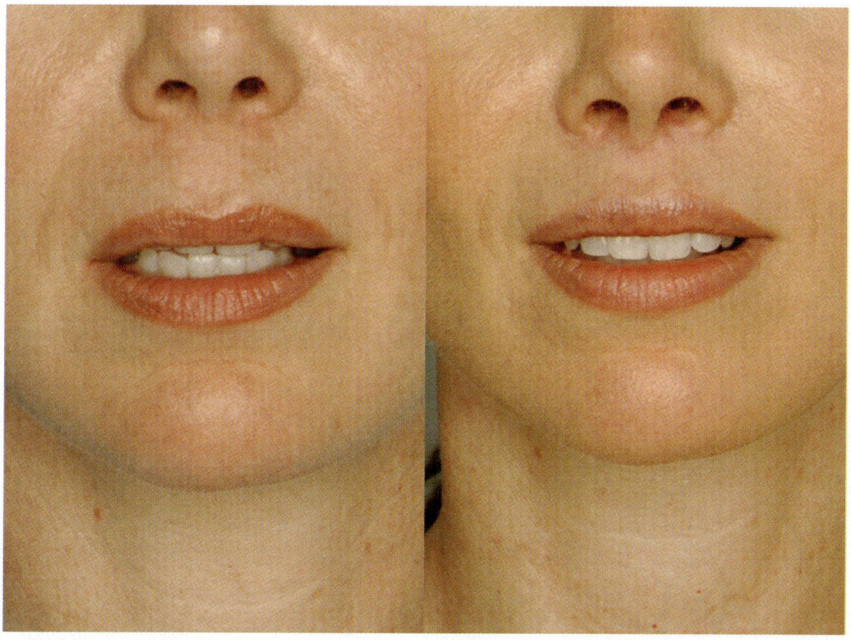

Figure 146.4. Frontal view. Observe the increase in the upper teeth showing at rest.

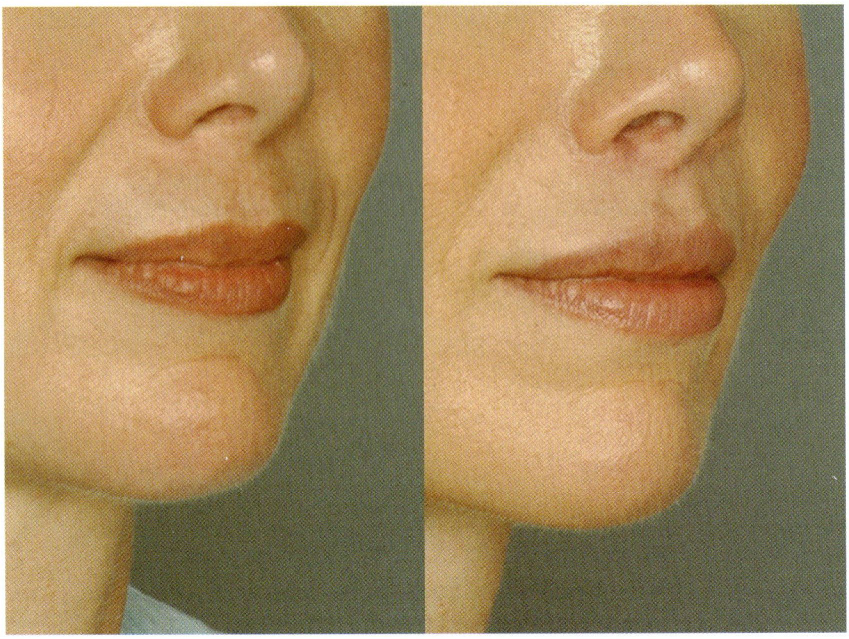

Figure 146.5. Three-quarter views: notice the decrease in the vertical height in the upper lip. Also notice the definition and outline of the philtrum columns.

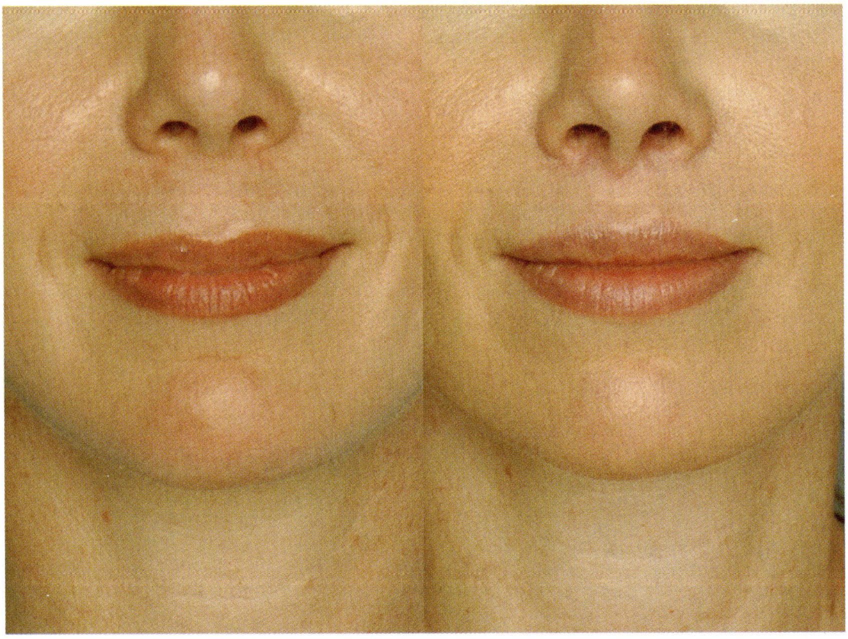

Figure 146.6. Frontal view: observe the shortening of the skin of the upper lip and the definition of the philtrum. The scar is barely noticeable.

Reference

Ramirez OM. The upper lip lift using the "bull's horn" approach. J Drugs Dermatol 2003;3:305–308.

147

SMAS Malar Fat Pad Lift with Short Scar Face Lift

Paul S. Nassif and Guy G. Massry

The malar fat pad lies superficial to the SMAS and the lip elevator muscles. It has a cheek and jowl portion. The buccal-maxillary retaining ligament courses through the fat pad. With age, there is anterio-inferior gravitational descent along with fat volume loss. Skeletal resorption of anterior facial skeleton also contributes to descent. Finally, loss of the retaining ligament occurs (zygomatic and buccal-maxillary support contribute to descent).

Aging of the malar fat pad and midface fat can cause a deep nasolabial groove, a heavy nasolabial fold, cheek folds, skeletonized appearance of the cheekbone, and a submalar hollow. Other effects of aging include a sad mouth, commissural lines, jowls (midfacial descent settles behind the mandibular retaining ligaments), marionette lines (labiomandibular groove), and lower cheek lines.

The principles of the SMAS malar fat pad lift (SMFPL) are that it elevates the malar fat pad to a more youthful position, elevates the anterior superficial SMAS, effaces the nasolabial folds, corrects the sad mouth, softens commissural marionette and lower cheek lines, and elevates the jowls. The anatomic basis of the SMFPL is the fact that the malar fat pad is adherent to the SMAS, which invests the lip elevators (zygomatricus major and minor), the zygomatic retaining ligaments (McGregor's patch is divided, and the buccal-maxillary ligaments are partially divided.)

Marking for the SMFPL is as follows: From the tragus to the inferior border of the zygomatic arch/zygoma (6 cm), from the tragus to the lateral commissure (7–8 cm), anterior to the mandible angle, from the tragus to the anterior border of the sternocleidomastoid (6 cm), and a postauricular short scar (Figures 147.01–3).

The anterior superficial SMAS and superior posterior malar fat pad is plicated in a vertical vector. With the SMAS elevation, the zygomaticus major and minor are elevated. With division of the retaining ligaments, the cheek skin flap and malar fat pad elevate easier. It is important to preserve the fat on the skin flap posterior to the malar fat pad. The fat on the skin flap at the malar fat pad should be minimal so that the malar fat pad is elevated with the SMAS.

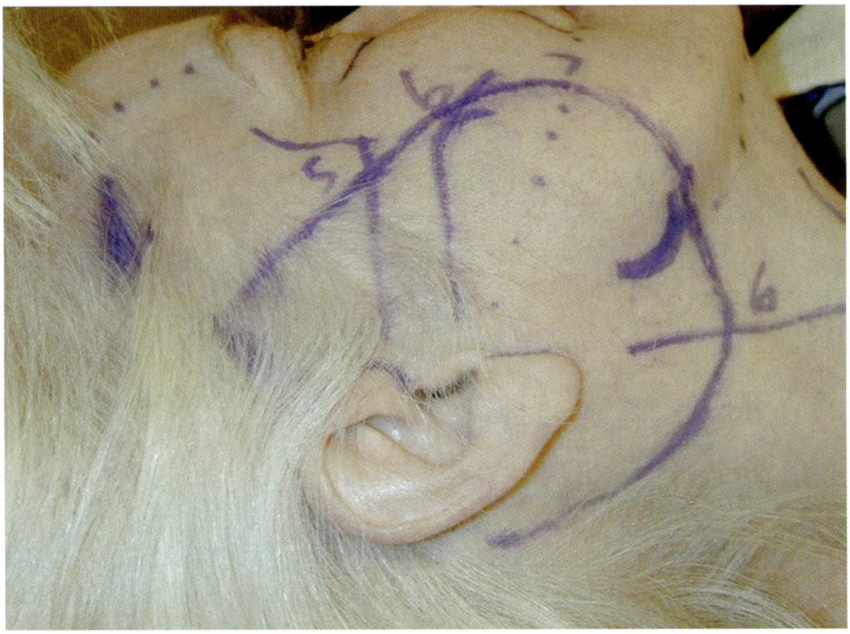

Figure 147.1. SMFPL markings

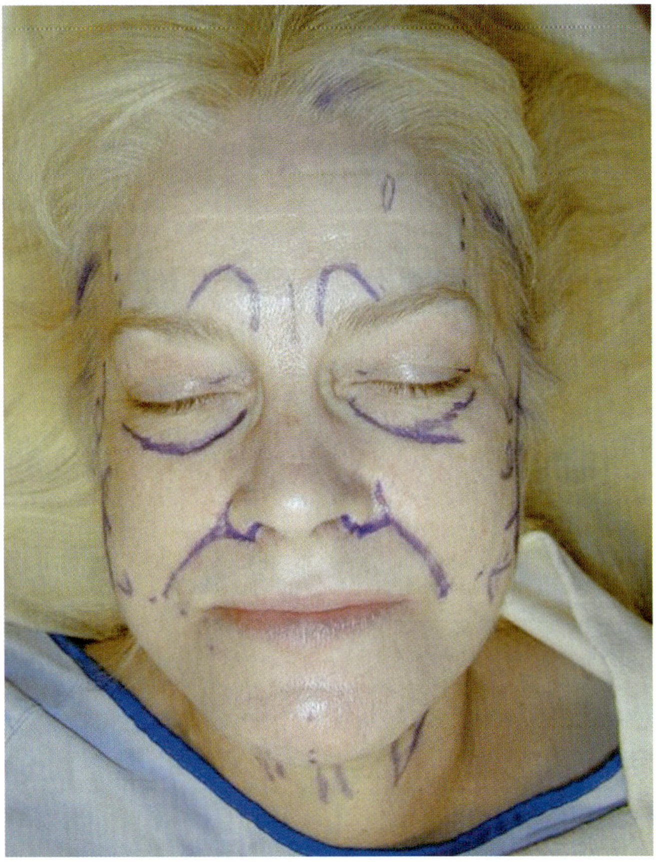

Figure 147.2. SMAS into nasolabial fold markings

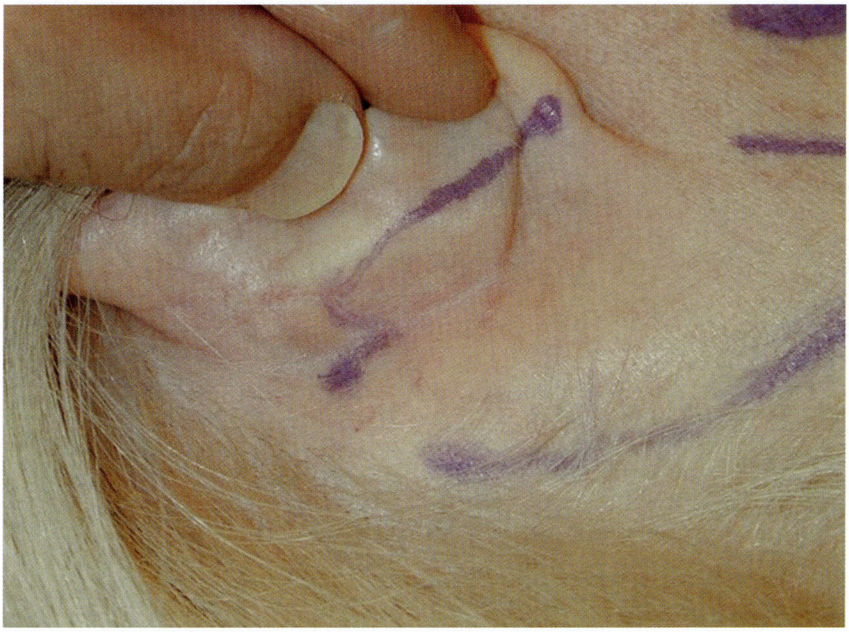

Figure 147.3. Short scar post-auricular markings

148

Ten Tips for a Reliable and Predictable Deep Plane Facial Rhytidectomy

David E.E. Holck, Jill A. Foster, Kevin A. Kalwerisky, and O. Bailey Robertson

Introduction

Facial rhytidectomy surgery is a reconstructive/cosmetic procedure to restore anatomic changes to the lower third of the aging face and neck. It is a surgery of planes. Understanding safe dissection planes allows the surgeon to maximize his or her results in a reliable fashion.[1,2] Facial rhytidectomy may also be considered a surgery of opportunity and compromise in which soft tissue dissection and redraping take advantage of the facial blood supply while predictable and desirable wound healing provide the rejuvenated appearance. Mastery of facial anatomy and the relationships of the superficial and deep facial layers, muscles, nerves, and vasculature are of paramount importance in performing rhytidectomy surgery safely, effectively, and with confidence.[3,4] We have noted 10 areas in which attention to detail offers a predictable and reliable rhytidectomy procedure and avoids some of the stigmata of rhytidectomy surgery.[5]

Tip 1. Marking (Figure 148.1)

Marking the skin under slight anterior traction decreases the risk of medial incision migration. The markings should be optimally camouflaged in the hairlines to avoid visible incisions. Placing a back-cut at the inferior border of the temporal hair tuft minimizes the risk of posterior temporal hair migration. Further inferiorly, the incisions may be placed posttragal in women and pretragal (to avoid mobilizing hair bearing skin on the tragus) in men (though we find both incisions heal well). Additionally, the retroauricular incision is placed onto the conchal bowl to avoid postoperative migration onto visible retroauricular area. The marking is carried into the hair-bearing scalp at an angle bisecting the posterior hairline and its tangent. We also gently score the markings with an 18-gauge needle tip to avoid erasure or distortion of the markings during infiltrative anesthesia or skin cleansing. The inferior lobule and the posterior hairline, which are useful landmarks for skin flap redraping later in the surgery, are also scored.

Tip 2. Skin Flap Dissection (Figure 148.2)

Tumescent anesthesia allows inflation of the subcutaneous layer and allows safer flap dissection. This also permits performance of rhytidectomy surgery under local anesthesia. Creation of the skin flap using a gentle spreading motion (gentle pushing of hand-locked scissors) with sparing cutting motion allows a safer dissection plane. We also utilize the mechanical advantage offered by the skin flap by keeping the skin on the conchal cartilage and mastoid attached until the posterior auricular dissection is complete. This acts as a second pair of hands holding gentle tension on the flap. The same may be done anteriorly with the preauricular skin. With an assistant applying gentle anterior/inferior traction on the facial soft tissue, the dissection is continued inferiorly over difficult dissection areas, including the mastoid and sternocleidomastoid muscle. Transillumination through the skin flap allows precise determination of flap thickness, keeping a cobblestone pattern of fat on its undersurface. Anteriorly, the dissection proceeds to the zygomatic osseocutneous ligament (McGregor's patch) and mandibular osseocutaneous ligament.

Tip 3. Marking the Zygomatic Arch (Figure 148.3)

To avoid injury to the temporal branch of the facial nerve, the inferior border of the zygomatic arch is indicated with a marking pen. This allows situational awareness throughout the surgery. The inferior border may easily be palpable at the level of the superior aspect of the external auditory canal. Medially the notch in the body of the zygoma is also marked, indicating the origin of the zygomaticus major muscle. This will be useful to identify the origin and remain superficial to this muscle as the superficial musculoaponeurotic (SMAS) flap dissection proceeds medially.

Tip 4. SMAS Flap Creation (Figure 148.4)

We mark a "J-shaped" 1-cm strip of SMAS from the angle of the mandible to the inferior border of the zygomatic arch at the anterior portion of the parotid to start our dissection. This allows a relatively safe position to start the SMAS flap and allows a fixed cuff of SMAS anterior to the tragal cartilage for suturing the mobilized SMAS flap. While excising the strip of SMAS, the surgeon stays superficial to the parotid capsule.

Tip 5. Creating the SMAS Flap (Figure 148.5 and 148.6)

Care must be taken in dissecting the SMAS flap to avoid creating a tenuous or button-holed flap. The flap is developed using scissors in a horizontal spreading motion with judicious cutting. A No. 10 blade may be used in a push down technique to further develop the flap. A Peanut may also be used for more blunt dissection more medially. Using countertraction and a headlight, the SMAS flap with platysmal fibers above is developed, with the masseteric fascia below. Branches of the facial nerve are easily seen on the surface of the masseter muscle covered by loose areolar masseteric fascia. The dissection is continued near but not crossing the inferior border of the mandible to the mandibular osseocutaneous ligament to avoid trauma to the marginal mandibular branch of the facial nerve. Superiorly, the previously marked notch on the body of the zygoma allows a dissection point to find the superficial surface of the zygomaticus major. Care is taken to avoid aggressive dissection under the zygomaticus major muscle to avoid trauma to the zygomatic and buccal branches of the facial nerve. Once the superficial surface of the zygomaticus major muscle is identified, the dissection plane is connected to the inferior sub-SMAS dissection. The flap is then dissected medially to the nasolabial fold, the cheek fat pad, and modioulus. It is critical to maintain a well developed SMAS flap to mobilize the lower face soft tissues.

Tip 6. SMAS Flap Fixation (Figure 148.7)

The optimal vector of pull for the SMAS flap is vertical. This optimizes the rejuvenative appearance without creating the "wind-blown" facelift look of lateral mobilization. The SMAS flap at the angle of the mandible is advanced superiorly to the tuft of SMAS adjacent to the inferior tragus. The SMAS flap at the angle of the mouth is advanced to the superior tragus. The inferior platysmal flap at the neck is advanced in a superolateral vector and fixed to the mastoid fascia. All sutures are placed with the knots buried in a "vest over pants" fashion. This vertical elevation creates a triangular overlap of SMAS above the zygomatic arch. This excess SMAS flap is excised and the remnant sutured to the SMAS attached to the inferior edge of the zygomatic arch. This elevates the malar fat pad.

Tip 7. Skin Flap Fixation (Figure 148.8)

After elevation of the SMAS flap, the excess skin drapes superiorly and laterally. The excess skin is trimmed and is attached at three key fixation points: the superior conchal cartilage and the posterior hairline (in the retroauricular area) and the temporal tuft anteriorly. The previously scored inferior lobular skin is advanced superoposteriorly and sutured to the superior most portion of the posterior conchal cartilage. The posterior hairline is reapproximated along the previously placed score and overlapped as needed. The skin along the hairline is back-cut to maintain the natural hairline and avoid a step-off. The anterior hairline is overlapped at the temporal back-cut and excess overlap is excised. Undermining of the temporal tuft may be necessary to avoid dog-ear deformities in this area.

Tip 8. Addressing the Earlobe (Figure 148.9)

Once the key fixation points of the facial skin flap are fixed, excess skin covering the earlobe remains. The inferior lobule of the earlobe is marked through the skin covering it. The skin overlying the outer curve of the helix is cut approximately two-thirds the distance to the inferior lobular mark. The inferior lobule is pulled out over the skin and its position evaluated. The skin flap should be slightly "bunched" up against the inferior lobule (if excessive bunching is present a few more millimeters may be cut and the inferior lobule reevaluated). This avoids inferior scar migration and the pixy-ear deformity. The inferior lobule and bunched skin is closed with a mattress suture.

Tip 9. Skin Excision Tips (Figure 148.10)

The retroauricular skin is evaluated for overlap and excess skin is backcut and excised with care taken to maintain the posterior hairline. We advocate minimal excision of posterior hair-bearing scalp. Maintaining the posterior hairline and elevation of the inferior lobular skin superoposteriorly to the superior conchal cartilage may lead to pleating of the retroauricular skin. This relative skin excess often smoothes out in the early postoperative period, but may be secondarily removed with an elliptical excision if it does not smooth out. The skin over the conchal cartilage is conservatively trimmed in the retroauricular area. The remaining skin overlying the pretragal portion of the ear is back-cut with care taken to follow the curvature of the cartilage. Conservative undermining of some subcutaneous fat may be indicated to avoid a too thick pretragal flap. Hair-bearing incisions are closed with 35R staples, and the skin is closed with a running 5–0 suture. Prior to wound closure, the contralateral side is trimmed. This allows a "second look" at both sides prior to closure to cauterize any small bleeders and place drains to avoid postoperative hematoma formation.

Tip 10. Addressing the Neck (Figure 148.11)

We frequently perform neck liposuction at the end of the surgical procedure, as early aggressive liposuction may result in unexpected skeletonization of the inferior border of the mandible after aggressive vertical SMAS repositioning. After neck tumescence, a 1-cm submental incision allows insertion of 3- and 4-mm single port cannulas. The cannulas connect the neck dissection to the facial flaps. As needed, midline platysmal plication is accomplished after liposuction. Alternatively, direct subcutaneous fat dissection from the platysma may be accomplished from the temporal facial flap and the submental incision prior to closure. Postsurgical dressing is accomplished using multiple layers of gentle compression. An ABD dressing works well and may be removed in 24 hours.

As our individual techniques in rhytidectomy surgery have evolved, we have found that respecting these fundamental tenants has allowed reliable and predictable results in our patient population (Figures 148.12 and 148.13). Certainly there are multiple other steps critical in the rhytidectomy procedure, and each surgeon needs to become aware of his or her own technique to provide predictable, optimal results for their patients.

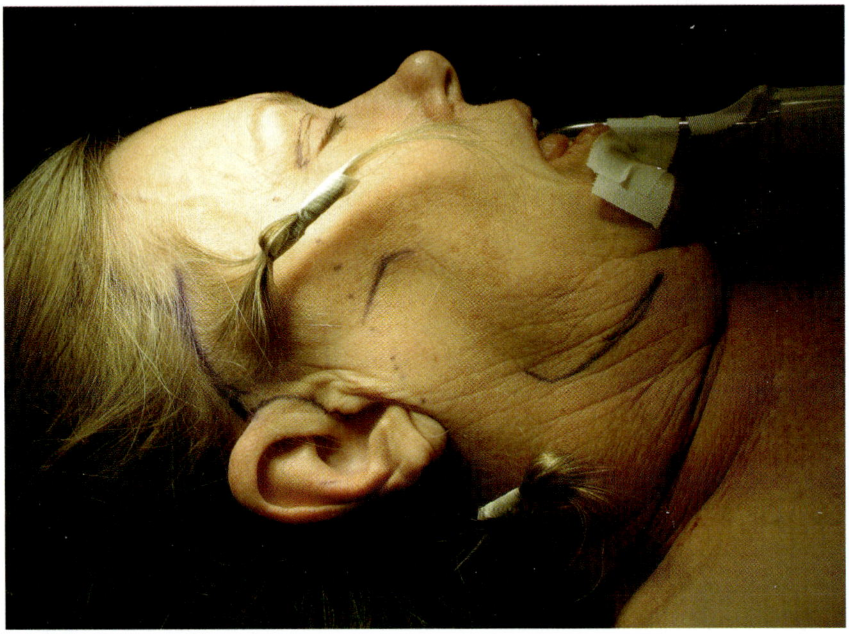

Figure 148.1. Marking the rhytidectomy patient. In addition to the incisional markings, labeling the inferior border of the zygomatic arch, the angle and inferior border of the mandible is useful to maintain situational awareness during skin flap creation.

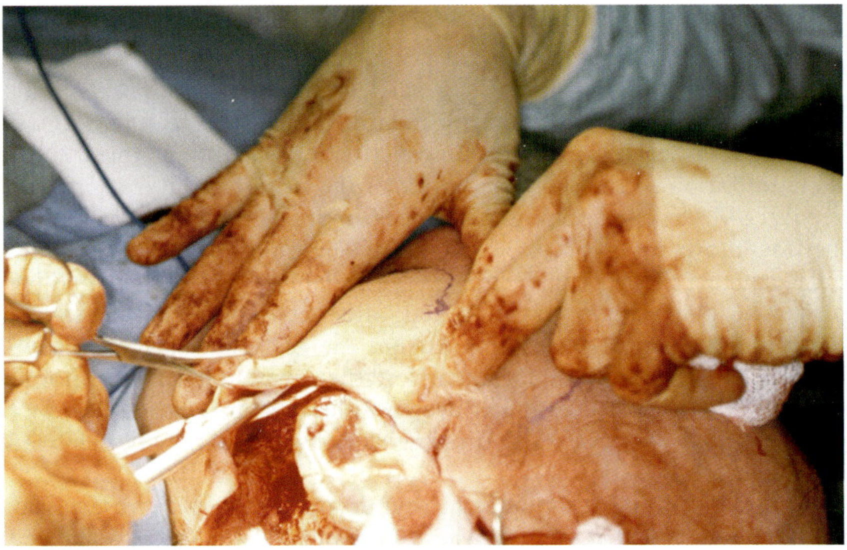

Figure 148.2. Countertraction and tumescence facilitates creation of the skin flap.

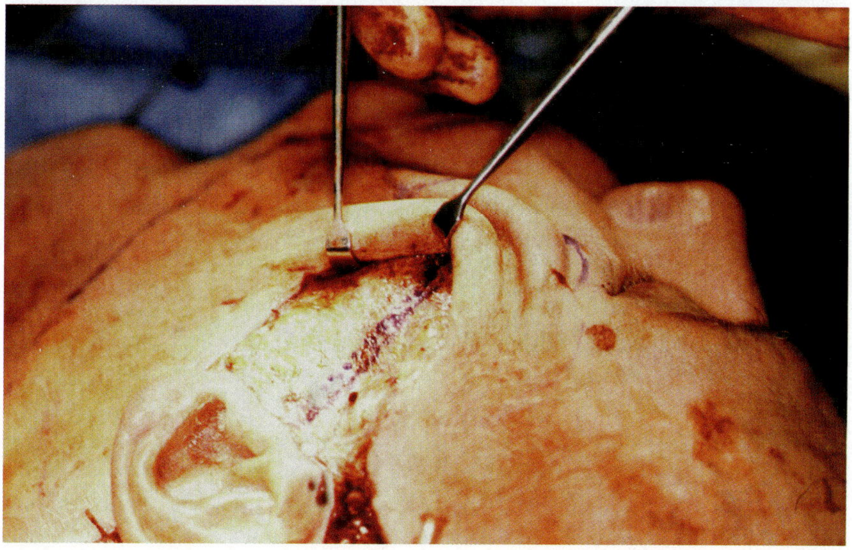

Figure 148.3. Marking the inferior border of the zygoma is critical for maintaining operative situational awareness and prevents inadvertent injury to the temporal branch of the facial nerve.

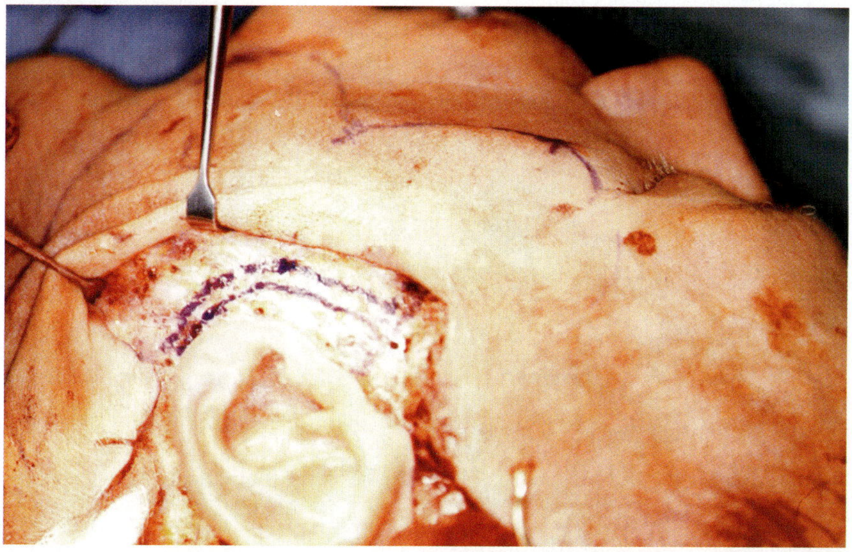

Figure 148.4. Excising a J-shaped piece of SMAS at the anterior border of the parotid allows safe entry into the deep plane while leaving a tuft of SMAS adjacent to the tragus to fixate the SMAS flap.

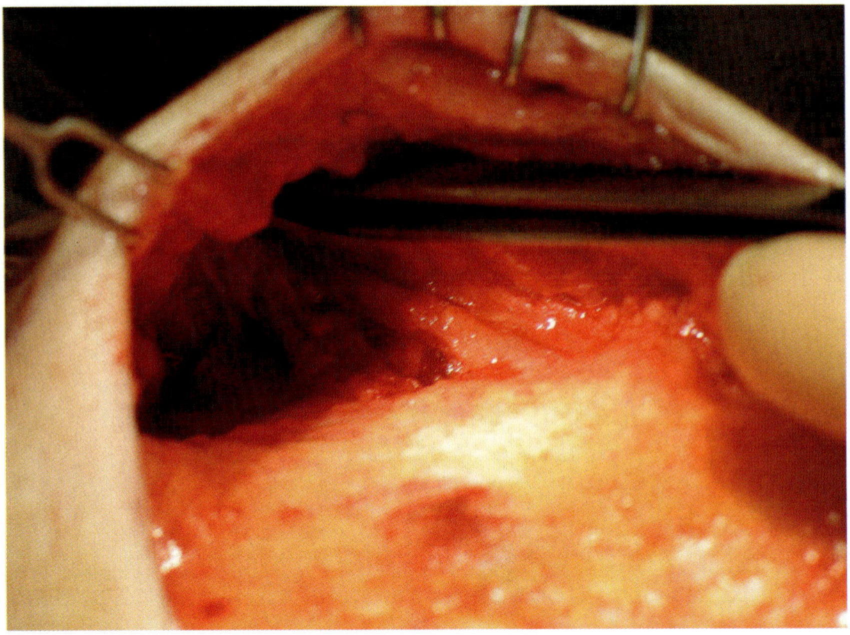

Figure 148.5. The SMAS flap is developed superiorly over the body of the zygoma to expose the zygomaticus major muscle (arrow demonstrates zygomaticus major on the left facial dissection). SMAS flap dissection should avoid dissecting beneath the zygomaticus to avoid trauma to the zygomatic and buccal branches of the facial nerve. Once dissected, the SMAS flap is connected to the inferior flap and continued medially to the nasolabial and melolabial folds.

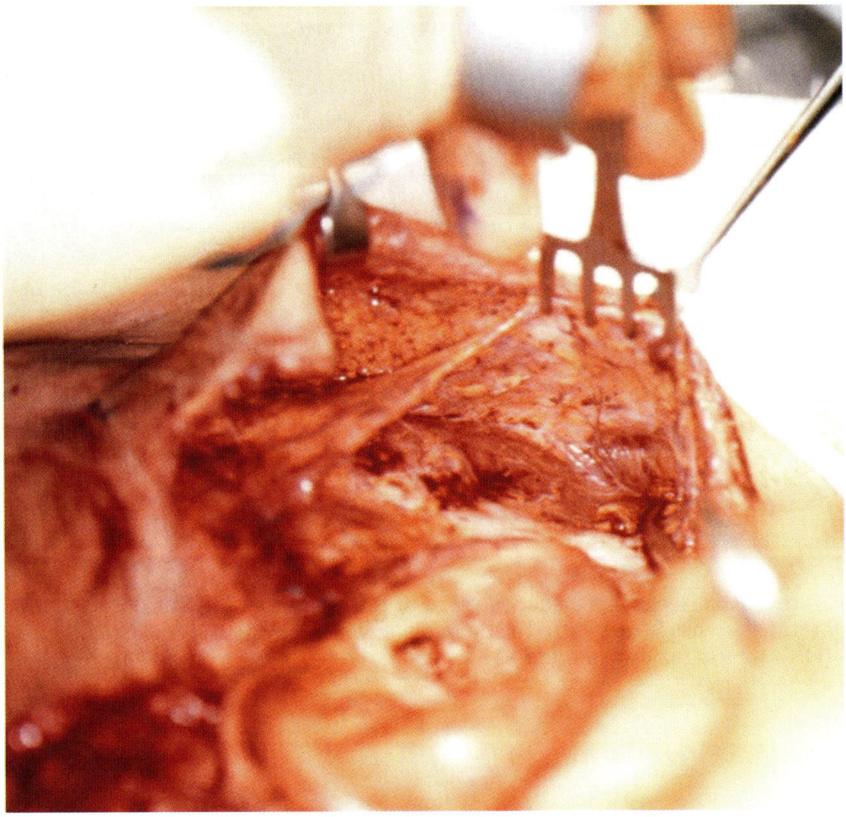

Figure 148.6. After dissection of the deep plane, the SMAS flap is easily mobilized for redraping and fixation.

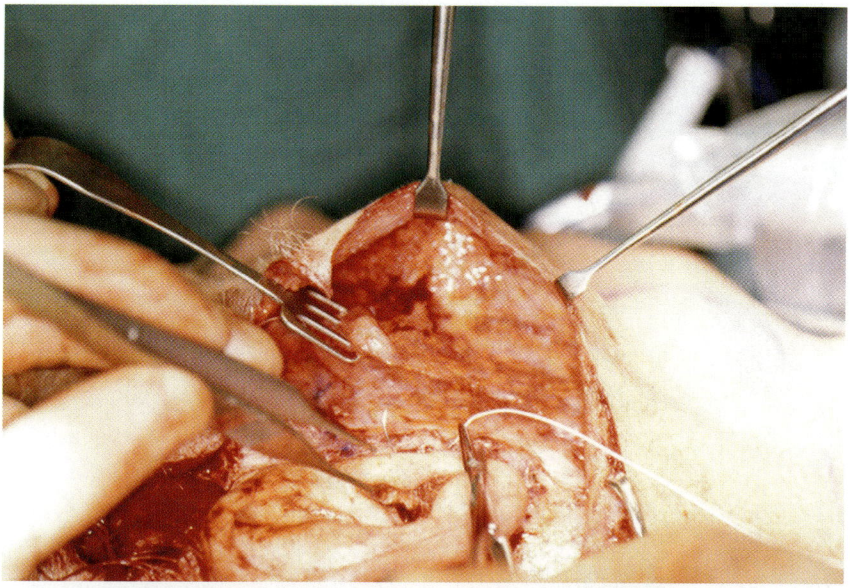

Figure 148.7. The correct vector for SMAS repositioning is vertical as the retractor is demonstrating. Fixing the SMAS flap from the angle of the mandible to the fascia at the inferior tragal border and from the angle of the mouth to the superior tragal border offers the desired vertical soft tissue redraping.

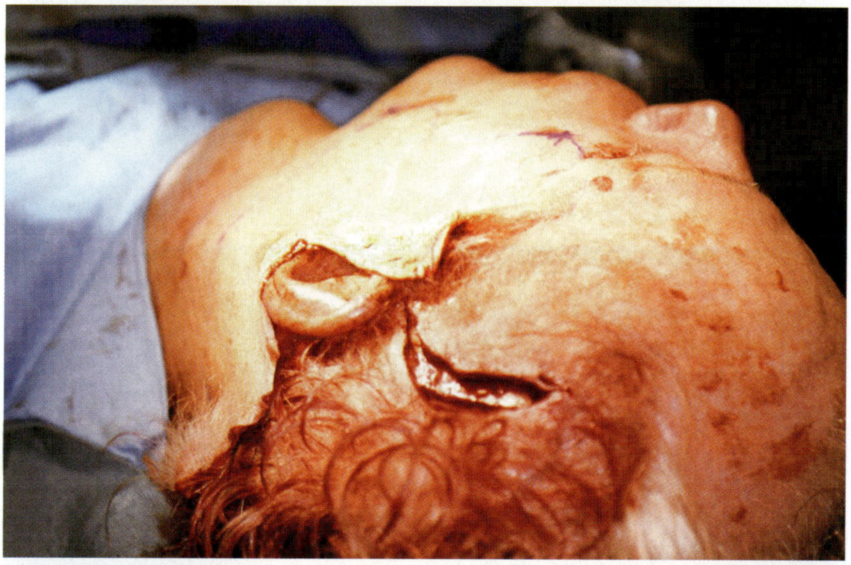

Figure 148.8. After SMAS fixation, a significant amount of excess skin is available for trimming. The previously scored the inferior lobule and posterior hairline offers landmarks for proper skin redraping.

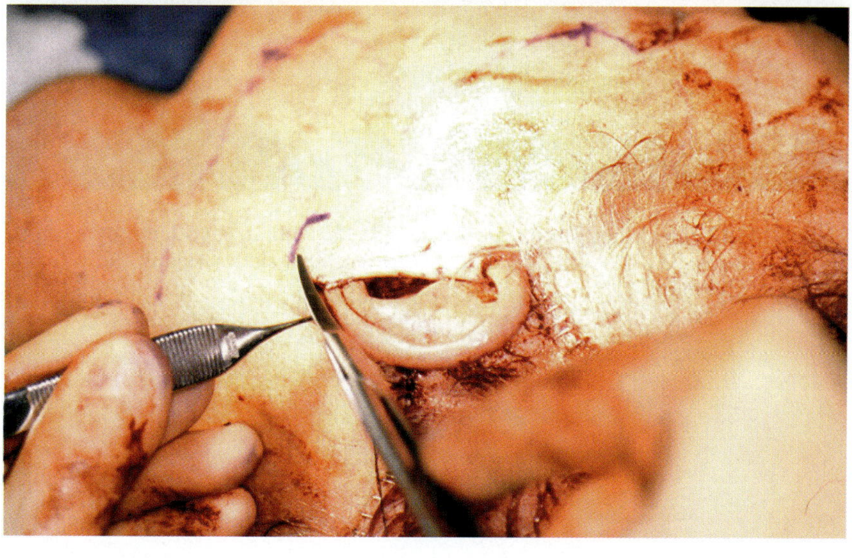

Figure 148.9. Marking the inferior lobule through the excess skin and cutting on the outer helical two-thirds the distance to the distal lobule mark allows slight bunching of the inferior lobule to prevent the pixy-ear deformity.

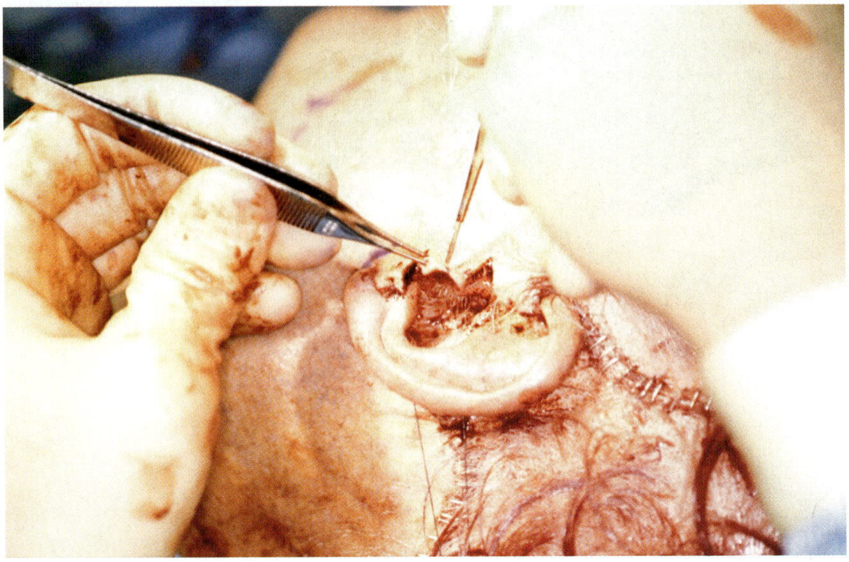

Figure 148.10. Conservative back-cutting excess skin on the tragus allows adequate skin removal without traction on the tragus.

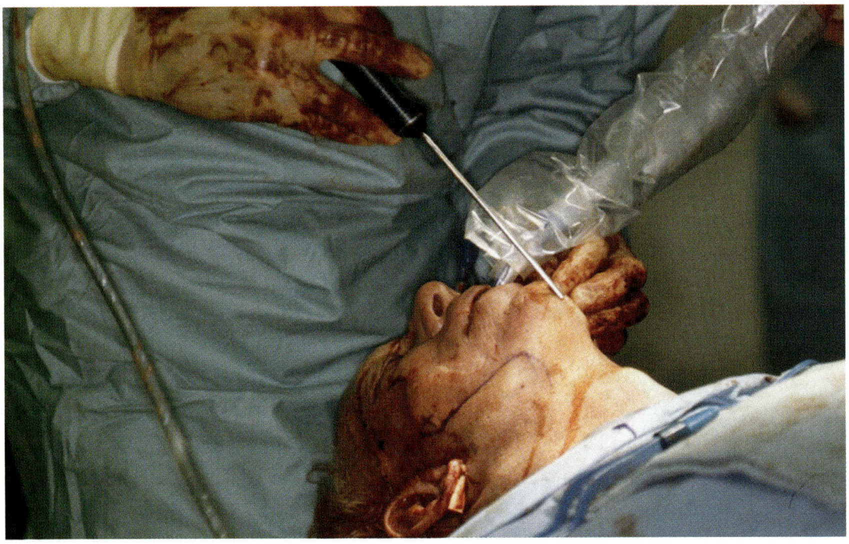

Figure 148.11. Neck liposuction performed at the end of rhytidectomy surgery allows tailoring the amount of fat removed to avoid skeletonizing the inferior border of the mandible.

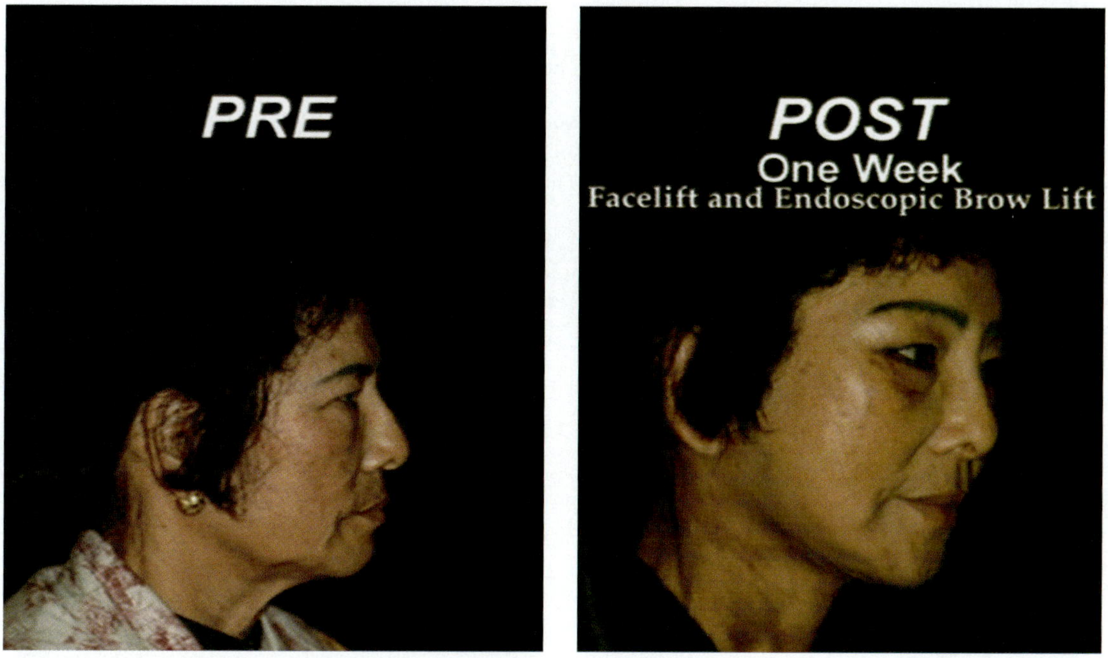

Figure 148.12. With a shorter skin flap, the deep plane lift may have less bruising than longer skin flaps.

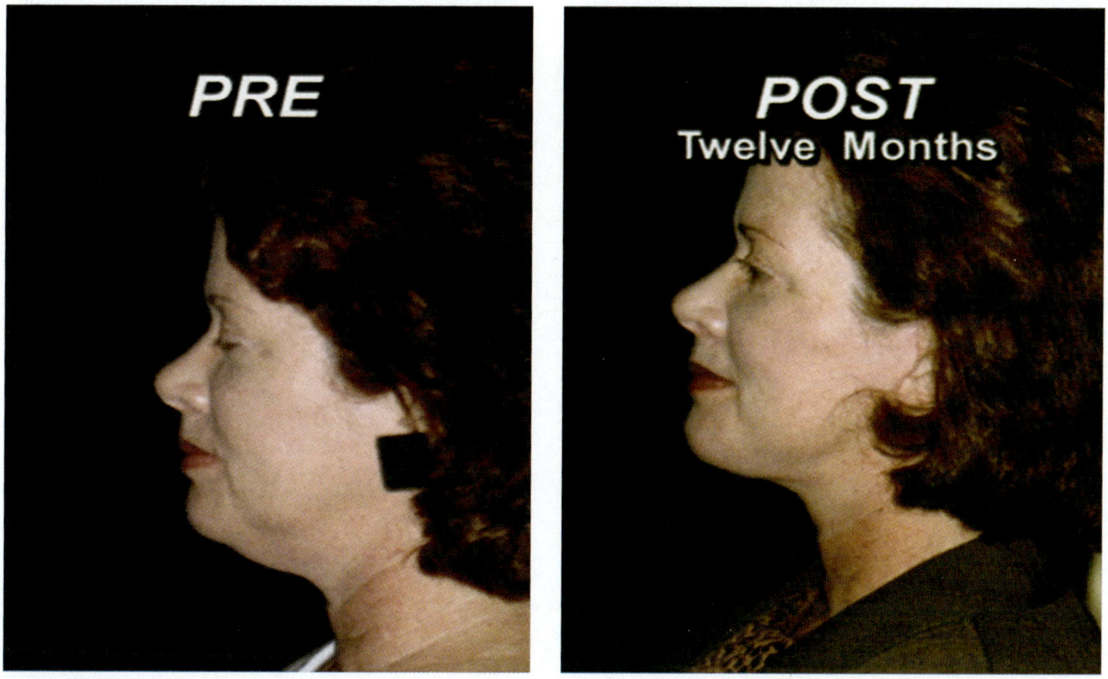

Figure 148.13. Pre- and 1-year postoperative lateral views after rhytidectomy and endoscopic browlift.

References

1. Larrabee WF. Facelift anatomy. Facial Plast Surg Clin North Am 1993; 1:415–426.
2. Baker DC, Conley J. Avoiding facial nerve injuries in rhytidectomy. Plast Reconstr Surg 1979;64:781–795.
3. Alsarraf R. Johnson C. The facelift: technical considerations. Facial Plast Surg 2000;16:231–238.
4. Baylis HI, Goldberg RA, Shorr N. The deep plane facelift: a 20 year evolution of technique. Ophthalmology 2000;107:490–495.
5. Franco T. Face-lift stigmatas. Ann Plast Surg 1985;15:379–385.

Part XII

Functional Lid Malpositions

Section One

Ptosis: Anterior Approach

149

Advantages of Sequential Versus Simultaneous Bilateral Levator Advancement Surgery

Herbert J. Glatt

Theoretical Advantages to Unilateral Surgery

1. Surgical catastrophes. Blindness after eyelid surgery is very rare, but it does happen. Bilateral blindness is exponentially worse than unilateral blindness. Despite rigorous preoperative screening, patients can occasionally sneak into your operating room with previously undiagnosed bleeding diatheses or undisclosed use of aspirin, nonsteroidals, or alternative medicines such as ginkgo biloba. Bilateral severe bleeding is exponentially worse than unilateral severe bleeding.
2. Decreased operating time per session. The longer a patient lies there, the more things can go wrong. An elderly male with prostatic hypertrophy may develop urinary urgency leading to hyptertension and consequent bleeding. If a patient's back starts to hurt after a while, his or her blood pressure may go up and they may bleed. Sequential surgery lets you get the patient out of the operating room faster.
3. Patching vs. ice packs. My preference is to patch unilateral cases and use ice packs in bilateral cases. A patch provides continuous pressure, whereas an ice pack provides only intermittent cooling. It is my impression that patients ooze less with a patch.

I prefer to do levator advancements combined with upper lid blepharoplasties as sequential rather than bilateral procedures. I have had a few cases over the years where the first and originally more ptotic side was a little undercorrected but still better than preop and the patients were happy. In these cases I have done blepharoplasties and omitted the levator advancements on the second eyelid. By staging the procedure, I have the flexibility to alter my plan when approaching the other side. With this sequential approach, the vast majority of my patients do well and I only rarely have to reoperate for asymmetry. I adjust the upper lid height without sedation. After adjustment, I ask the anesthetist to administer sedation for the fat resection and closure. Since some patients are nervous during the first half of their levator advancements in which they are unsedated, unilateral surgery decreases the minutes they have to lie there without sedation.

150

Considerations in Simultaneous vs. Sequential Bilateral Levator Repair

Robert A. Mazzoli*

When faced with a patient with bilateral true ptosis, the question arises as to whether to operate on both lids simultaneously at one sitting, or sequentially, separated by weeks or months. Sound arguments can be made to support each approach, especially if contemplating bilateral external levator procedures. Less of an argument for sequential surgery might be made if considering bilateral conjunctival-muellerectomy (Putterman procedure), since active patient participation for lid height adjustment is not as critical in this operation as opposed to levator surgery.

For the sake of this discussion, financial implications of surgical cost and reimbursement of single- or multiple-episode surgery are not considered.

Bilateral simultaneous surgery is no doubt more convenient for the patient—one anesthetic episode, one trip to the surgery suite, one operative and convalescent period away from work. It may also be more efficient and convenient for the surgeon. Theoretically, the surgeon can set one lid at the desired height and immediately use it as a guide for the fellow lid (i.e., complete one lid and then start the next). Alternatively, some surgeons may alternate from one lid to the other, doing similar steps on both lids simultaneously and adjusting both lids simultaneously—this is a relatively more advanced technique and requires expert knowledge of anatomy, precise dissection, and economy of movement. Speed is critical in this approach, as in less-than-expert hands the local anesthetic may wear off prior to completion, requiring supplemental injections, often into the deeper tissue planes: these injections may then pharmacologically paralyze the levator, making subsequent height adjustment all the more difficult.

Regardless of technique, balancing the advantages of simultaneous surgery are the real-life possibilities of asymmetric intraoperative lid

*The views expressed in this chapter are those of the author and do not reflect the official policy of the Department of the Army, the Department of Defense, or the U.S. Government.

swelling and edema of one lid, or dyspraxia of the lid (usually as a result of local anesthesia diffusing into levator), which complicates the adjustment of the fellow eyelid. This might also occur with longer operative times, as in the case of the occasional or infrequent ptosis surgeon—the longer the operation, the more likely the intraoperative swelling will become significant. Some surgeons would then advocate ignoring the height of the first lid and independently placing the second lid at the desired height (i.e., place each lid at the desired anatomic height as separate efforts). While this approach is generally reliable, it does not adequately address the additional possible intraoperative contribution of Hering's law on lid height. In actuality, of course, the possibility of Hering's contribution occurs regardless of the state of edema and swelling. In either case, the surgeon may then be faced with unexpected postoperative asymmetry and the prospect of having to reoperate one lid or the other at a later date. Most oculoplastic surgeons will admit to some percentage of postoperative asymmetries that require revision.

Of course, any operation through previously traumatized tissues complicates the subsequent surgery for a variety of reasons: landmarks are distorted; bleeding may be more profuse; scarring and cicatrix are unpredictable; and cicatrix is difficult to anesthetize, often requiring larger anesthetic volumes, which may then further distort anatomy or color the surgical endpoint. Most surgeons, if given the choice of operating on virgin anatomy vs. reoperating, would choose the former. Consequently, if any surgeon has an x% chance of postoperative asymmetry necessitating revision (in his or her own hands), the surgeon must frankly ask him- or herself whether that percentage of reoperation is outweighed by the convenience of simultaneous surgery. Intuitively, the more experienced the surgeon, the smaller x should be (and conversely, the higher (1-00 – x) the chance for success with a single surgery—should be). In less experienced hands, however, the prospect of performing a second and ostensibly more difficult operation may mitigate to sequential surgery, wherein one lid is operated and allowed to heal and is then used as a gauge for matching the virgin fellow lid at a second, separate surgery.

I discuss these scenarios preoperatively with patients and solicit their thoughts and desires. I have found most patients understanding of the difficulties and subtleties of ptosis surgery and willing and appreciative participants in the decision of how to proceed in their own medical care. Many factors weigh into their individual decisions. Some are understandably anxious about surgery and want it over with as quickly and painlessly as possible, often saying "Doc, you've got me once. . . . I'll take my chances and live with a little asymmetry." Others, dreading the possibility of unsightly asymmetry and the prospect of a second, more difficult surgery, will opt for sequential surgery. In any case, I now involve the patient in the discussion and decision and proceed as the patient desires.

151

Unilateral Levator Resection for Jaw-Winking Ptosis

Stuart R. Seiff

While some surgeons have reported good experience with bilateral levator release and frontalis sling surgery for unilateral jaw-winking ptosis, I feel unilateral levator resection provides good results and that is all I have ever done on these patients. It turns out that most parents (or patients) are unwilling to sacrifice the normal muscle. I typically wait until the child is 3 or 4 years old, but if you can do the surgery sooner, I suspect the results might be even better. In my experience, the younger kids tend to try harder to elevate a ptotic lid.

The levator resection surgery should be based on the most ptotic position and function, not the "jaw-winked" position or function. With the "jaw-wink" movements, these kids typically produce good levator function (10 mm and more). However, the isolated levator function without jaw movements is generally poor and the ptosis severe. I have had the most success setting the intraoperative lid height approximately where I want it when the child is awake with eyes open. This generally requires a levator resection of 17–23 mm. This way we don't have to rely on the limited levator function to achieve symmetry.

It has been rumored that the jaw-wink becomes more obvious after levator resection. I have not found this to be at all true. With the affected lid already in an elevated position, the excursion of the wink is limited and less noticeable.

Kids with dissociated du=issociated vertical deviation (DVD) present a special problem. When fixing with the affected eye, the lid position can look great. However, when they fix with the normal eye, the affected eye drifts upward and the lid appears ptotic. I have had some success managing these patients with postop patching, but strabismus surgery may be necessary.

Suggested Reading

Bowyer JD, Sullivan TJ. Management of Marcus Gunn jaw winking synkinesis. Ophthal Plast Reconstr Surg 2004;20:92–98.

Callahan MA, Beard C. Beard's Ptosis, 4th ed. Birmingham, AL: Aesculapius, 1990:115–116.

Seiff SR. Re: Management of Marcus Gunn jaw winking synkinesis. Ophthal Plastic Reconstruct Surg 2004;201–402.

152

Ten Steps to Making Ptosis Surgery More Predictable

Russell S. Gonnering

There is many a boy here today who looks on war as all glory, but, boys, it is all hell.

—General William Tecumseh Sherman
August 11, 1880
Columbus, Ohio

Ptosis is hell.

—Richard K. Dortzbach, MD
Summer of 1981
Madison, Wisconsin

In training, I did not fully appreciate the words of my mentor, Richard K. Dortzbach, M.D., when he first uttered this concise description of one of the most common operations we perform. Now, several thousand procedures later, I understand what he was saying.

I am sure that there exists a precise, mathematical model for ptosis repair: take this much ptosis, this much levator function, this set of anatomic parameters, and perform this degree of surgery to get this result. While the equation no doubt exists, the constants and variables that would allow one to use it remain a mystery.

It is very difficult to fully teach external levator repair. Results are very predictable, but those results are dependent upon exactly duplicating a multitude of steps, some of them unconsciously performed. For this reason, it is not surprising that one can read a description of an operative technique, attempt to duplicate it, and then be disappointed when the results are very different from those described by the author.

With that caveat, the following maneuvers have proven to be helpful to me in external levator surgery:

1. In virtually all cases, I confine my surgery to the aponeurosis. I do not like the idea of sacrificing sarcomeres for shortening an already weakened muscle. I want all of those elements lifting the eyelid. For levator function of less than 6 mm, I often use a frontalis sling instead of a maximum levator recession.

2. Note the position of the lid margin relative to the corneal limbus and levator function with the patient supine on the operating table before any sedation is given. Also assess the position of the lid margin in downgaze, and if there is any lagophthalmos. periodically retest that at points during the surgery, to assess how the sedation and the local anesthetic have affected the baseline measurements.

3. Use a small amount of local anesthetic—usually a 1:1 mixture of 0.75% bupivacaine with 2% lidocaine with 1:100,000 epinephrine—to produce a final epinephrine concentration of 1:200,000. I inject approximately 1 cc in the eyelid directly under the incision. I prep, then mark, and inject.

4. Make the incision slightly below the intended upper eyelid crease. In an Asian eyelid, this may only be a few millimeters above the lid margin.

5. After waiting at least 5 minutes, I make my incision with the fine point electrocautery needle. Put the lid on downward stretch with a traction suture, and then dissect with scissors, in both a sharp and spreading fashion, until the orbital septum is reached. If there is a levator disinsertion, I can see it before I open the septum.

6. Mobilize the levator as gently as possible to avoid bleeding and use the bipolar cautery to limit hematoma formation. If a hematoma forms, take this into account when setting the lid position.

7. I use a 5-0 suture, most often nylon on a $^1/_4$ circle spatula needle, and pass it first in a partial thickness bite of the tarsus, approximately 2 mm inferior to the superior border. Then pass it up through the aponeurosis, and then down through the aponeurosis, so the knot will be covered by the aponeurosis. Tie in a slip knot, and assess height and contour. This is the most difficult part of the operation. In most instances, I do not try for an "overcorrection," as the lid usually stays where I set it, using this technique. If the levator function is markedly diminished from sedation, local, bleeding, or some other cause, I may set it a bit higher, but then look at where the lid margin is in downgaze to make sure the ptosis is not overcorrected.

8. When performing bilateral surgery, open both sides until reaching the step above, and then correct the dominant eye first, as this can affect the position of the nondominant eye.

9. I may then add a suture either medial or lateral to my central suture, more to aid in obtaining a strong attachment more than to get additional lift.

10. Once satisfied with the lid position, trim off the redundant aponeurosis, taking care to leave enough behind so the sutures do not "cheese wire" through. Closure involves a few absorbable sutures, taking inferior orbicularis to levator to superior orbicularis to reform the lid crease. Use orbicularis rather than skin so the crease is normally effaced in downgaze. I then run the skin, usually with a 6-0 fast-absorbing plain suture.

153

Adjustable Suture Technique for Levator Surgery

Morris E. Hartstein and John J. Woog

Externalized adjustable sutures allow for early postoperative adjustment of lid height and contour.

The predictability of levator surgery both for ptosis repair and for recession for eyelid retraction may be influenced by several factors, including: variable orbicularis muscle and Müller muscle response to local anesthetic injection, intraoperative hemorrhage involving orbicularis, Müller, or levator muscle, and variable patient cooperation when surgery performed under intravenous sedation. These factors may confound efforts to achieve the desired postoperative result, even when eyelid position and contour are satisfactory at the time of intraoperative adjustment. In certain cases, adjustable sutures may be a useful adjunct in eyelid surgery.[1]

Surgical Technique

Ptosis repair is carried out in standard fashion. A double-armed 5-0 prolene suture is passed partial thickness through the anterior surface of tarsus, and both arms are brought up through the edge of levator aponeurosis. A second set of 5-0 prolene sutures is passed around the first set and the ends left untied (Figure 153.1). The lid crease incision is then closed in standard fashion with interrupted and running 6-0 plain gut. The prolene sutures are then taped to the forehead (Figure 153.2). If there is persistent ptosis at 5–7 days postop the levator-tarsal sutures are tied with a single throw and carefully tightened until the eyelid position is satisfactory. An additional throw is placed to create a square knot, after which the ends of the suture are cut short and tucked beneath the edges of the incision. However, if eyelid position is satisfactory at 5–7 days postoperatively, then the supplemental levator-tarsal suture is pulled out and removed.

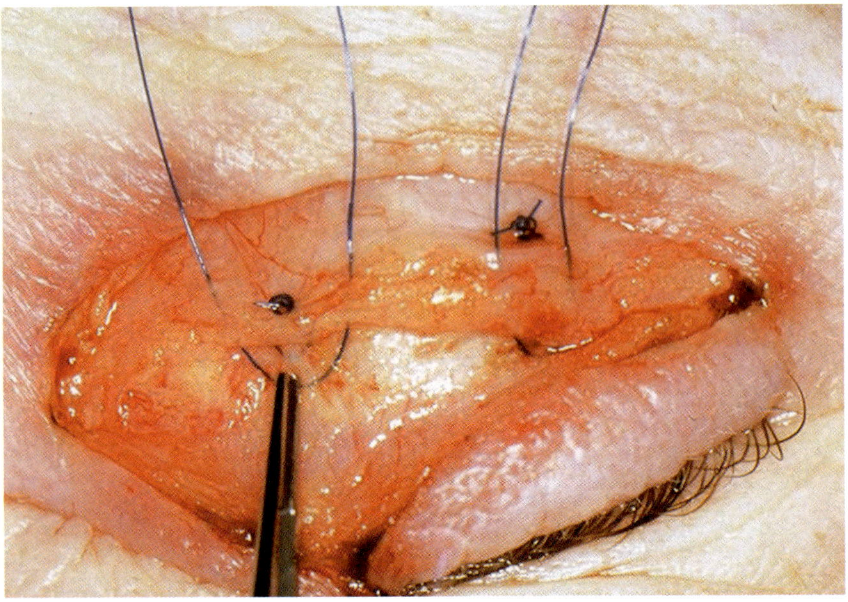

Figure 153.1. Permanently tied polyproplyene sutures for levator advancement, with adjustable sutures passed in similar fashion around them in a hang-back fashion.

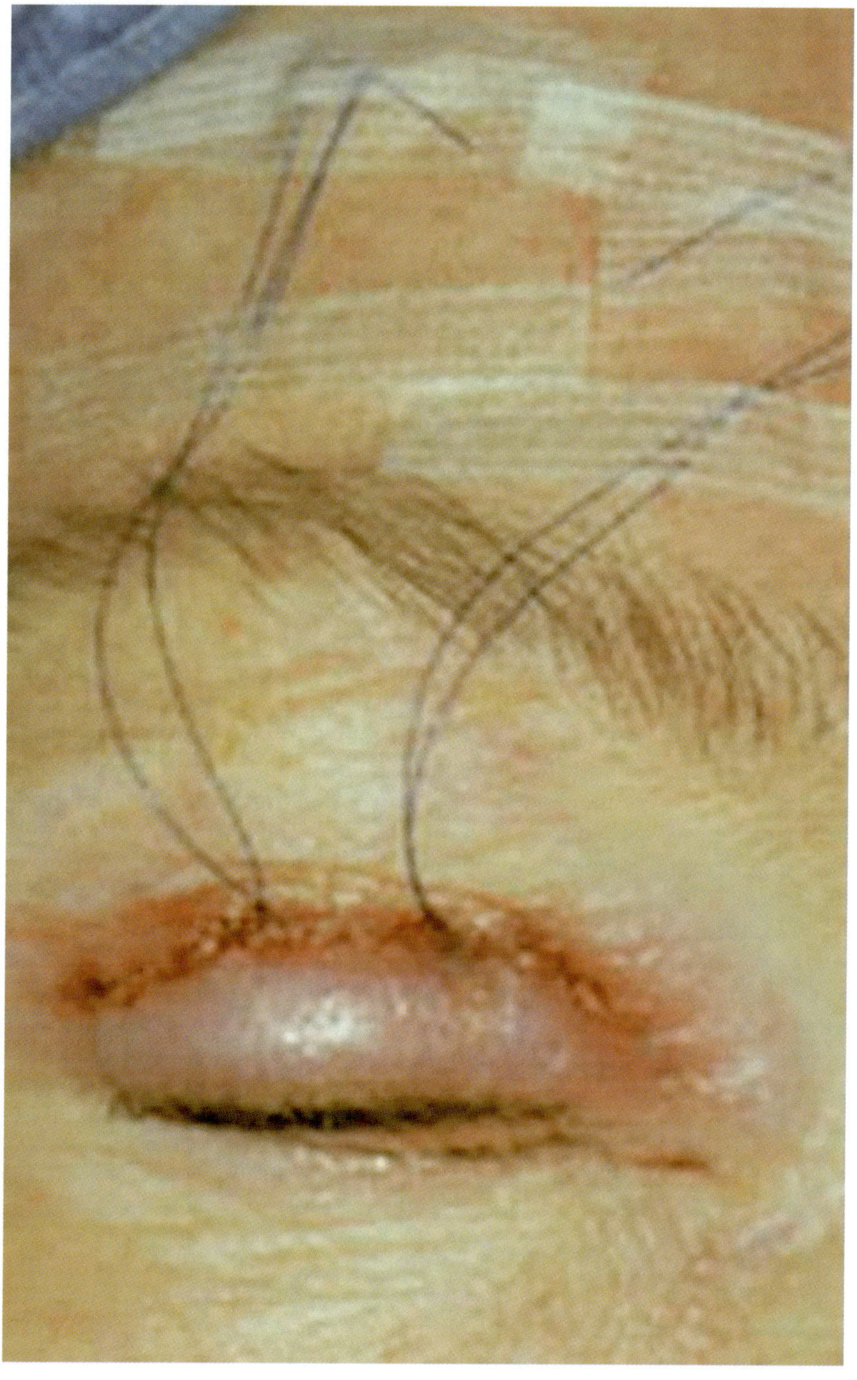

Figure 153.2. Following incision closure, the adjustable sutures are loosely taped to the forehead for 5–7 days.

Reference

1. Woog JJ, Hartstein ME, Hoenig J. Adjustable suture technique for levator recession. Arch Ophthalmol 1996;114:620–624.

154

Tarsal Switch Levator Resection for the Treatment of Myopathic Blepharoptosis

Sheri L. DeMartelaere, Todd R. Shepler, Sean M. Blaydon, Russell W. Neuhaus, and John W. Shore

Progressive myopathic ptosis is often associated with fair to poor levator function. These patients usually adopt a head-back/chin-up position with heavy recruitment of the frontalis muscle to see, resulting in chronic neck pain and visual fatigue. In addition, these patients often have a poor Bell's phenomenon and the orbicularis muscle can be weak, resulting in poor eye protective mechanisms. Surgical procedures to correct blepharoptosis in patients with poor eye-protective mechanisms are associated with an increased incidence of postoperative lagophthalmos and corneal exposure.

The goal in these patients is to lift the eyelid to a level that allows them to see without placing them at risk for lagophthalmos/exposure keratopathy and without having to tilt their head back. We describe a tarsal switch-levator resection procedure that predictably raises the upper eyelid a predetermined amount and elevates the lower eyelid to almost the same distance. This essentially shifts the patient's palpebral fissure cephalad, thereby unmasking their visual axis in primary gaze (Figure 154.1).

Surgical Technique

The skin to be excised from the upper eyelid is marked as is done for a conservative upper eyelid blepharoplasty surgery, leaving 2.5 cm of skin for eyelid closure. A corneal protective shield is placed in the eye. The upper eyelid skin is incised and skin only is removed, leaving the orbicularis muscle in place. The orbicularis oculi muscle is divided at the upper border of the wound to expose the orbital septum. The orbicularis is dissected free from the underlying septum, which is then opened horizontally. Preaponeurotic fat is liposculpted or retracted superiorly. The upper anterior surface of tarsus is exposed by dissecting in the suborbicularis fascial plane, creating a flap of orbicularis muscle hinged inferiorly. Centering on the superior border of tarsus, a 6 × 20 mm ellipse is marked on the surface of levator aponeurosis and tarsus. The ellipse is excised resulting in a composite graft resection of 3 mm of tarsus/conjunctiva and 3 mm of levator aponeurosis/Müller's muscle/conjunctiva (Figures 154.2 and 154.3). The graft is preserved in a saline-soaked gauze.

The elliptical defect in the posterior lamella of the upper eyelid is closed with 7-0 polyglactin 910 sutures (Vicryl™; Ethicon, Inc.) placed partial thickness through the upper border of tarsus and through the distal end of the levator aponeurosis/Müller's muscle complex. Care is taken to ensure that the sutures do not protrude through the conjunctival surface posteriorly. The orbicularis muscle is then closed with interrupted 7-0 polyglactin 910 sutures (Vicryl™; Ethicon, Inc.) with the knot buried. Skin is closed with a running suture of 6-0 silk or 6-0 polypropolene.

Attention is directed to the lower eyelid. A 6-0 silk traction suture is placed and the lid is everted. A horizontal conjunctival incision is made at the inferior tarsal border extending from the punctum to the lateral canthus. The lower eyelid retractors are dissected free from the conjunctiva to the level of Lockwood's ligament and are excised (Figure 154.4). The composite graft taken from the upper eyelid is positioned in the lower lid with the tarsal edges abutting and the conjunctival surface of the graft directed toward the globe. The graft is sutured in position with a running suture of double-armed 6-0 polypropolene externalized and tied on silicone bolsters (Figure 154.5). The corneal protective shield is removed. Suture tarsorrhaphies of 6-0 polypropolene are placed medially and laterally and tied over bolsters. These tarsorrhaphies are removed at 1 week postoperatively.

Figure 154.6 illustrates a typical patient with oculopharyngeal muscular dystropy. He underwent the surgical technique described in this chapter. At one year postoperative follow-up (Figure 154.7), he has a clear visual axis and improved head position.

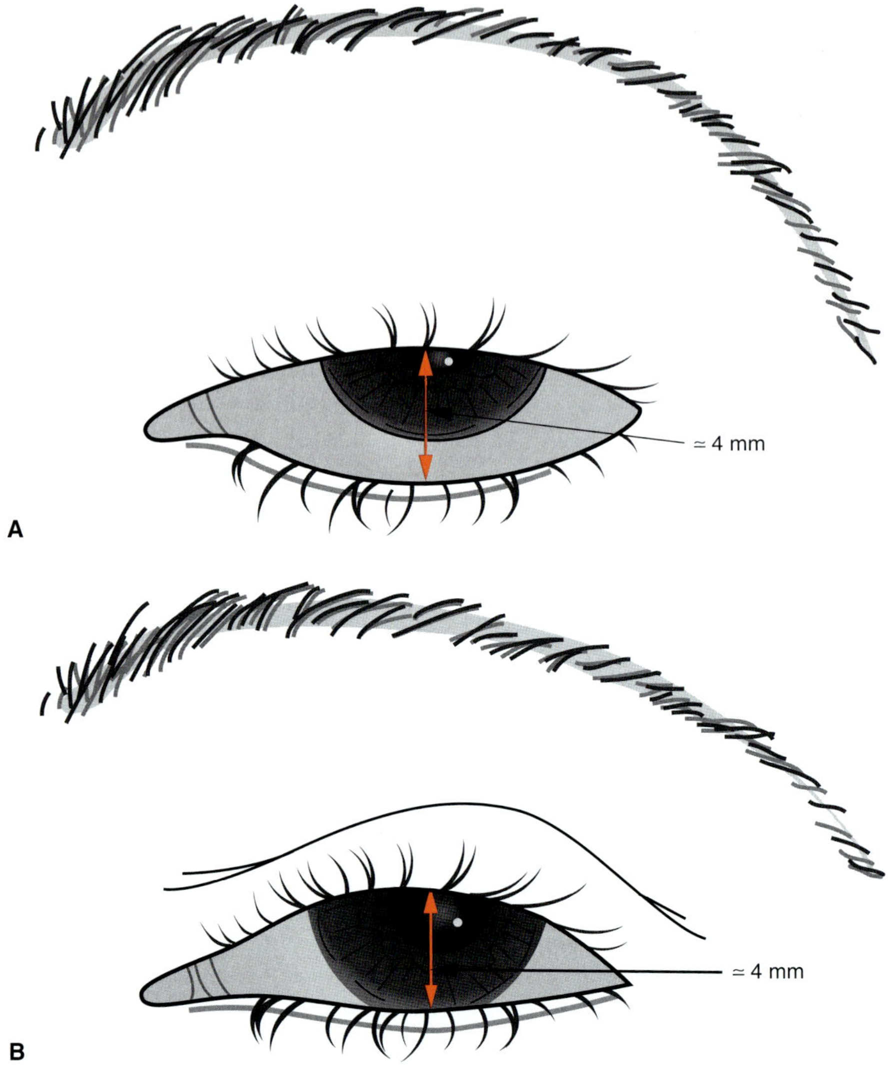

Figure 154.1. Artist sketches depciting movement of palpebral fissure cephalad. (A) Before surgery. (B) After surgery.

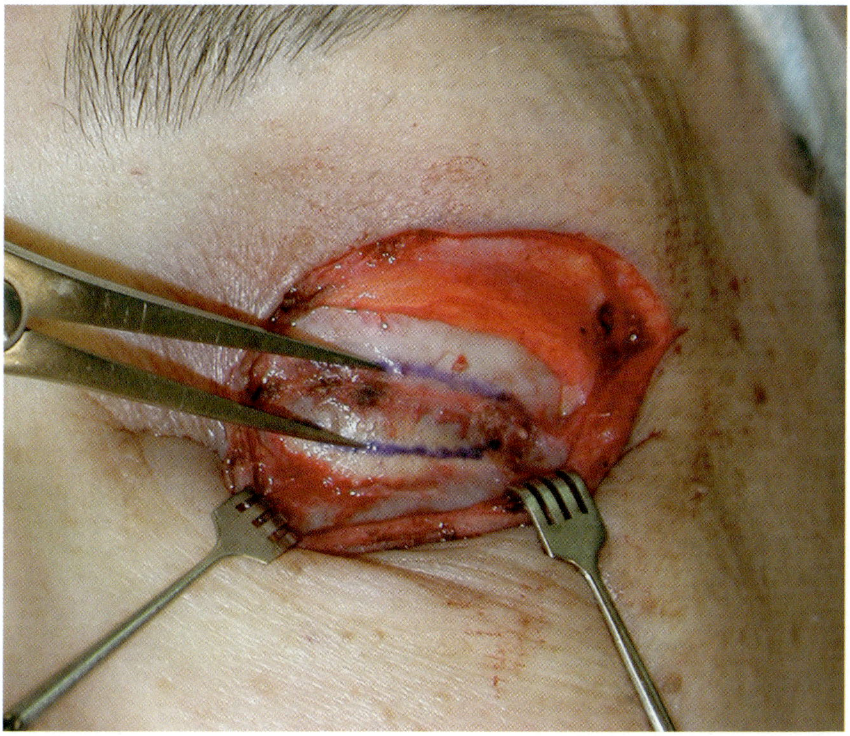

Figure 154.2. Demarcation of free graft.

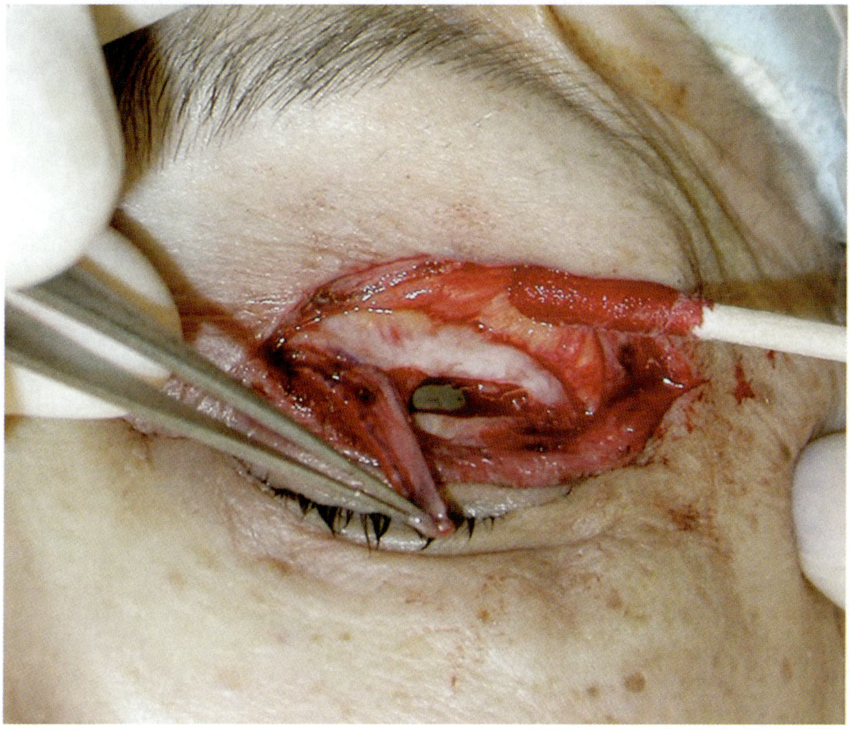

Figure 154.3. Excision of free graft.

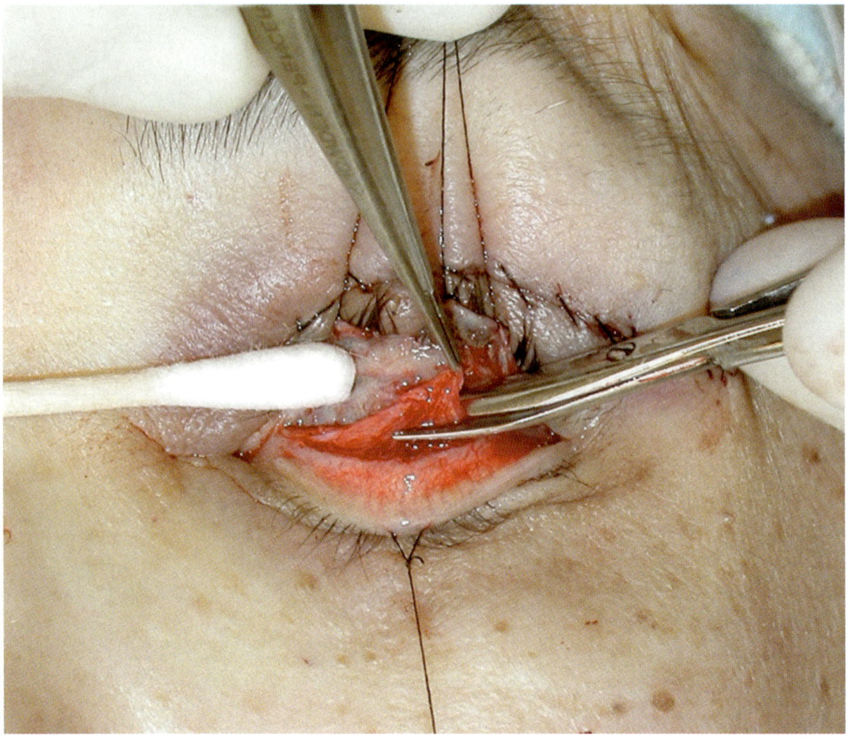

Figure 154.4. Excision of lower eyelid retractors.

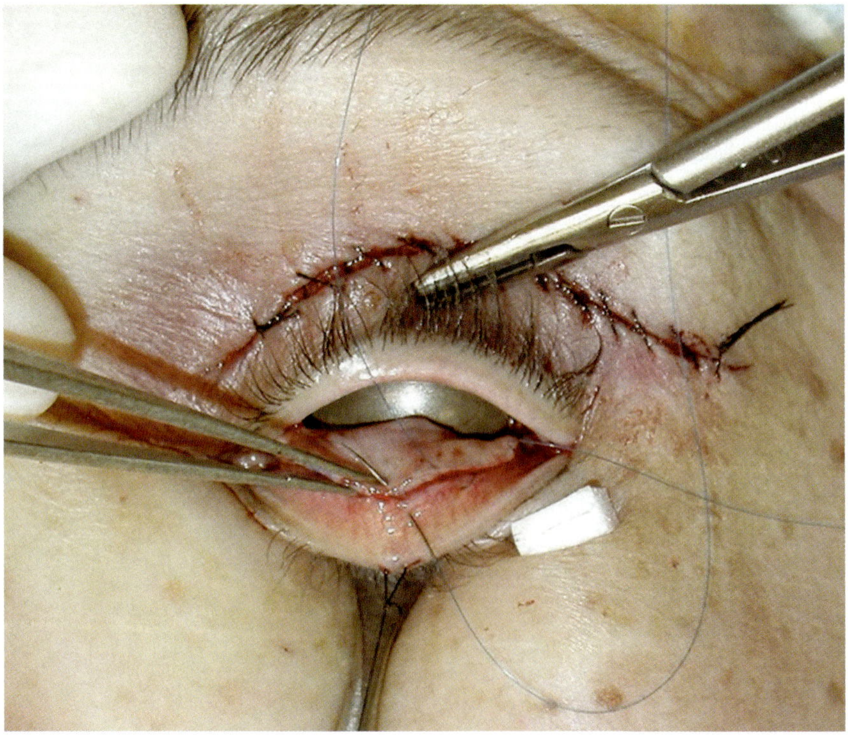

Figure 154.5. Placement of lower eyelid graft.

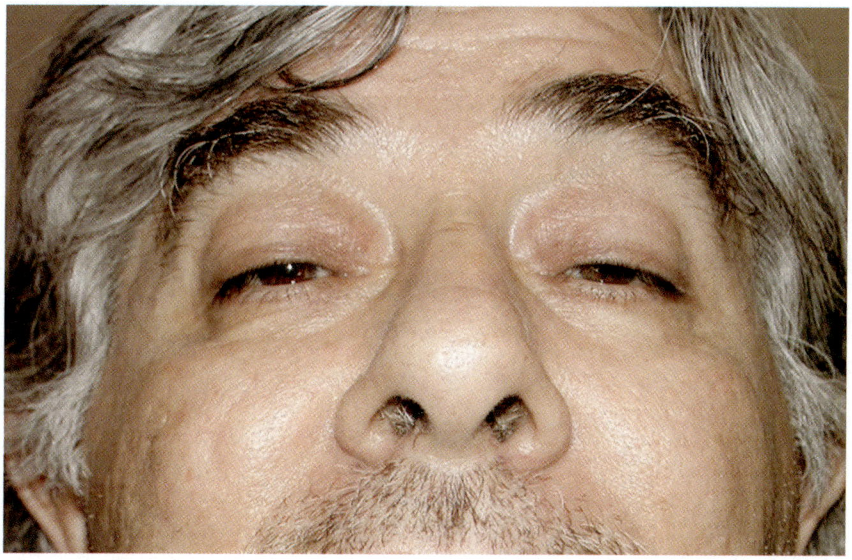

Figure 154.6. Preoperative photo; had to lift chin to see.

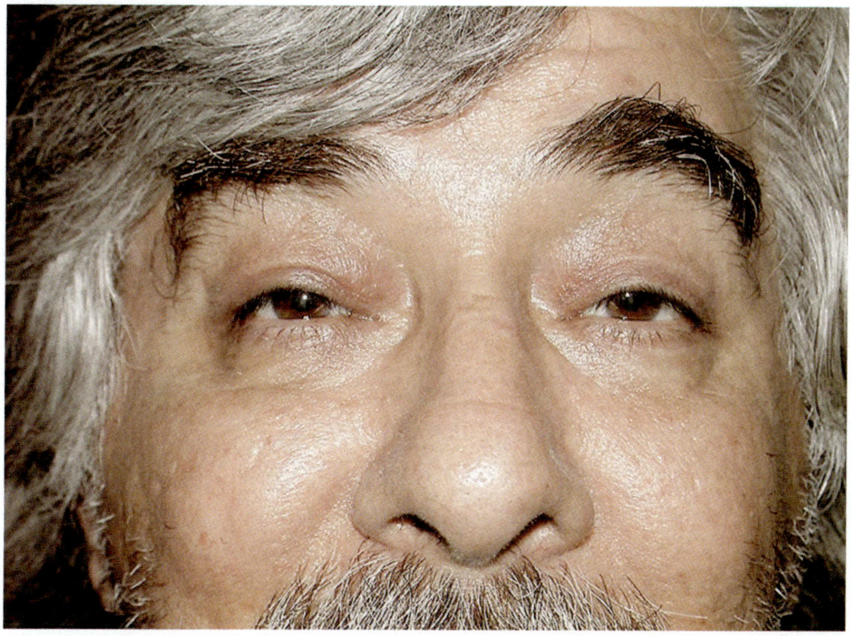

Figure 154.7. Twelve-month postoperative photo, chin normal.

Suggested Reading

DeMartelaere SL, Blaydon SM, Shore JW. Tarsal switch levator resection for the treatment of blepharoptosis in patients with poor eye protective mechanims. Ophthalmology 2006;113:2357–2363.

155

Modified Levator Advancement Ptosis Technique

Rona Z. Silkiss

A preferred technique for the repair of ptosis is a modification of a levator advancement technique.

In this modified technique, a blepharoplasty is performed if needed, after which the levator aponeurosisis reflected from its insertion from underlying tarsus and Müller's muscle. Two or three double-armed 5–0 Dexon sutures on a SS2 spatulated half-circle needle are then placed in a lamellar fashion through tarsus. These sutures are placed in the midline as well as medially and occasionally laterally. There is a "sweet spot" just medial to the midline that provides for an optimal eyelid configuration. These sutures are then placed in a mattress fashion through the levator aponeurosis superior to the area of relative thinning. All the double-armed sutures are then held with a snap and tied and cut. The advanced aponeurosis may or may not be trimmed. The skin is then closed in the usual fashion.

156

Minimally Invasive Ptosis Repair

Francesco P. Bernardini

Minimally invasive ptosis surgery offers many advantages—a less visible scar, a reduced surgical time, and an improved postoperative period—and it is as effective and reliable as the traditional surgical approach. I have been delighted with the minimally invasive approach in aponeurogenic ptosis.

Mini-invasive Ptosis Surgery

When dealing with a patient affected by aponeurogenic ptosis, where an upper eyelid blepharoplasty is not required and the levator function is normal (i.e., >12 mm), I make a 1-cm incision in the eyelid crease and perform a routine levator advancement through that minimal skin incision. What makes this procedure very fast is the simple exposure of the orbital septum after opening the orbicularis muscle (Figure 156.1). With the surgeon holding the superior skin\orbicularis edge apart with one rake retractor in one hand, the orbital septum can be identified by gently moving the rake up toward the brow with minimal dissection in the suborbicularis plane. After opening the orbital septum, the dissection is carried between the levator aponeurosis and the fat so that the aponeurosis and levator muscle will be clearly visualized (Figure 156.2). A single suture between the tarsal plate and the aponeurosis will give an excellent contour in the vast majority of cases. A slight overcorrection of 1–2 mm is required to achieve an optimal final result and two or three individual sutures are used to close the skin (Figure 156.3). The technique requires an injection of a very small amount of local anesthesia in the eyelid (<1 ml), limiting its impact on the eyelid position; in my hands the procedure takes usually 8–10 minutes at most and postoperative swelling and bruising are also greatly reduced.

Suggested Reading

Lucarelli MJ, Lemke BN. Small incision external levator repair: technique and early results. Am J Ophthalmol 1999;127:637–644.

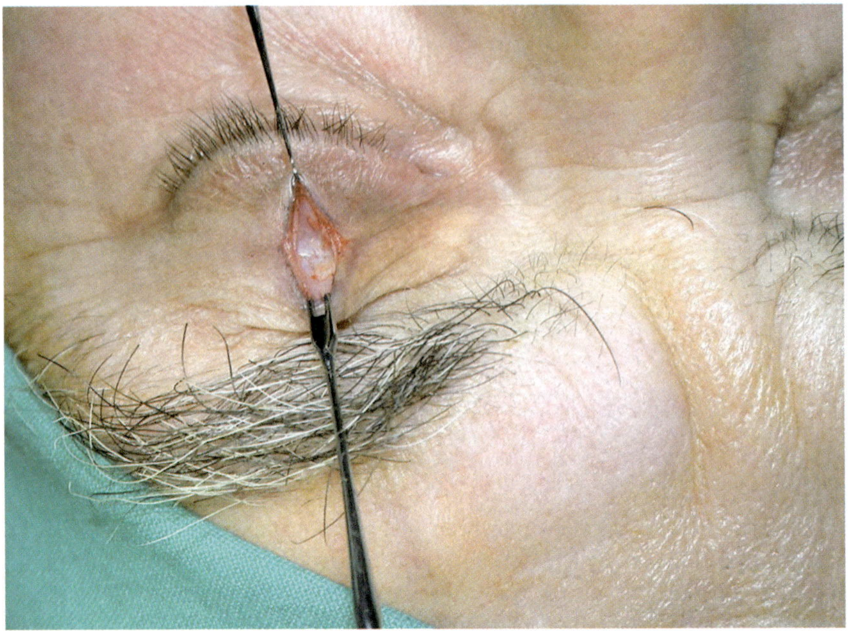

Figure 156.1. Exposure of the septum.

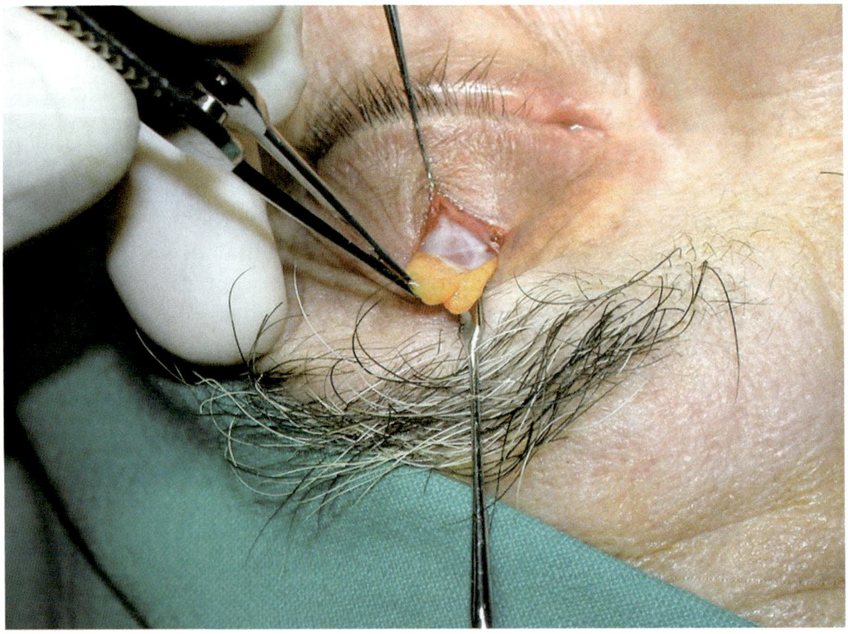

Figure 156.2. Exposure of the pre-aponeurolic fat and levator aponeurosis.

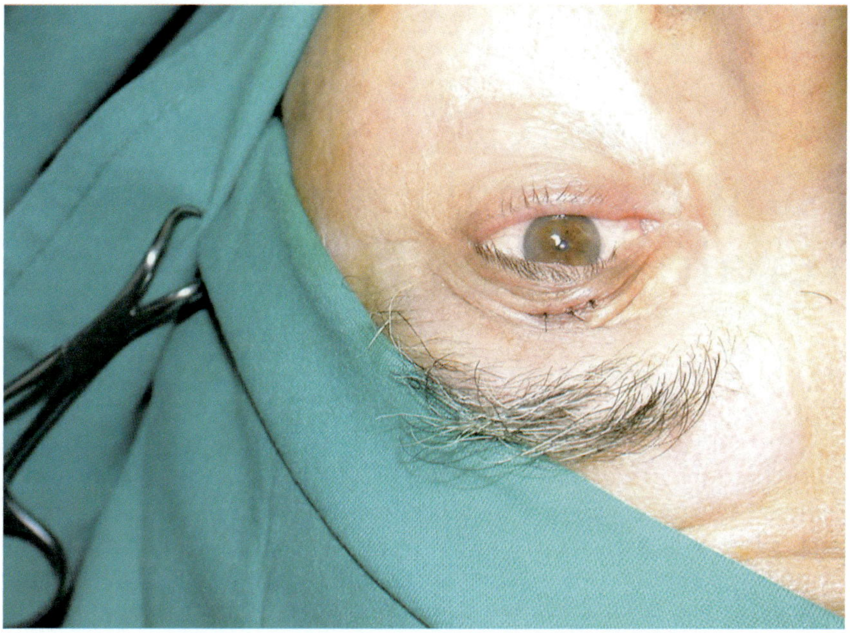

Figure 156.3. Final intra-operative aspect.

157

Small Incision External Levator Repair

Mark J. Lucarelli

External levator repair is a time-honored method of correcting ptosis. Such surgery is performed frequently by specialists who specialize in significant amounts of eyelid surgery. Achieving predictable, aesthetically appealing results can sometimes, however, be challenging. Hence, alternatives such as the conjunctival muellerectomy have found an important place in the surgical eyelid armamentarium. This section provides a number of guidelines that have been helpful to me in achieving more consistent results with an external levator repair utilizing a smaller incision and limited dissection.

1. As with other procedures, proper patient selection is key. In order to achieve excellent results, this operation must be restricted to patients with minimal dermatochalasis. The best candidates are patients with dermatochalasis ratings of 0–1+ on a scale of 0–4+.
2. If the patient's ptosis is unilateral, a phenylephrine test is helpful. This is done by placing on drop of 2.5% phenylephrine on the ocular surface of the ptotic side Q 5 minutes × 2. The phenylephrine test will help determine if the patient is a good candidate for internal ptosis repair (conjunctival muellerectomy). It will also help reveal asymmetric, subclinical ptosis on the supposedly normal side (Hering's effect).
3. The upper eyelid position (margin reflex distances) should always be evaluated with the brow relaxed. Significant brow recruitment can dramatically alter the true position of the upper eyelid margin.
4. This procedure can be readily performed in the office under local anesthetic or using monitored anesthesia care. If intravenous sedation is used, propofol is an excellent agent, as its effects wear off nearly completely in 10 minutes.
5. Although our previously published description of this procedure recommended an 8-mm incision, I have found that a slightly larger incision of approximately 12 mm that extends from the medial limbus to the lateral limbus allows the procedure to remain minimally invasive yet affords considerably better surgical exposure. These markings are always placed before the patient is sedated so that the ideal horizontal position of the incision can be marked without concern for any deviation of the ocular position owing to sedation. In women, the relevant segment of

the lid crease is typically marked at 9 or 10 mm superior to the lash line. In men, the position is often marked slightly lower at 7–8 mm. In Asian patients, lower lid positions are indicated.

6. 0.6 ml of local anesthetic is used superficially into the lid at the site of the lid crease marking. 2% lidocaine with 1:100,000 units of epinephrine mixed in equal parts with 0.5% bupivicaine with epinephrine is a reliable combination and aids with hemostasis.

7. After incision of the skin, gentle retraction inferiorly by an assistant is often helpful during dissection to identify the levator aponeurosis. A microdissection needle on an electrosurgical monopolar unit is my preferred means of dissection. Other surgeons favor the Ellman radiofrequency surgical unit. Gentle blunt dissection is also sometimes helpful in identifying the levator aponeurosis.

8. The preaponeurotic fat pad and the musculo-aponeurotic junction should be identified. No dissection on the underneath side of the levator aponeurosis is necessary.

9. The anterior superior surface of the tarsus is exposed in a standard fashion. Dissection on the tarsus is limited to the central portion overlying the cornea. This degree of dissection allows for two levator-tarsus sutures to be placed without any difficulty.

10. A 6–0 Prolene suture is passed in a horizontal mattress fashion, first through the levator complex at the level of the aponeurotic-septal junction and then partial-thickness through the superior third of the tarsus, and finally back through the levator complex at the level of the aponeurotic-septal junction. Restricting the tarsal bites to the superior third of the tarsus minimizes the likelihood of contour abnormalities. The suture is temporarily tied.

11. The patient is placed in a seated position. Eyelid height and contour are then carefully inspected in primary gaze, up-gaze, and down-gaze. The Prolene suture is then adjusted as desired. If desired, an additional medial or lateral suture may easily be placed.

12. The Prolene sutures are tied permanently. Eyelid crease reformation is not recommended in this procedure. The orbicularis is reapproximated with one or two buried interacted sutures of 7-0 Vicryl. The skin is usually then closed with a running fashion using 6-0 fast-absorbing plain gut suture.

13. The patient is seen 7–10 days postoperatively. Although rarely necessary, adjustment of the operated eyelid can easily be performed in the office in the 10-day period following the first postoperative week.

Further Reading

Lucarelli MJ, Lemke BN. Small incision external levator repair: technique and early results. Am J Ophthalmol 1999;127:637–644.

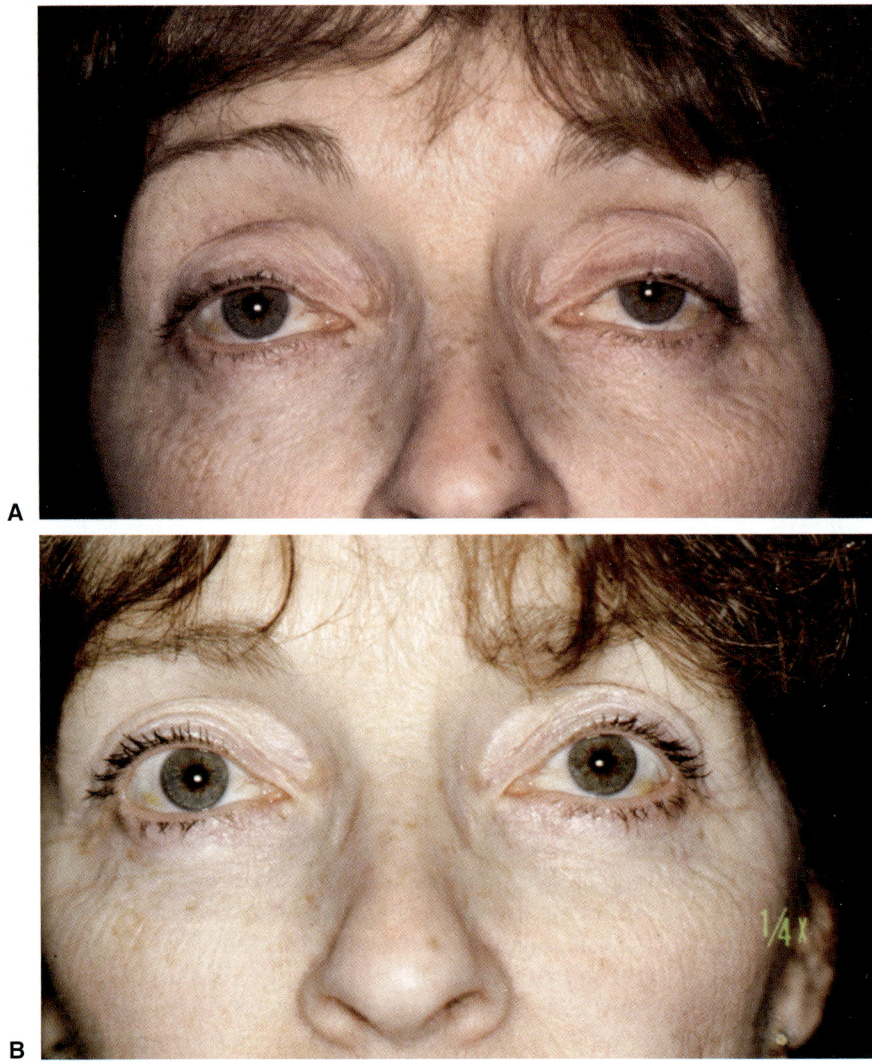

Figure 157.1. (A) Preoperative and (B) postoperative appearance of patient who underwent bilateral small incision external levator repair. Note improvement of the superiod sulcus defect.

158

Ptosis Repair by a Single-Stitch Levator Advancement

Don Liu

This versatile, simple technique for ptosis repair can be used to correct most cases of involutional, traumatic, and postsurgical ptosis of 1–5 mm. Patients must have at least 8 mm of levator function. It may be performed with local injection only or with additional intravenous sedation. The steps for performing this procedure are as follows:

1. Identify, mark, and inject the lid crease with no more than 0.5 ml of 2% lidocaine with epinephrine. (An anesthetic injection of more than this amount would distort the anatomy and affect the function of various extraocular muscles.) Allow 10–15 minutes for hemostasis.
2. Use a No.15 blade to make the skin incision and a curved Stevens scissors and 0.5 forceps to perform dissection. Undermine the orbicularis superiorly for about 10 mm.
3. Identify the orbital septum by grasping and tugging the tissue in question with the forceps and placing a finger at the superior orbital rim. The orbital septum is identified when your finger feels the tug. This helps in the identification of all the relevant structures throughout the procedure.
4. Open the orbital septum with the scissors 5 mm above the skin incision to avoid injuring the aponeurosis (Figure 158.1). If this incision is too low, the aponeurosis and conjunctiva could be inadvertently incised. Prolapse of orbital fat into view serves as an indication that the incision is indeed of orbital septum. In patients with little fat, the aponeurosis comes directly into view.
5. Spread and tease aside the orbital fat with the curved Stevens scissors (Figure 158.2). Apply a Desmarres retractor superiorly to get the fat out of the way. Do not perform this dissection too vigorously as it may iatrogenically create aponeurosis dehiscence.
6. To better expose the deeper portion of the aponeurosis, roll a cotton-tipped applicator on the apeneurosis while the patient looks downward. The applicator is gently rolled, not pulled or pushed. This maneuver is a key to a successful repair.

7. Place a 6-0 nylon suture high up in the aponeurosis centrally (Figure 158.3). This suture may be used as a traction suture if the initial placement is not high enough. Rarely a patient feels minor momentary discomfort.

8. Anchor the suture in the anterior surface of the superior tarsus and place a temporary slip-knot. This suture should be 1–2 mm medially displaced from the mid-pupillary line. Observe the lid curvature and height and make appropriate adjustment as necessary.

9. As the knot is being tied, watch the lid move up and aim for a 1 to 2 mm overcorrection with 2-mm lagophthalmos upon gentle lid closure.

10. When the position of the lid is satisfactory, tie the nylon suture permanently and cut its ends short. Double-check the lid curvature and height before skin closure. Close the skin with 6-0 nylon suture.

11. Instruct the patient to apply ice-cold compress over the operative eyelid for 3 days and to avoid any rubbing or squeezing of the lid.

12. If overcorrection is seen postoperatively, it can easily be eliminated by early institution of downward massage of the lid. Undercorrection and recurrence of ptosis may require a repeat operation. Since anatomy is least disturbed, a reoperation is usually very simple. Over- and undercorrection rarely occur with this technique, however.

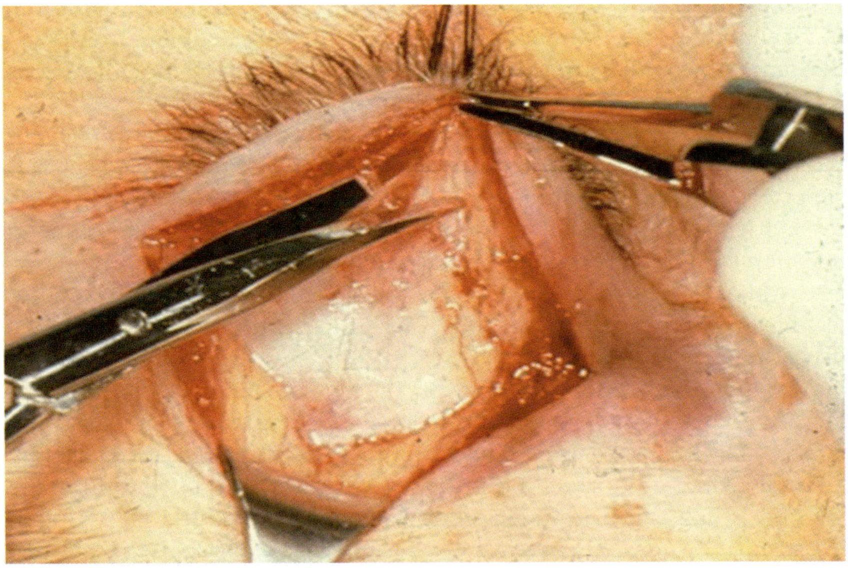

Figure 158.1. Open the septum 5 mm above the skin incision to avoid injury to the aponeurosis.

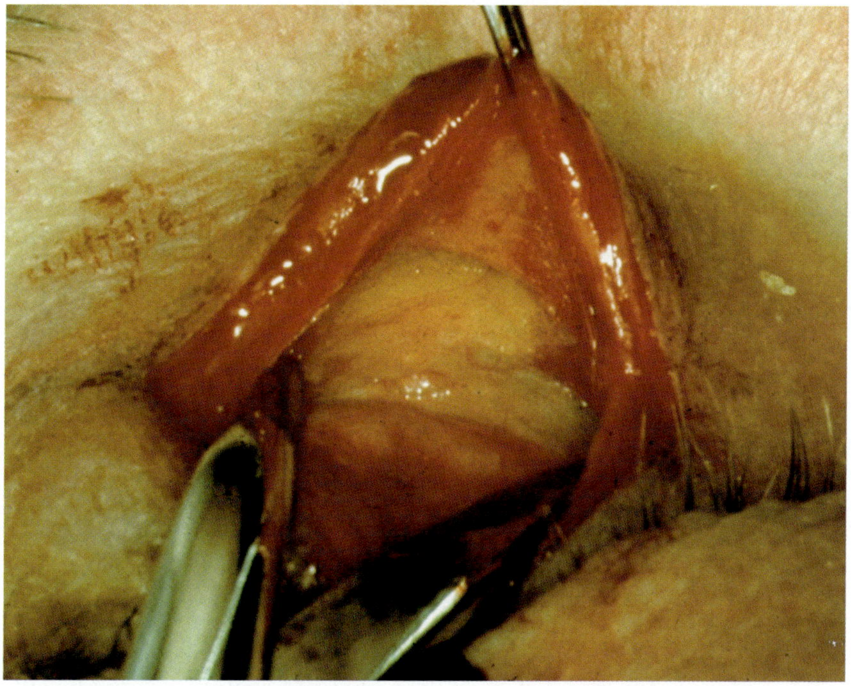

Figure 158.2. Spread and tease aside the orbital fat with a curved Stevens scissors.

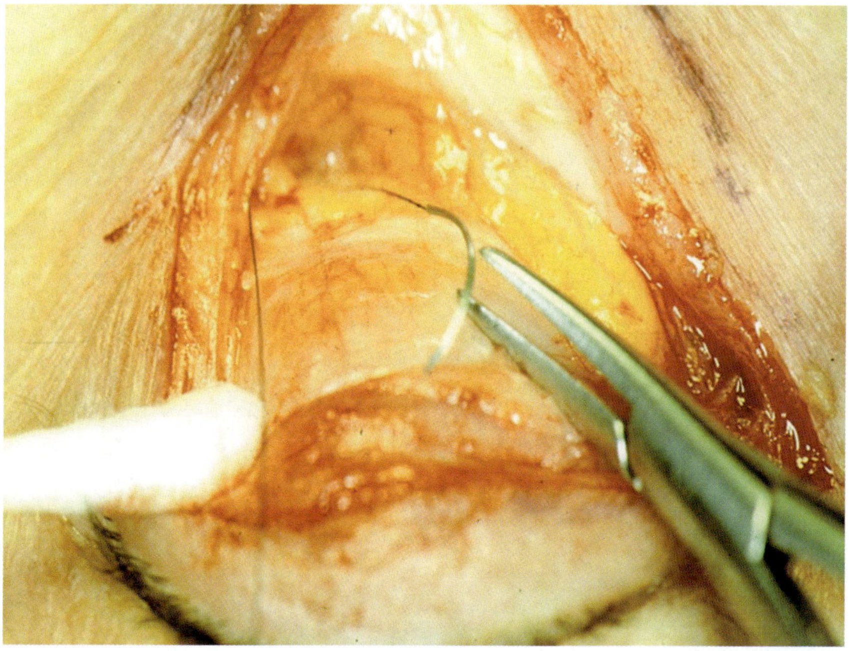

Figure 158.3. A 6-0 nylon suture is passed high up in the aponeurosis centrally.

Reference

Liu D. Simplified ptosis repair: single suture aponeurotic tuck. Ophthalmology 1993;100:251–259.

159

Postoperative Care in Ptosis Surgery

Edsel Ing

In patients with immediate postoperative lagophthalmos, an Opsite (Smith & Nephew) or Tegaderm (3M) plastic dressing can be used until local anesthetic effect on the orbicularis resolves or overnight in patients who have difficulty instilling eyedrops or if they have compromised corneas. The inferior portion of the plastic dressing can be crimped to make a channel for blood to seep through. Cold compresses can be still applied through this thin plastic dressing.

Section Two

Ptosis: Posterior Approach

160

Pearls for Müller's Muscle–Conjunctival Resection–Ptosis Procedure Combined with Upper Blepharoplasty

Allen M. Putterman

The Müller's muscle–conjunctival resection ptosis procedure is a relatively simple means of relieving upper eyelid ptosis in patients whose upper eyelids elevate close to a normal level when phenylephrine drops are placed in their upper fornix.[1-3] Although the procedure is fast to perform, there are pearls to know and pitfalls to avoid in order to achieve optimal results.

- A frontal nerve block is performed to provide sensory anesthesia of the upper eyelid without infiltrating the lid, which can make the procedure more difficult to perform. The $1^1/_2$-inch retrobulbar needle is placed centrally and hugs the roof of the orbit during insertion. The surgeon should aim toward the temporal roof of the orbit rather than the nasal roof to avoid penetration of the supraorbital artery, which could cause a retrobulbar hemorrhage. Also, the surgeon should withdraw the syringe before injecting the anesthetic to make sure that the needle has not been passed into a blood vessel.
- A scratch incision is made over the area of excessive upper eyelid skin outlined in ink. If this is not done, the marked areas could smear and disappear on eversion of the upper eyelid.
- Usually a medium-sized Desmarres retractor is employed, but occasionally it is necessary to use a large retractor.
- The 6-0 black silk marking suture is placed only through conjunctiva. If it penetrates Müller's muscle, a subconjunctival hemorrhage can occur, which could interfere with the resection of both conjunctiva and Müller's muscle.
- The clamp made for this procedure (Bausch & Lomb Storz Instruments, Manchester, MO) that has three teeth on each side seems to work the best.

- The amount of resection is determined preoperatively by the patient's response to phenylephrine. If the amount of ptosis differs on each side, usually the difference in the amount of resection is double the difference in ptosis. For example, if the MRD1 preoperatively is 0.5 mm on one side and 1.5 mm on the other side, then a 2-mm difference in the amount of Müller's resection is accomplished. For example, a 9 mm resection on the 0.5 mm side and a 7 mm resection on the 1.5 mm side.
- An attempt is made to clamp only conjunctiva and Müller's muscle. If tarsus is included, it is slipped out of the clamp. Occasionally, if the eyelid level does not go up to the desired position with phenylephrine, a few millimeters of tarsus are included in the clamp along with Müller's muscle and conjunctiva.
- A 5-0 plain catgut suture with a spatula needle is used. This needle will not sever the mattress suture when the running suture is passed through conjunctiva.
- The mattress suture bites are placed close together through tarsus and slightly farther away on the conjunctival surface. This minimizes postoperative keratopathy from the suture rubbing on the eye.
- Each arm of the 5-0 plain catgut suture needle is passed through the temporal conjunctiva into the wound so that the knot will fall into the subconjunctival space and not rub on the eye. The surgeon leaves the first needle in place while passing the second needle to avoid cutting the suture.
- The suture needles are taped to the surgical drapes to avoid a needle stick.[4]
- Pull the upper lid downward with the traction suture placed through central upper eyelid skin, orbicularis oculi muscles, and tarsus while pulling the skin above the central incision site upward and outward allows penetration of Westcott scissors into the suborbicularis space. This avoids cutting the levator, Müller's muscle, and orbital septum. The 5-0 plain gut sutures are tied after removal of skin and orbicularis on the upper eyelid and after cautery. It is best not to tie them before this to avoid breaking the internal 6-0 plain gut sutures.
- The eyelid crease is formed by attaching orbicularis muscle to levator aponeurosis with polyester fiber (Mersilene) sutures, as well as 6-0 polyglactin (Vicryl) sutures that pass through skin, levator aponeurosis, and skin.[5,6]

References

1. Putterman AM, Urist MJ. Müller's muscle-conjunctival resection: technique for treatment of blepharoptosis. Arch Ophthalmol 1975;93:619.
2. Putterman AM. Müller's muscle-conjunctival resection-ptosis procedure combined with upper blepharoplasty. In: Putterman AM (ed.). Cosmetic Oculoplastic Surgery, 3rd ed. Philadelphia: W.B. Saunders Co., 1999: 137–149.
3. Putterman AM, Fett DR. Müller's muscle in the treatment of upper eyelid ptosis: a ten-year study. Ophthalmic Surg 1986;17:354–356.
4. Putterman AM. Avoidance of needle stick injuries during reuse of surgical needles. Plast Reconstr Surg 2003;112:333–334.

5. Putterman AM. Treatment of upper eyelid dermatochalasis with reconstruction of upper eyelid crease: skin-muscle flap approach. In: Putterman AM (ed.). Cosmetic Oculoplastic Surgery, 3rd ed. Philadelphia: W.B. Saunders Co., 1999:91–100.
6. Putterman AM, Fagien S. Müller's muscle-conjunctival resection-ptosis procedure combined with upper blepharoplasty. In Fagien S (ed.). Putterman's Cosmetic Oculoplastic Surgery. Longon, Elsevier, 2008; pp.123–133.

161

Müller's Muscle–Conjunctival Resection Pearls: Phenylephrine and Resection Considerations

Melanie H. Erb and Steven C. Dresner

The goal of blepharoptosis repair is to elevate the eyelids to an acceptable level while maintaining proper contour, lid crease, and final symmetry of eyelid height to within 0.5 mm. Müller's muscle-conjunctival resection (MMCR) [1] predictably attains these goals because the correction is consistently titratable according to published [2] or personal nomograms. MMCR is the preferred approach to raise an eyelid by 2.5 mm or less in patients with a positive phenylephrine test.

Patients with good levator function who do not respond to phenylephrine are better served with either a modified Fasanella-Servat or a levator aponeurotic repair. Occasionally, one can get a good result with a MMCR in a patient with a negative test; however, the result is not predictable. The Fasanella-Servat works well in patients with a negative phenylephrine test, so we recommend it for patients with 2 mm or less of ptosis. For greater than 2 mm of ptosis with a negative test, we usually perform a levator aponeurotic repair.

The idea is to always use the operation which is most predictable for the condition. One has to have a number of tools in one's armamentarium.

Pearl 1. The Phenylephrine Test

The phenylephrine test is used to determine whether the patient is a candidate for MMCR. We perform the 2.5% phenylephrine test in only one eye—the more ptotic eye or an arbitrary eye, if ptosis is equal. This serves three purposes: it determines whether a patient is a candidate for MMCR, demonstrates to the patient what he or she may look like after surgery, and unmasks contralateral ptosis in the fellow eye secondary to Hering's law of equal innervation.

If the patient is a candidate for MMCR and has bilateral ptosis, the resection amount of both eyelids is calculated from the MRD1 to the desired final eyelid height from the nomogram below. If contralateral ptosis is revealed with the uniocular phenylephrine test, either a smaller resection is performed on the previously ptotic eyelid or bilateral surgery is planned.

Pearl 2. The Resection Nomogram

If the patient is a candidate for MMCR with a positive phenylephrine test, then the amount of resection is planned according to the preoperative MRD1 and the desired final eyelid position. Dresner [2] has reported his full nomogram, which will be briefly summarized here. Generally, for every 1 mm of desired elevation, 4 mm of Müller's muscle and conjunctiva are resected. Modifications to this nomogram are made for 3 mm of desired elevation, positive phenylephrine response of only 1.5 mm instead of 2 mm, and congenital ptosis.

Level of Phenylephrine Response

There is not a direct correlation between the level of phenylephrine response and the amount of MMCR resection. If the response to phenylephrine is 2 mm, one uses the nomogram as described above. If the response is slightly less than 2 mm, such as 1.5 mm, the resection amount can be increased by 1 mm. If the response is larger than 2 mm, the nomogram remains unchanged. In Horner's syndrome, sometimes the response can be 4 mm or greater. We still will resect about 8 mm for 2 mm of Horner's ptosis. However, we rarely use MMCR for congenital ptosis. In our hands, a modified Fasanella-Servat is more predictable than a MMCR for 2 mm of congenital ptosis.

Nomogram for MMCR[2]

Elevation desired (mm)	MMC resection (mm)
1.0	4
1.5	6
2.0	8
3.0	10

References

1. Putterman AM, Urist MJ. Muller muscle-conjunctiva resection. Technique for treatment of blepharoptosis. Arch Ophthalmol 1975;93(8):619–623.
2. Dresner SC. Further modifications of the Muller's muscle-conjunctival resection procedure for blepharoptosis. Ophthal Plast Reconstr Surg 1991; 7(2):114–122.

162

Avoiding Lid Contour Abnormalities in Müller's Muscle–Conjunctival Resection: Recognizing the Lateral Shift

Michael E. Migliori

Müller's muscle–conjunctival resection (MMCR) has gained in popularity as a quick, reliable and predictable surgical approach to carefully selected patients with ptosis.

I have found that surgeons can sometimes get into trouble with contour abnormalities with nasal peaking and central flattening. For this reason, I think it is important that one recognizes a lateral shift in the tarsal plate in many older patients. It is important to center the locking Putterman ptosis clamp over the tarsus and not center the clamp over the pupil. This prevents asymmetric advancement of the overlying levator muscle in cases in which the tarsus has shifted laterally. Figures 162.1 and 162.2 demonstrate centering of the clamp over the tarsus.

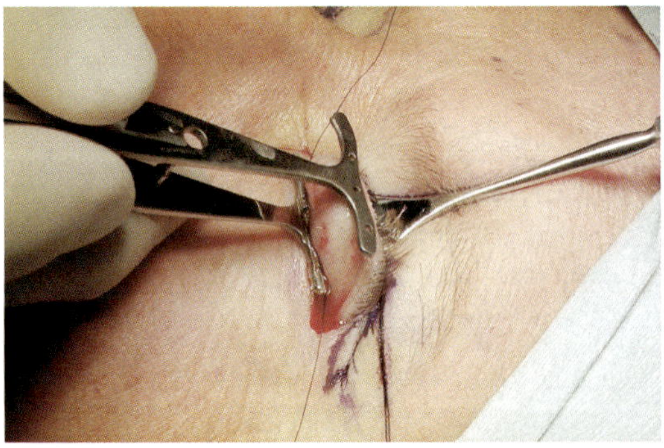

Figure 162.1. Lateral view showing placement of clamp centered over the tarsus.

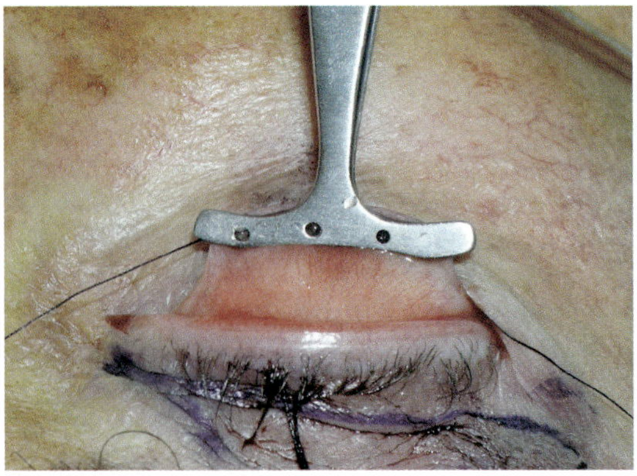

Figure 162.2. Clamp positioned correctly centered over the tarsus.

163

Müller's Muscle–Conjunctival Resection Procedure Tips

Melanie H. Erb and Steven C. Dresner

Pearl 1: Marking the Pupillary Axis

Preoperatively, with the patient sitting up, the center of the pupillary axis is marked on the eyelid margin (Figure 163.1). Intraoperatively, this mark is used to align the Müller's muscle-conjunctival resection (MMCR) clamp. The clamp is centered above this mark, thus ensuring that the highest archpoint of the clamp is aligned above the pupil. This provides proper lid contour postoperatively.

It should be noted that, above the pupil, the upper eyelid moves slightly laterally upon eyelid closure. Thus, it is best to mark eyelid when patient is awake and sitting with eyelids open.[1]

Pearl 2: 6-0 Prolene Suture

We use 6-0 prolene suture instead of 6-0 plain gut for MMCR closure. The suture is started from the skin and passed full-thickness through the eyelid to the conjunctival surface in the superior fornix. The suture is then passed under the Putterman MMCR clamp in standard, running, horizontal mattress fashion. At the end of the clamp, the prolene suture is brought out, full-thickness, to the skin surface. Müller's muscle and conjunctiva are excised with 15 blade in standard fashion. The eyelid is everted back into its anatomic position, and the medial and lateral ends of the prolene suture are tied together atop the skin in the pretarsal area (Figure 163.2). The suture is removed in 5–7 days. The use of prolene suture decreases the risk of suture keratopathy.

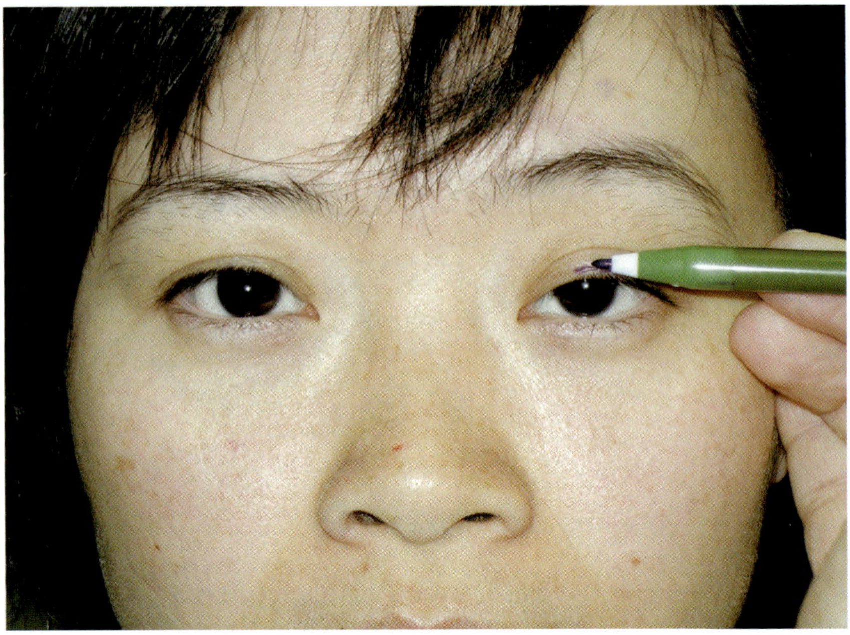

Figure 163.1. Preoperatively, with the patient sitting up, the center of the pupillary axis is marked on the eyelid margin.

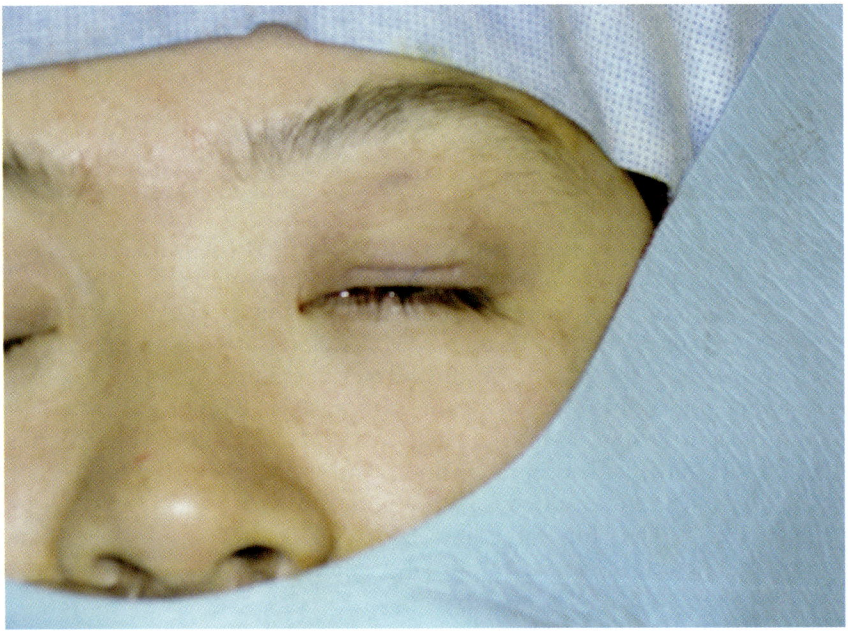

Figure 163.2. Prolene suture is run in horizontal mattress fashion and the medial and lateral ends are tied together atop the skin in the pretarsal area.

Reference

1. Frueh BR, Hassan AS, Musch DC. Horizontal eyelid movement on eyelid closure. Ophthal Plast Reconstr Surg 2005;21(2):109–111.

Section Three

Entropion

164

Minimally Invasive, Three-Step, Transconjunctival Entropion Repair

Francesco P. Bernardini

The surgical treatment of involutional entropion requires the correction of the three anatomic causes: lower eyelid laxity, lower eyelid retractors disinsertion, and preseptal orbicularis override.

This can be accomplished through a transconjunctival approach, without opening the conjunctiva all the way across the lower eyelid. After preparing the lateral tarsal strip in the usual fashion and anchoring the strip to the periosteum temporarily (without tying the sutures down), the lower eyelid is everted on an iris hook. The conjunctiva and lower eyelid retractors of the lateral third of the eyelid (after the lateral canthopexy) are incised for 1 cm at the inferior tarsal border with Westcott scissors. The edges of the conjunctiva are retracted superiorly with an iris hook and the dissection is carried in the suborbicularis plane down to the orbital septum. The orbicularis muscle is easily identified and a 3- to 4-mm strip of the preseptal orbicularis muscle is excised (preseptal orbiculectomy) for most of the entire length of the eyelid (Figure 164.1). At this stage the eyelid retractors will lie just posterior to the conjunctiva and are easily identified without opening of the orbital septum. The upper edge of the retractors is attached to the lower tarsal edge with a single 6-0 nylon suture and the conjunctival edges are approximated with 7-0 vicryl suture. Now the lateral tarsal strip can be tied permanently and the skin closed (Figure 164.2).

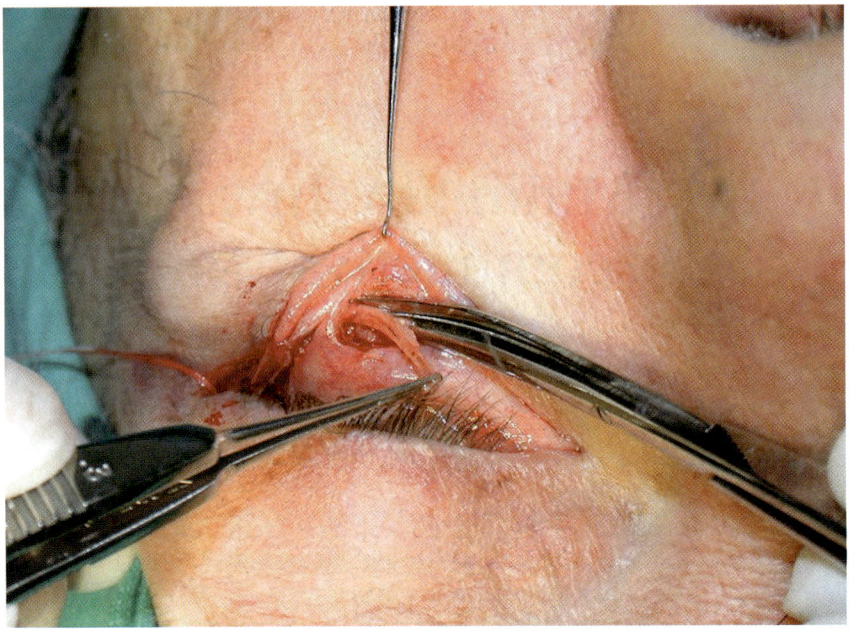

Figure 164.1. Orbiculectomy (surgeon's view) through subtarsal incision.

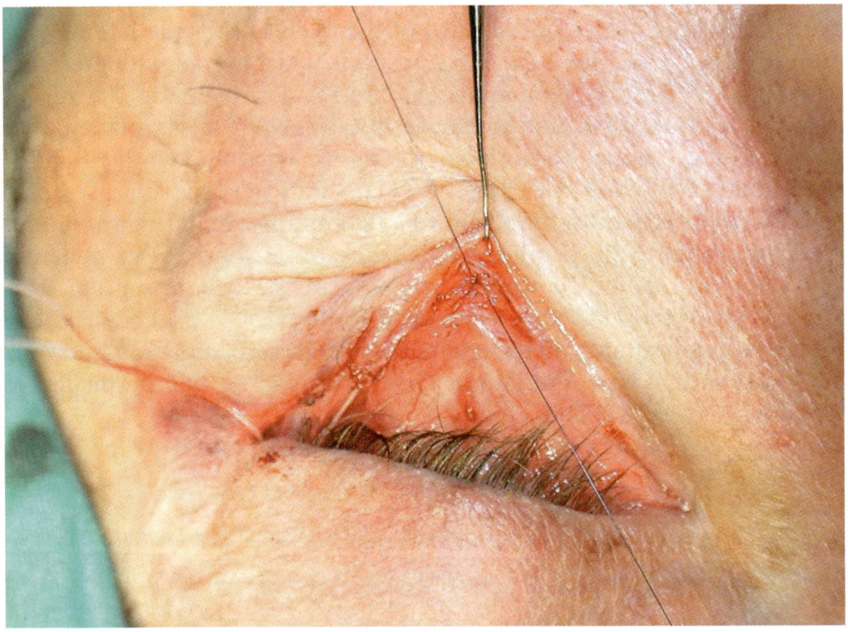

Figure 164.2. Retractors reinserted at lower tarsal border.

165

Simple Entropion Repair Using the Orbicularis Strip

Don Liu

This technique is one of the simplest and most effective methods of entropion repair. It allows the surgeon to address all of the major anatomic causes of involutional entropion. The steps for performing this technique are as follows:

1. Mark and inject the lower eyelid with 2% lidocaine with epinephrine as for lower lid blepharoplasty. No more than 1 ml of anesthetic solution is necessary.
2. Make a subciliary incision with a No. 15 blade. Use a blunt-tipped scissors to undermine the skin widely and carefully, down to the inferior orbital rim.
3. Use a muscle hook and scissors to fashion a pretarsal orbicularis muscle strip that is 5–7 mm wide. The muscle strip spans from the punctum to the lateral orbital rim, with both ends of muscle insertion left undisturbed. The muscle is not denervated.
4. Inspect the lid's position. If dehiscence or disinsertion of the lower lid retractor is evident, it can be corrected now. If there is horizontal lid laxity, it can be corrected at this time with a pentagonal resection or any other lower eyelid-tightening procedure.
5. Displace the muscle strip inferiorly 7–11 mm, depending on the severity of the entropion.
6. Place a double-armed 6-0 chromic suture in the center of the lower lid, in the fashion typical of a Quickert suture. The first arm enters deep in the fornix, emerges 2 mm below the tarsus muscle, and goes through muscle strip superiorly. The second arm also enters deep in the fornix but emerges 5 mm below the tarsus and goes through muscle strip inferiorly.
7. Tie these two arms of suture over the muscle strip so that the muscle strip is fixated in a new and inferiorly displaced position.
8. Place one double-armed 6-0 chromic suture 5 mm on each side of the center suture to displace and fixate the muscle.
9. Ask the patient to close the lids tightly and observe the position of the lids. If the position is satisfactory, proceed with skin closure.

10. Drape skin over the wound with minimal or no skin excision. Close the skin with 6-0 absorbable suture.

11. Instruct the patient to apply ice cold compress to the involved eyelid for 1–2 days and antibiotic ointment for about one week.

Because of its versatility and simplicity, this technique rarely fails to correct entropion. Although recurrence is extremely rare, if it does occur, reoperation can be simply performed, since the anatomy is minimally disturbed and the muscle strip is not denervated. The muscle strip may be relocated and fixated easily during a repeat procedure.

Suggested Reading

Hsu WM, Liu D. A new approach to the correction of involutional entropion by pretarsal orbicularis oculi muscle fixation. Am J Ophthalmol 1985; 100:802–805.

Liu D, Wu L. Involutional entropion. Geriatr Ophthalmol 1987;3(3):28–31.

166

Simple "Bedside" Cautery Entropion Repair

David J. Singer

This is a simple and effective "bedside" procedure for someone unwilling or unable to undergo surgery in the operating room. Following injection of local anesthetic (lidocaine/epinephrine) and topical anesthetic drops, insert a lid plate into the inferior fornix for globe protection. Using your finger, downwardly displace the roll of orbicularis adjacent to the lid margin, rolling the lid outward. With a disposable hand-held cautery, make multiple vertical stab incisions through the lid down to the lid plate so that, when finished, you have six or so vertical stab incisions charred burns longitudinally along the middle part (over the tarsus) of the lid, from medial towards the lateral canthal area. Apply your favorite antibiotic/steroid ointment. No patch is required, but patients need reassurance that the burn marks will totally disappear.

What you are doing is creating multiple thermal scars that involve skin, subcutaneous tissue, orbicularis and tarsus, and a bit of conjunctiva, which, when healed, will prevent the palpebral orbicularis from rolling inward and bringing the lid with it, thereby preventing entropion.

The vertical "burns" are only as long as the heating element at the end of the handheld cautery. The cautery is turned on to red/white hot, then the skin and orbicularis pulled inferiorly while a plunge of the cautery is made, with the heating element perpendicular to the eyelid margin, through the entire substance of the eyelid, down to the lid plate, then withdrawn. This is repeated as "parallel vertical" burns are made along the horizontal length of the lid, putting in five or six (or less) burns from medial to lateral. The burns initially have a dark crust at the surface, but that sloughs off, with time, and the wounds heal without scarring.

I have used this procedure numerous times, with the resolution of the entropion. In a few cases, a year or more later the entropion recurred, but this treatment can be repeated, if desired. The beauty of this is that it is simple, effective, and can be done anyplace.

Section Four

Ectropion

167

"Simple-Dimple" Lateral Tarsus Fixation

William L. Walter

This procedure is useful in entropion repair when there is a small amount of lid laxity that does not warrant a tarsal strip. I will describe a suture-fixation technique that stabilizes the lateral aspect of the tarsus to the firmly attached pretarsal muscle at the lateral orbital rim. I use this technique whenever there is minimal lid laxity.

After the pretarsal orbicularis muscle has been excised and the lower eyelid retractors have been advanced to the lower edge of the tarsus, the lateral aspect of the exposed tarsus is stabilized with an undyed 6-0 vicryl suture. The suture is passed through the lateral portion of the exposed tarsus, and the needle is directed deep either to catch the periosteum or pass under the tendon attachments of the pretarsal orbicularis muscle at the lateral orbital rim area. The needle is then directed in an upward and outward direction to exit the skin above the lateral canthal area (Figure 167.1). The needle is redirected back along the same pathway and finally out through the tarsus (Figure 167.2). The suture is tightened until a dimpling of the skin of the lateral canthal area is apparent. After the suture has been tied, the lateral aspect of the lower lid will be found to be well stabilized (Figure 167.3).

This procedure is effective and stable in entropion with minimal lid laxity.

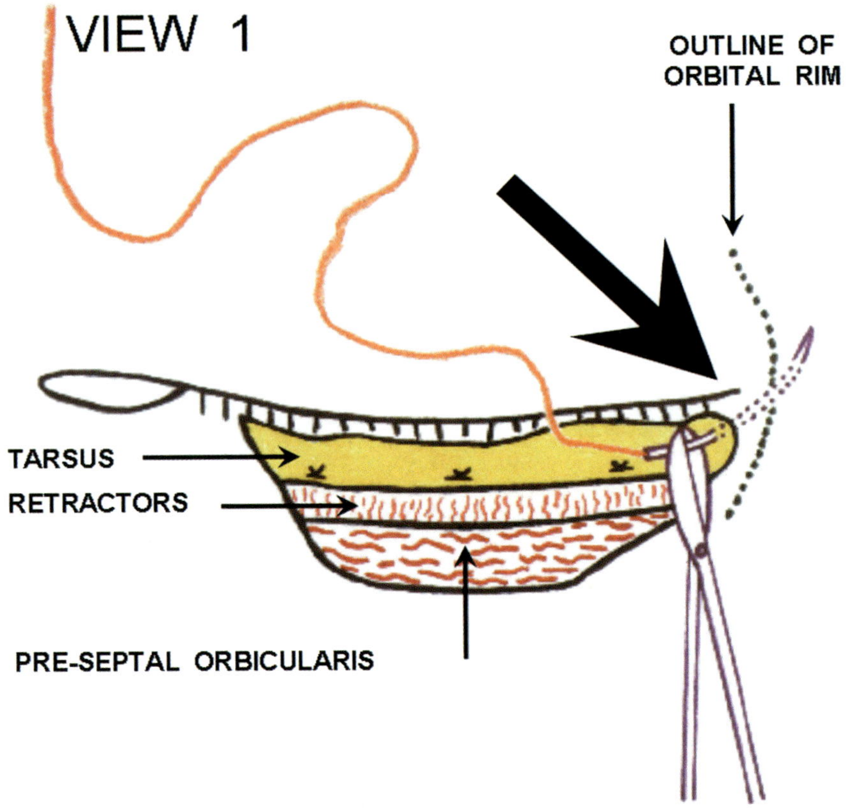

Figure 167.1. Direction of first needle pass through lateral tarsus and orbital rim periosteum.

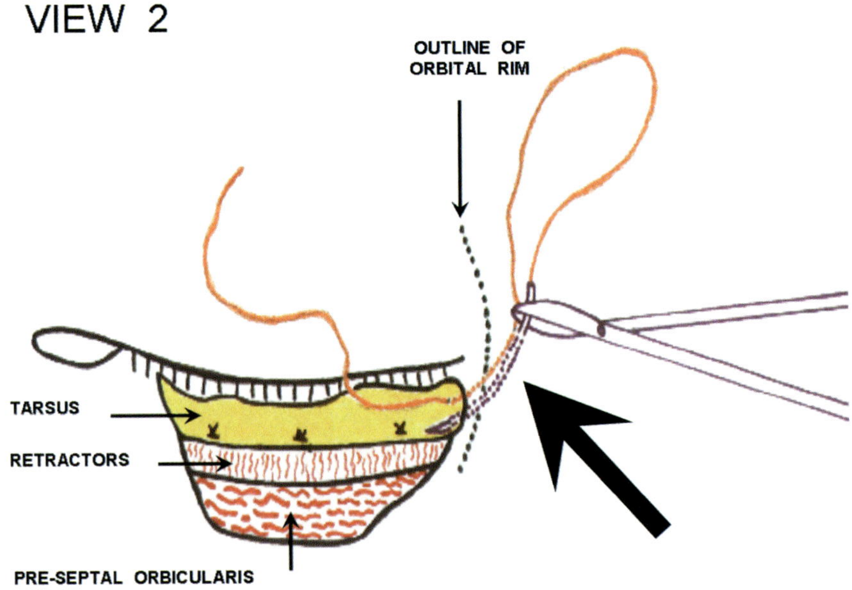

Figure 167.2. Second suture pass reenters first suture exit site (the dimple).

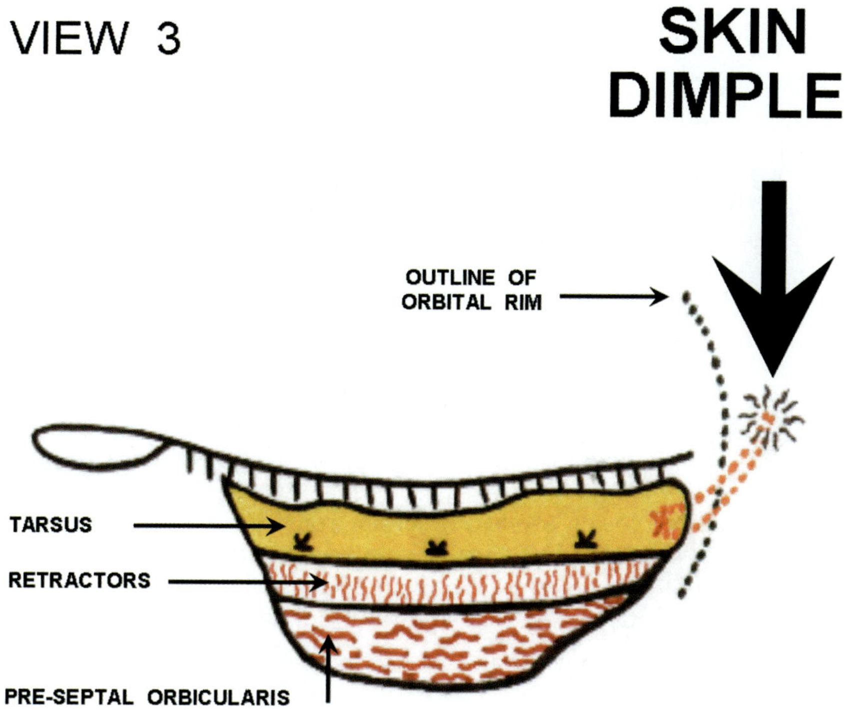

Figure 167.3. Suture tied after second pass through tarsus.

168

Lower Lid Retractor Dissection

Jeffrey P. Edelstein

When dissecting lower eyelid retractors from the conjunctiva, inject anesthetic (I use 2% lidocaine with epinephrine between the conjunctiva and retractors to "hydrodissect" a plane). This makes the sharp dissection easier and reduces the chance for buttonholing the conjunctiva. It works!

169

Simple Lower Lid Tightening Without Tarsal Strip

Don Liu

Lower lid laxity may be a component of entropion, ectropion, or lower eyelid retraction. To correct these problems completely, the lower eyelid often must be tightened. This technique for tightening the lower lid produces consistent and long-lasting results. It is much simpler than a pentagonal resection or a tarsal strip procedure. There is no potential lid notch or prolonged lower eyelid edema. Rarely, transient point tenderness may be encountered. The steps for performing this surgical technique are as follows:

1. Inject about 1 ml of 2% lidocaine with epinephrine into the lateral canthus and the lateral one third of the lower eyelid.
2. Perform a lateral canthotomy in the usual fashion.
3. Pull the lateral portion of the lower eyelid laterally to estimate the amount of excess tissue to remove.
4. Mark the excess tissue to be removed.
5. Place a straight Stevens scissors at the lower lid margin and aim laterally. Excise a narrow, triangular-shaped, full-thickness eyelid wedge laterally. The scissors should not be placed in the usual vertical direction as in Bick's triangle or the pentagonal resection. It is placed almost horizontally to avoid prolonged lid edema.
6. Slightly undermine the superior canthotomy wound using the scissors.
7. Retract the tissues superiorly and place a 6-0 nylon suture in the periosteum of the lateral orbital rim superiorly, allowing 2 mm of overcorrection. This step is a key to successful repair.
8. Place the same suture in the tarsus of the lower eyelid laterally. With the assistant's fingers holding the tissues together, tie this nylon suture tightly and cut the end short. The lower eyelid should now be tight and slightly overcorrected.
9. Close the wound with absorbable 6-0 plain suture.
10. Apply ice-cold compresses for 1–2 days and antibiotic ointment for a week.

Further Reading

Liu D. Lower eyelid tightening: a comparative study. Ophthal Plast Reconstr Surg 1997;13(3):199–203.

170

Technique for Medical Canthal Flap to Correct Lid Retraction/Medial Ectropion

Kathleen M. Duerksen

This is a variant of other procedures described in the past to correct medial lid retraction.

It's simple, avoids the need for a graft, and is generally aesthetically acceptable.

Place Bowman probes in upper and lower canaliculus for protection.

Denude skin layer overlying the upper and lower canaliculi, medial to the puncta along the length of the medial canthal tendon (MCT) (Figure 170.1). Suture these denuded inferior and superior limbs of the MCT together with running or interrupted 6-0 vicryl on an S-14 needle (Figure 170.2). Take care not to damage the canaliculi!

Create skin/orbicularis muscle flaps from the tissue above and below and lateral to the MCT. Suture these together over the MCT, again using 6-0 vicryl or 6-0 plain suture (Figure 170.3). All of these sutures are *medial* to the puncta. A backcut just lateral to the puncta may be needed to prevent webbing.

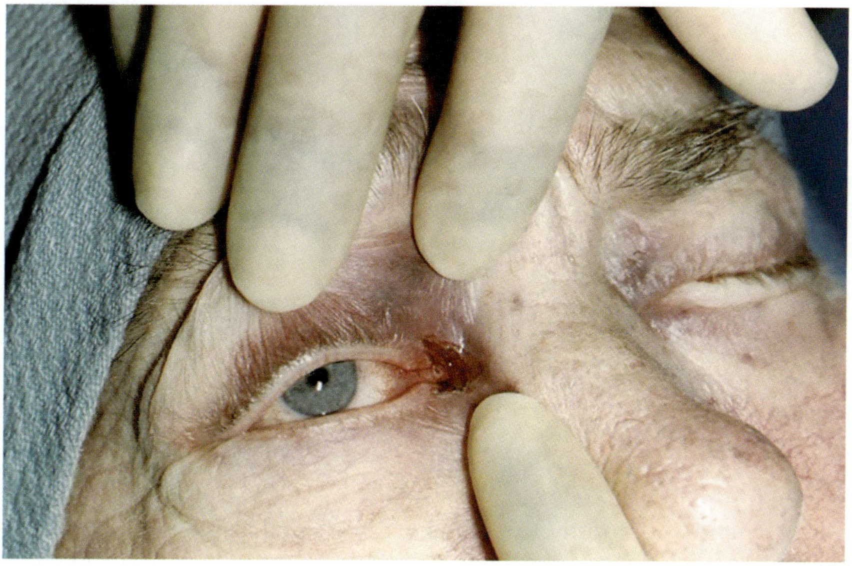

Figure 170.1. Skin denuded from MCT limbs.

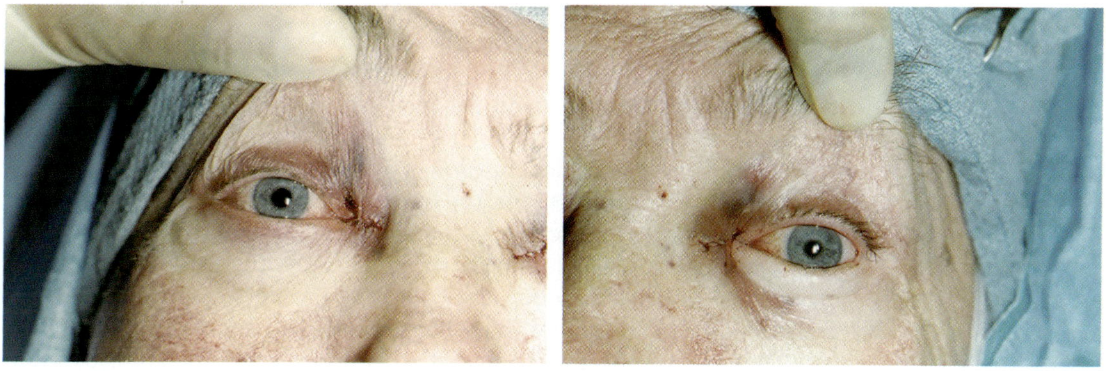

A B

Figure 170.2. Skin/muscle flaps sutured together.

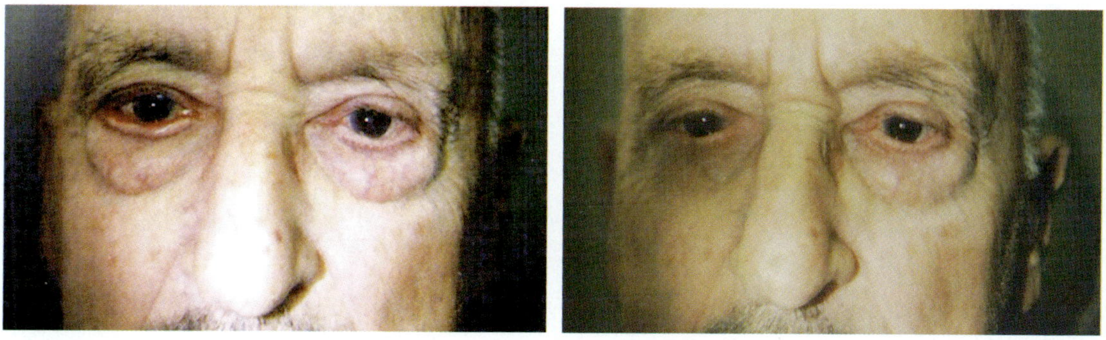

A B

Figure 170.3. Results. (A) preoperative. (B) postoperative.

171

Medial Canthorraphy

Francesco P. Bernardini

This technique is useful to stabilize the medial canthal tendon and prevent medial migration of the lower punctum when performing a lateral tarsal strip for involutional ectropion with marked medial tendon laxity. It is also useful in the treatment of inferior scleral show/ectropion in case of VII nerve palsy, along with a lateral tarsal strip.

The canalicular system is protected by the insertion of 00 Bowman's lacrimal probes in the upper and lower canaliculus. A 4-mm-long incision is made parallel to the eye lid margin, 3–4 mm above and below, respectively, the superior and inferior canaliclum (Figure 171.1). The superficial fibers of the orbicularis muscle are bluntly dissected with Wescott scissors in a vertical fashion, perpendicular to the eyelid margin; using a pair of toothed forceps, the deep orbicularis oculi that surrounds and attaches to the inferior and superiror limb if the medial canthal ligament is grasped. A horizontal mattress suture with 7-0 vicryl is passed through the bulk of the deep orbicularis in the upper and lower eyelid (Figures 171.2–171.4). The skin flaps overlying the muscle flaps are closed with three interrupted 7-0 vicryl sutures. No extra skin is excised, and the canalicular system is checked to verify its patency at the end of the procedure.

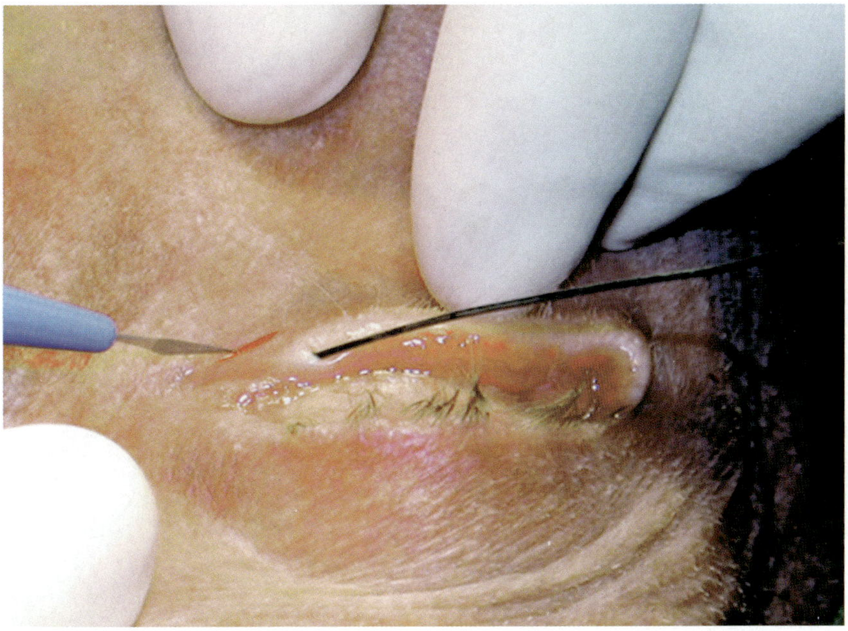

Figure 171.1. A 4 mm incision below the inferior canaliculus.

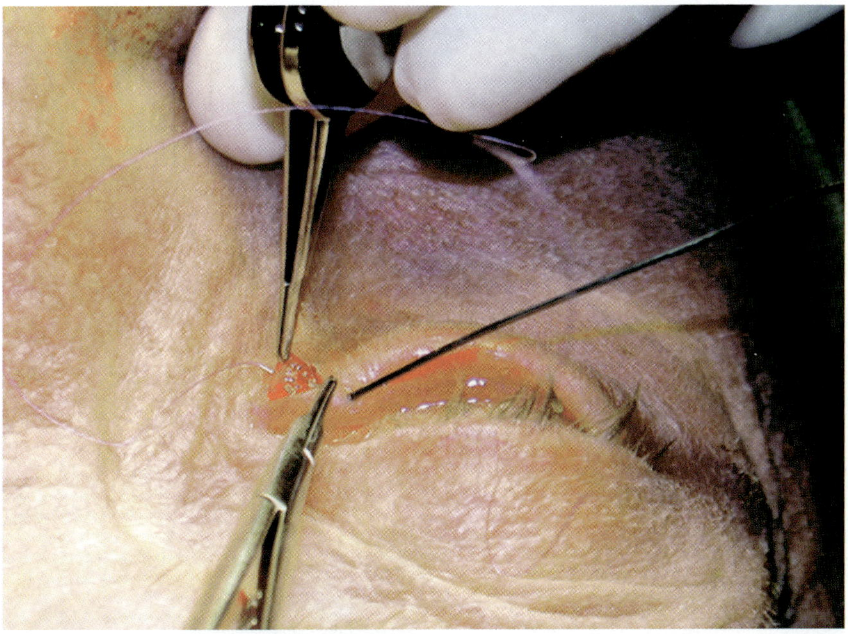

Figure 171.2. Suture passing through the deep medial orbicularis muscle fibers.

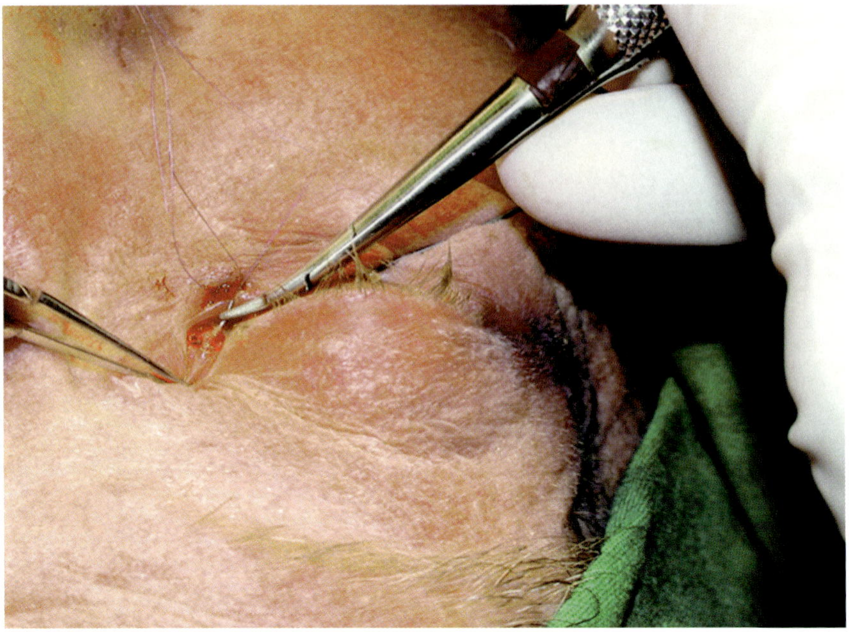

Figure 171.3. Mirros image suture of the deep medial orbicularis muscle in the upper lid.

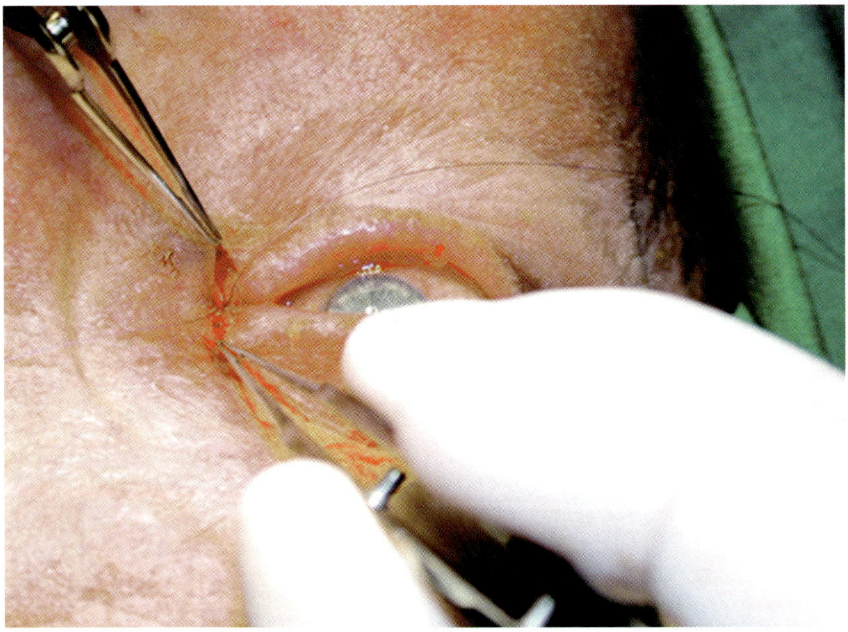

Figure 171.4. Suture knot tied between the opposite orbicularis muscle.

172

Myocutaneous Flaps and Canthopexy for Repair of Severe Cicatricial Ectropion

James Leong and Raf Ghabrial

In selected cases, the particular combination of myocutaneous flaps with canthopexy is an effective technique for repair of severe cicatricial ectropion. It incorporates the well-known benefits of myocutaneous flaps with a canthopexy suspension suture, thereby avoiding some of the potential complications of full-thickness horizontal shortening procedures.

Local myocutaneous flaps provide good cosmesis as they maintain their original color and texture after their transfer and, if made to follow the relaxed skin tension lines, should result in inconspicuous scars.

The incorporation of a canthopexy suspension suture to correct horizontal laxity has a number of potential advantages over the commonly used lid-shortening procedures such as wedge resection and canthotomy. In particular, canthopexy avoids the possibility of lid notching, lateral displacement of the punctum, phimosis of the lid, and distortion of the canthal angle.

Suitable patients must have sufficient upper eyelid dermatochalasis to allow for an adequate myocutaneous donor flap. Depending on the nature of the ectropion, medial, lateral, or bipedicle myocutaneous flaps may be used.

Bipedicle myocutaneous flaps in particular have the functional advantage of forming a sling supported by the upper lid. The passive inward and upward propensity of the sling and a dynamic mechanical support provided by the orbicularis muscle both work to counteract the downward and outward effect of the ectropion.

One constraint associated with this technique is its dependency on a certain degree of upper lid redundancy. Additionally, unilateral procedures may result in less cosmetically acceptable asymmetrical unilateral blepharoplasty.

Overall, however, this procedure provides excellent results in patients with severe cicatricial ectropion with accompanying upper eyelid dermatochalasis and horizontal lid laxity (Figures 172.1 to 172.3).

Figure 172.1.
Lateral ectropion.

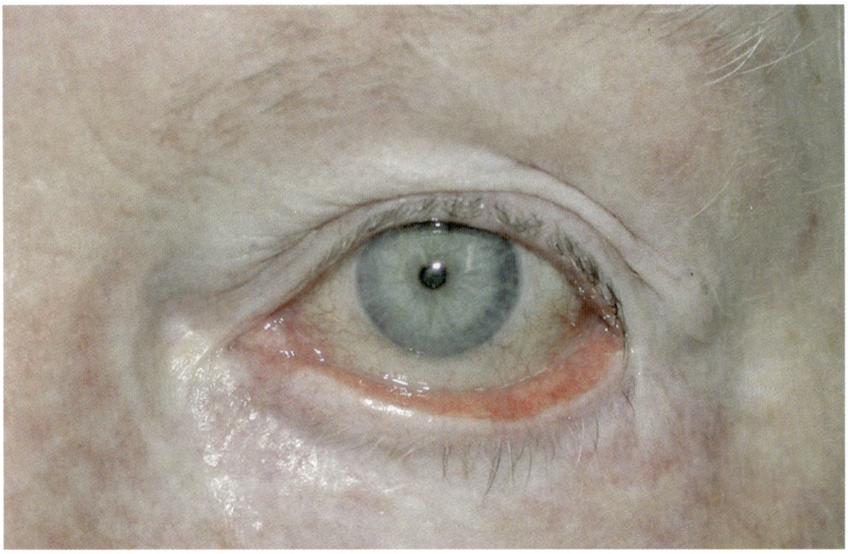

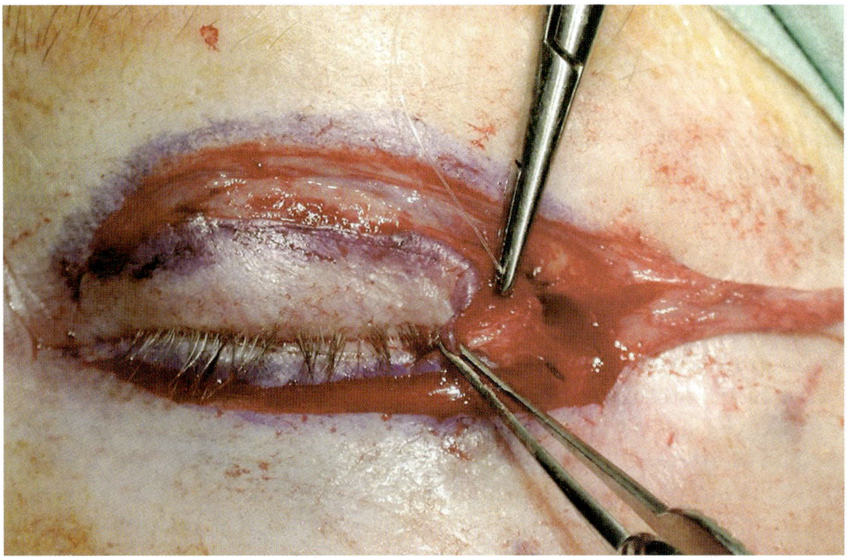

Figure 172.2.
Myocutaneous flap and canthopexy suture.

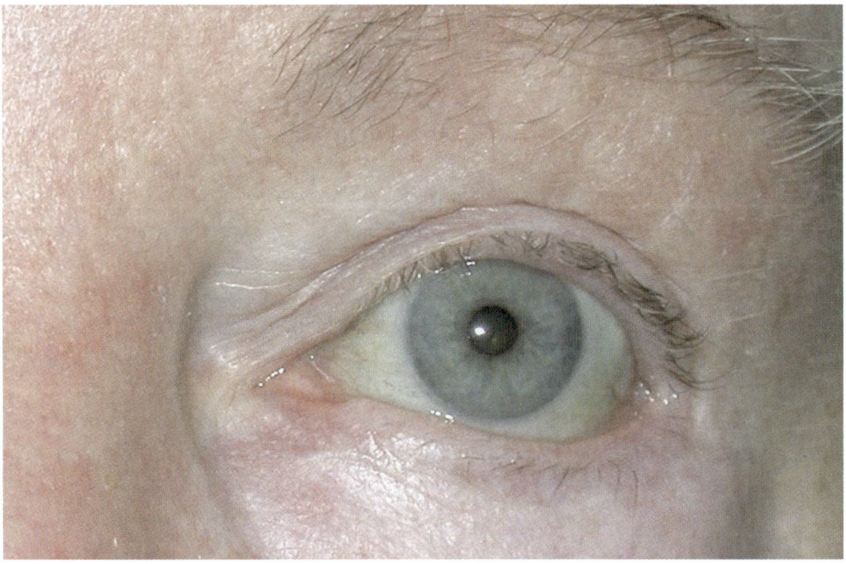

Figure 172.3.
Postoperative appearance at 12 months.

Index

Printed in the United States of America